Workbook for

MRI and CT of the Head and Neck

Second Edition

Workbook for

MRI and CT of the Head and Neck

Second Edition

Anthony A. Mancuso, M.D.
Professor of Radiology
Clinical Director, Magnetic Resonance Imaging
The University of Florida
College of Medicine
Gainesville, Florida

with contributions by

H. Ric Harnsberger, M.D.
Associate Professor
Department of Radiology
The University of Utah
School of Medicine
Salt Lake City, Utah

William P. Dillon, M.D.
Associate Professor
Department of Radiology
University of California, San Francisco
San Francisco, California

WILLIAMS & WILKINS
Baltimore • Hong Kong • London • Sydney

Editor: Timothy H. Grayson
Associate Editor: Carol Eckhart
Copy Editor: Megan Westerfeld
Design: Bob Och
Illustration Planning: Lorraine Wrzosek
Production: Anne Seitz

Williams & Wilkins
428 East Preston Street
Baltimore, Maryland 21202, USA

Accurate indications, adverse reactions, and dosage schedules for drugs are provided in this book, but it is possible that they may change. The reader is urged to review the package information data of the manufacturers of the medications mentioned.

Printed in the United States of America
First Edition 1984

Library of Congress Cataloging in Publication Data

Mancuso, Anthony A.
Workbook for MRI and CT of the head and neck / Anthony A. Mancuso, H. Ric Harnsberger, William P. Dillon. — 2nd ed.
p. cm.
Rev. ed. of: Introductory workbook for CT of the head and neck / William Hanafee, Anthony Mancuso. © 1984.
Includes bibliographies and index.
ISBN 0–683–05478–3
1. Head—Radiography. 2. Neck—Radiography. 3. Tomography. 4. Head—Tumors—Diagnosis. 5. Neck—Tumors—Diagnosis. I. Harnsberger, H. Ric. II. Dillon, William P., 1952– . III. Hanafee, William N., 1926– . Introductory workbook for CT of the head and neck. IV. Title.
[DNLM: 1. Head—radiography—problems. 2. Head and Neck Neoplasms—radiography—problems. 3. Magnetic Resonance Imaging—problems.—4. Neck— radiography—problems. 5. Tomography, X-Ray computed—problems. WE 18 M269w]
RC936.M35 1989 617'.510757—dc 19 88-14357
DNLM/DLC CIP
for Library of Congress
ISBN 0-683-05478-3

88 89 90 91 92
1 2 3 4 5 6 7 8 9 10

To all of my teachers
but especially
Bill Hanafee and
Donald Hewitt

Thank you

A.A.M.

Preface to Second Edition

This book has four main goals: 1) to be an educational resource for those who wish to learn the anatomy and basic pathology of the head and neck as seen on CT and MRI, 2) to serve as a technical manual for those wishing to produce consistently high quality CT and MR images of the head and neck, 3) to provide guidelines for the effective use of MRI and CT in the complex clinical problems that affect this region and for the interpretation of the equally complex images, and 4) to serve as an interim update between editions of our major textbook on these topics, entitled *CT and MRI of the Head and Neck*.

The *Workbook* was originally Bill Hanafee's concept. It was an outgrowth of teaching methods he experimented with at post-graduate seminars in the early 1980s. The feedback I have had over the years from medical students as well as residents and practitioners of radiology, otolaryngology, and radiation oncology has been overwhelmingly positive and enthusiastic about both the method and the content of the workbook. So Bill Hanafee had another good idea and there is little question that the first workbook fulfilled its educational mission.

Any projects such as this can be improved. Over the years it became apparent that despite major technological advances CT and MRI are being underutilized relative to their ability to produce high quality, highly informative images of the head and neck. In this edition two means of improving image quality are offered. First is Chapter 1. It is new and important. It relates image quality to the technical parameters under operator control in MRI and CT. Second are the imaging protocols. These took hundreds of man hours to prepare (I hope they will save you the trouble). These two sources describe all of the "tricks" I use to get excellent images in 90–95% of my studies. However, such quality is only possible with a strong commitment to high level, consistent physician interaction during the planning and execution of CT and MRI studies. I think such a commitment combined with the two resources just mentioned will help accomplish the second goal of the *Workbook*.

Since the last edition of the *Workbook,* MRI has assumed a role equivalent in importance to that of CT in head and neck imaging. The studies are inherently complimentary because of their relative technical advantages and disadvantages. Over the years of MRI development, I have tried to maintain a balanced attitude toward relative value of the studies, hoping to avoid the natural tendency to become an advocate for either exam. The main theme of this book is, in fact, how to exploit the strengths of MRI, CT, or both in specific clinical situations. Numerous algorithms are presented describing not only which imaging study to use but also how to ensure that they are incorporated into logical schemes of clinical triage. We must become advocates of patients rather than of tests. The commitment to helping our clinical colleagues care for their patients combined with the use of the diagnostic algorithms and checklists provided should help achieve the third goal of the workbook.

It is obvious that some material in books becomes dated not long after the books are published. In the future "E books" may become the equivalent of "E mail" (electronic mail). For now, however, we are largely limited to slower, traditional (print) means of information transfer. This *Workbook* is meant to be an update of and companion to the third edition of our text *CT and MRI of the Head and Neck.* It contains timely information about MRI reflecting the state of the art up to February 1988. However, new software and hardware arrive every 3–6 months and it's pretty hard to write a book that often. Education is a continuum. These books are a continuum. Their basis, however, is in the *clinical practice* and pathoanatomic concepts related to head and neck disease. Keeping this in mind, it is hoped that you will agree that the fourth goal of the *Workbook* has been met.

A.A.M.

Acknowledgments

First thanks go to my professional godfather (no, he is not Italian), Bill Hanafee. This book was his original concept.

The MR images in the book range from those done at 0.15 T to 1.5 T. The excellent quality of the low field pictures is due mainly to the hard work of Jeff Fitzsimmons, Ph.D., who designed and supervised the building of the receiver coils used to make the images. This remainder of our physics group—Kate Scott, Raymond Andrews, Tom Mareci, Richard Briggs, and Jintong Mao—have given me so much personal teaching and advice about MRI over the years that I can't begin to thank them enough.

Throughout the book I suggest that MRI and CT *should* be physician intensive. I can guarantee that they are technologist intensive. Many technologists have contributed their skill and thoughtfulness in producing the images seen here. In particular I would like to thank Lori (Buck) Angus, Anna Wehle, Bob Googe, and Tony Litwiller for going well beyond the call of duty. You and your coworkers have my gratitude and utmost respect.

There are a number of people who have helped me a little (and a lot) everyday. Joy Wilcox, Patsy Rigdon, Leigh Levy, Deirdre Lawson, Linda Pigott, thanks to all of you. A special thanks to Candy Caputo, who did a great job preparing this manuscript.

Debra Neill-Mareci is a wonderful artist. It shows in her excellent medical illustrations. She is also responsible for the illustrations for the third edition of *CT and MRI of the Head and Neck* (our "big" textbook).

My clinical colleagues are a constant source of support and knowledge. Special thanks to the best clinicians anyone could hope to work with, including Rod Million, Nick Cassisi, George Singleton, Gerry Merwin, Jim Parsons, Bill Mendenhall, John Issacs, and Scott Stringer.

Finally (I always leave them for last), I have to thank the Williams & Wilkins crew. Tim Grayson, Carol Eckhart, and Anne Seitz—as always its been great working with you and your colleagues. Let's do it again!

A.A.M.

Contents

How to Use This Book

Usually you get a book and read it. No instructions are necessary. This book, however, is one with several different goals (see Preface to Second Edition) and it is worthwhile to consider some of the following suggestions.

1. For studying anatomy first copy the appropriate checklists in Appendix A. Then go to the appropriate chapter and find the normal images and line diagrams that they are keyed to. Be sure that you find each structure on the images. Keep the three-dimensional nature of the anatomy in mind by having other gross anatomic references handy while you look at the sectional images. From such study you will begin to form the basis for all image interpretation, a thorough three-dimensional knowledge of the anatomy under investigation. Also please note that some specific anatomic concepts are emphasized outside of the initial basic set of images. These include the anatomy of the cavernous sinus, middle meatus, and cranial nerves, among others. Anatomic concepts are also discussed in conjunction with the quiz cases in Chapters 2 through 9.

2. As a guide to performing, interpreting, and consulting on CT and MRI studies, some questions that may come up include:

   a. *Should I use CT or MRI first?* Read the brief introductory section of the appropriate chapter and consult the appropriate algorithm (if available). Decide how to proceed. Remember, more than one study may be necessary.

   b. *How exactly should the study be done?* General approaches to MRI studies are at the end of the "Technique" section in each chapter. Computed tomography protocols are in a table in each chapter. The spread patterns table in Appendix C may help in choosing the proper planes of section. Very specific instructions reflecting such techniques should be given to the technologists in written form. You should supervise each case.

   c. *I only see one or two of these studies per week (or month); how can I be sure I am not missing something?* Use the checklists in Appendix A to establish what anatomy is deranged. Spread patterns of cancers appear in Appendix C, and this table may prove to be a valuable interpretive aid. Work through a sample case, if one is available. Consult the tables for differential diagnosis when appropriate. Look at more comparable cases in other texts. If you have good images and you are still confused you can always ask someone with a little more experience for help.

The book is meant to serve many purposes. The most important is to help improve the quality of CT and MRI studies and the interpretation of those studies. Good luck. If you need help I can be reached at (904) 395-0106.

A.A.M.

perceived as separate from one another. The image contrast for those two objects can be thought of as setting the threshold for spatial resolution. Both contrast and spatial resolution are affected by altering voxel size or more fundamentally the protons per voxel (MRI) or electrons per voxel (CT). This is discussed in detail later. The two concepts are interrelated in a very complex manner that has relatively recently led to the development of the concept of relative resolving power (T). This concept is a useful one and is fully discussed in some of the suggested reading sources. In the following discussions image contrast and spatial resolution are dealt with separately so as to emphasize the operator-dependent variables that may be used to improve the overall resolving power of the CT or MRI unit.

COMPUTED TOMOGRAPHY

At the outset it is useful to consider what optimal CT technique might be, assuming that a "fully loaded" (software and hardware) system is available. Units capable of routinely excellent images of an entire region have been available from all major manufacturers since 1985. Older units with full projection scan times in the 9-sec range can do the work but image quality is variable, mainly as a result of motion artifacts in the upper aerodigestive tract. Some older units may also lack the tube-detector configuration to do very high-resolution work or to be capable of state-of-the-art "dynamic" vascular studies.

Basic requirements for good head and neck imaging include the following:

1. Slice thickness (SLT): 1.5 to 2 mm for high-detail work, 3 to 5 mm for routine studies
2. Field of view (FOV): 9 to 18 cm
3. Matrix: 512 × 512
4. Scan time: 2 to 3 sec routine; 4 to 6 sec for high-detail work
5. Capacity for dynamic vascular studies

These scan parameters are discussed in detail in the following sections.

Ultimately the limitations of spatial and contrast resolution in a CT system are profoundly influenced by original scan data measurements. Some factors influencing this are related to the dimensions of the imaging hardware; they include focal spot size, detector aperture width, sampling distance, and magnification (tube-object and object-detector distance). These parameters can be influenced during the purchase of the CT equipment. Other factors affecting spatial and contrast resolution are under operator control on a day-to-day basis, and these can profoundly influence the information content of the image if one pays attention to a few simple details during the planning stages of each exam (Table 1.1). These include SLT, matrix size, FOV, choice of reconstruction algorithm, exposure, and sampling detail (milliamperage and time) as well as strategic use of intravenous contrast enhancement.

Spatial Resolution

In CT anything that is done to reduce voxel size reduces the photon flux per voxel (i.e., decreases SNR). Reduced SNR decreases image contrast while the reduction in voxel size increases spatial resolution. In a given situation one must consider whether increasing the milliamperage or time (sampling frequency) is necessary to increase the photon flux per voxel to compensate for this loss in image contrast. This decision will largely depend on the inherent contrast and size of the region or pathology under study. The main cost of increased milliamperage and/or time is increased patient dose. For instance, a study of the temporal bone at 200 mA and 4 sec may look better than one done at 170 mA and 2 sec, but the latter may be as highly spatially resolved, contain the same diagnostic information, and be more appropriate in a pediatric patient. In fact, increased dose will have relatively little effect on improving resolving power for high-contrast structures such as the temporal bone once a certain threshold is reached. After that point, increasing the radiation dose may improve aesthetics but it probably will not alter diagnostic capabilities. The trade-off between spatial and contrast resolution, area under study, and dose should be determined in advance and protocols or guidelines established based on the individual equipment available and the perceived requirements for the degree

Table 1.1
Steps for Planning CT Examination

1. Adequate definition of clinical questions to be answered by the study
   a. From referring physician
   b. From talking with and examining the patient
2. Planning the study
   a. Proper positioning
   b. Preliminary view—select gantry angles, slice thickness
   c. Choose optimal FOV, matrix size
   d. Set technique factors according to demands of study and dose considerations
   e. Choose appropriate primary reconstruction algorithm
3. Execute study
   a. Reduction of motion artifacts—patient restraint, shoulders down, breathholding
   b. Proper use of I.V. contrast
   c. Constant physician supervision; repeat or add views as needed
4. Recording the data
   a. Proper photography
   b. Magnify areas of interest
   c. Save and reconstruct raw data whenever necessary

of clarity required in an image for diagnosis. The guidelines at the University of Florida are outlined in Table 1.2 and based on experience with a GE system. Fortunately, with the currently available tube-detector systems, excellent-quality, fast images are virtually routine at reasonable technique (dose) levels. Further improvements will no doubt occur. In the following sections it should become apparent that the factors affecting spatial resolution are largely under operator control and may be manipulated to greatly improve the clarity and content of the image.

Slice Thickness

Neurologic head and neck imaging was the driving force behind the move to thinner sections in the late 1970s. The need was based upon the desire to visualize increasingly small structures, some on the order of 1 to 2 pixels (at that time) in size, and a perceived need for highly resolved reformatted images.

It is known that with a thinner section comes higher contrast and better spatial resolution for objects not occupying the full thickness of the section; this is the result of diminished volume averaging. Reduced section thickness also reduces photon flux per voxel per unit of time, and the reduced SNR aggravates the tendency for the system to produce artifacts, such as the aliasing artifacts most commonly visually expressed as bright and dark streaks in the image. The disadvantages of thinner sections, then, are potentially noisier images with possibly less image contrast and more artifacts. In areas of high inherent (subject) contrast the increased noise poses no great problem because contrast in voxels at the edges of neighboring structures of interest is likely to be far above background noise. The air-bone–soft tissue interfaces of the temporal bone are an ideal situation for the use of thin sections; these interfaces occur between small structures that need to be resolved and all have very high inherent contrast. Therefore high-contrast images can be obtained using thin sections, without dramatically increasing radiation dose to the patient, so long as sampling frequency (detector density, time) is adequate to limit artifacts. When thin sections (1.5 to 2 mm) are used to study tissues of less inherent contrast (e.g., orbital apex) then more photon flux (milliamperage) may be required to provide the necessary SNR per voxel. If streak artifacts are the problem an increase in time (sampling frequency) may be more appropriate (Table 1.2). However, increasing the scan time will increase the risk of motion artifacts. Thus, with CT as well as with MRI the optimal image is a compromise between multiple factors that tend to work against each other.

Table 1.2
Basic CT Technique Chart

Area of Interest	Slice Thickness (mm)	mA	kV	Time (sec)
Head (adult)	10	200	120	2
Head (child)	10	140	120	2
	5	170	120	2
	3	200	120	2
Posterior fossa (adult)	5	170	120	3
	3	200	120	3
Temporal bone	1.5	170	120	4
Orbits, sinuses, nasopharynx	3	170	120	3
Oropharynx, larynx, neck	3	200	120	2

An equally important matter is the relationship between the overall cephalocaudad extent of the area under study and the SLT. It would be optimum to have 2-mm sections through the entire larynx and neck, but routine 75-section studies may be impractical. In the upper aerodigestive tract and neck contiguous 5-mm sections or sections 3-mm thick at 5-mm increments are adequate for survey and general usage. Three-millimeter contiguous sections are now always used over the portion of the anatomy likely to most critically affect diagnosis and management. Examples of areas where the thinner 3-mm sections are used include the true and false vocal cords and subglottic region of the larynx; the oropharynx in the region of primary tumor or other lesion; the nasopharynx and skull base; and the orbits, paranasal sinuses, and parotid gland. Three-millimeter sections are important in large lesions as well as small lesions since it is often a 3- to 5-millimeter margin between pathology and some critical piece of anatomy that will alter therapy. On modern CT equipment tissue contrast remains excellent with 3-mm sections with acceptable radiation dose levels. The temporal bone is almost always studied with 1.5- to 2-mm contiguous sections and sometimes these are done at 1-mm table increments. Overlapped sections in the axial plane should be avoided when increased radiation dose to the lens is likely, unless there is a strong indication that this will potentially alter patient management. Angling at 0° or 30° to the infraorbital-meatal line (IOML) during temporal bone work helps limit dose to the lens. Contiguous 1.5- or 3-mm sections always suffice even in the most demanding orbital case.

Pixel Size (FOV)

Recall that the spatial resolution in a CT image can be no greater than that provided by the display system (CRT) matrix. For this discussion it is assumed that the display system itself is not a limiting factor since this is true of virtually all CT systems nowadays. Because each pixel has a discrete attenuation value, there must be an adjacent pixel of a different value in order for an interface to be perceived. Put differently, two pixels of the same attenuation value must be separated by another of a different value in order for the two to be resolved. Because of averaging effects it is generally assumed that in order for two objects to be resolved they must be separated by slightly more than one pixel width. Improved array processors and increased memory in modern CT systems have made routine use of a 512 × 512 matrix possible, and this should be standard technique when feasible in both extracranial head and neck and body imaging.

The selection of the FOV is the second major factor affecting pixel size and, therefore, spatial resolution (Fig. 1.1). The *x,y* dimensions of a pixel can be derived by dividing the FOV by the matrix size. If a 512 × 512 matrix and a 12- to 18-cm FOV are used routinely one can see that about a 0.25- to 0.35-millimeter pixel size is now the rule in the head and neck. Of course, the pixel size is only partially related to spatial resolution, and from the prior discussion it should be clear that, at minimum, spatial resolution will be somewhat larger than a pixel width (usually said to be about 1.5 pixels). Actual spatial resolution needs to be measured because it also depends on tube-detector factors, inherent contrast, and which filter function (convolution kernel) is used in the reconstruction. Recall that thin section high-resolution CT scanning requires that the basic technique (peak kilovoltage, milliamperes per second) and sampling frequency (time, detector density) are high enough to allow the desired resolution to occur without significant degradation due to artifacts.

Every effort should be made to reduce the FOV to the smallest practical limit because of the improved spatial resolution (Fig. 1.1). On current (circa 1985 to 1987) systems this can be done easily. A FOV of 18 cm or less is always used except for unusually large patients or at the thoracic inlet when the supraclavicular fossae and/or axillae must be included. Our scanning routine begins with an axial section, following the planning "scout" projection radiograph, the former being used to set up the extent of the study and proper gantry angulation(s). Both are done before contrast infusion (Fig. 1.2 and Table 1.1). The FOV is then chosen with a circular cursor, making allowances for the anterior-to-posterior shift in anatomy of interest that occurs as one moves from the head to the neck region. This can be done retrospectively but requires saving the raw data as well as increased data manipulation and storage, resulting in decreased throughput on some systems. Currently if a 512 × 512 reconstruction/display matrix is used, one can do either prospective or retrospective (targeted) reconstructions with pixels as small as 0.25 mm. The logistics and exact mode of doing this vary with the vendor, but virtually all newer, "fully loaded" general-purpose scanners can perform this function.

Reconstruction Algorithm

The last major factor affecting spatial resolution is the choice of filter function (convolution kernel). Coarse filters enhance large changes in spatial frequency information along the beam path (e.g., bone

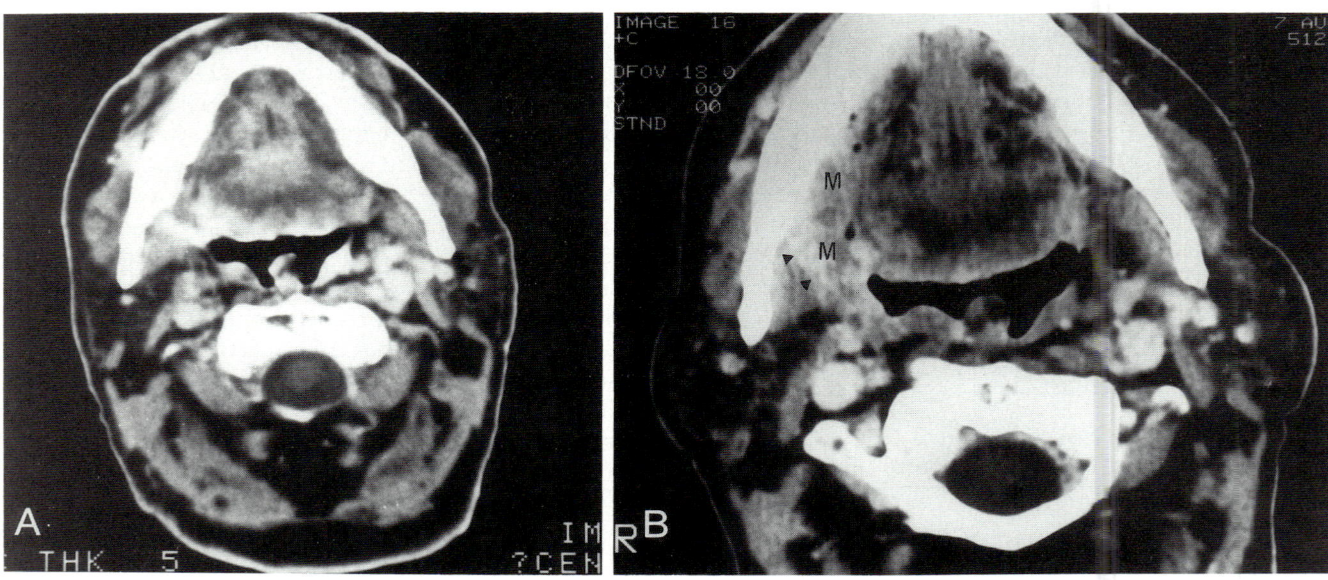

Figure 1.1*A* and *B*

Figure 1.1. Images from studies on the same patients made within 1 week of each other. The patient has a retromolar trigone carcinoma. *A*, from an outside institution—field of view is too large and the patient was not instructed to suspend respiration; the result is a diagnostically useless image. *B*, same patient restudied at the University of Florida—correction of the technical errors mentioned above leads to highly informative image showing aggressive, deeply infiltrating mass (*M*) invading medial pterygoid muscle *(arrowheads)*. Attention to technical detail is of paramount importance in head and neck imaging.

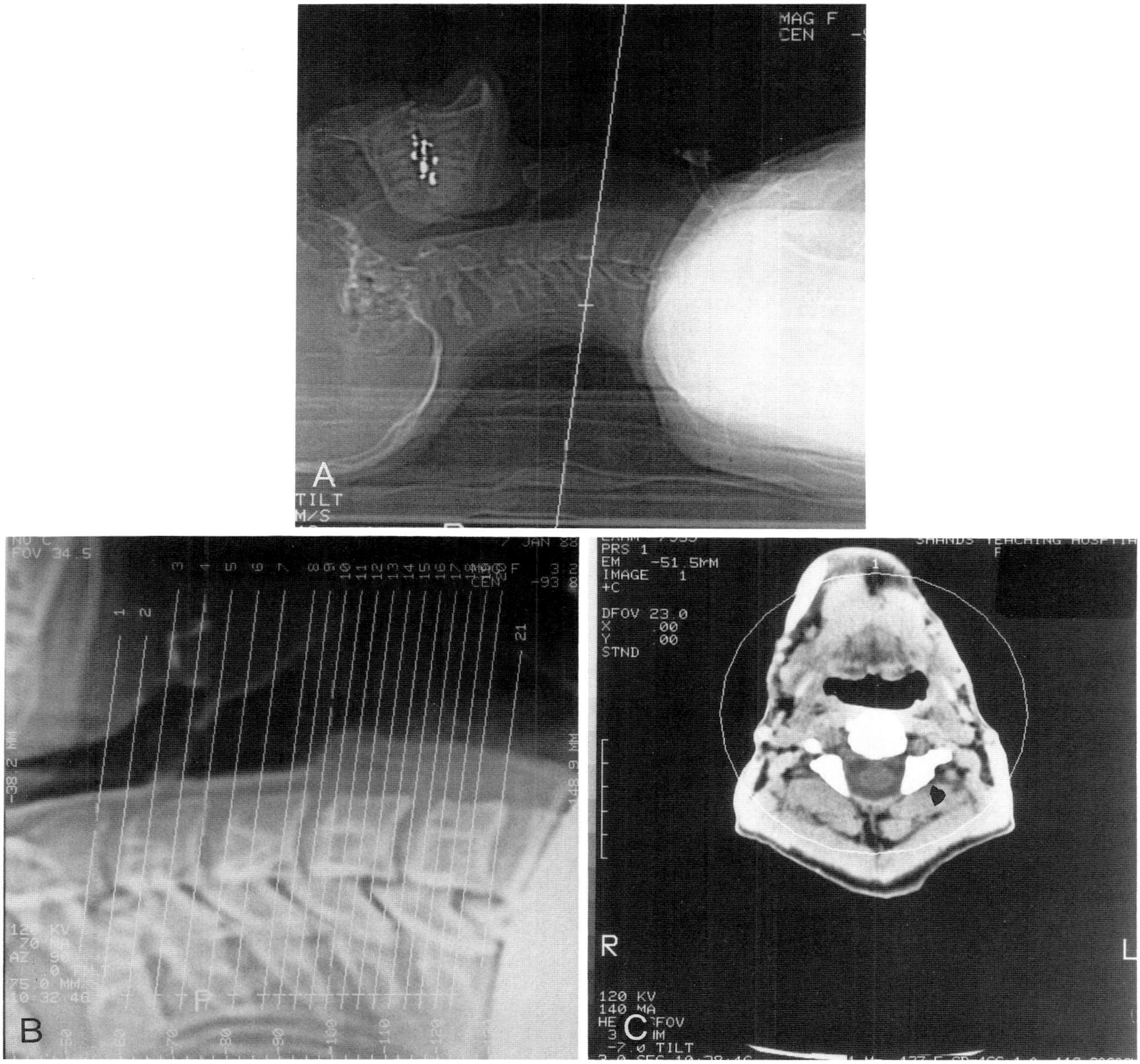

Figure 1.2*A–C*

Figure 1.2. Steps in planning CT study (also see Table 1.1). *A*, preliminary digital radiography is obtained and optimal gantry angle selected. In this case sections are parallel to the true vocal cords because the patient has laryngeal carcinoma. *B*, slice thickness, interval, and full extent of study are programmed according to highly site- and pathology-specific protocols. *C*, first axial section is obtained and optimal field of view chosen. This may be changed prospectively during or retrospectively after the study.

to air to cerebrospinal fluid to brain); the lower spatial frequency changes are somewhat "glossed over" in the reconstruction algorithm. This means that only a gross assessment of the brain is possible and some loss of contrast in other soft tissue results. In general at least four choices will exist in most manufacturers' software. Before selecting a coarse or sharp (bone) algorithm the structures of major interest should differ from each other by about 100 Hounsfield units. The air, soft tissue (pathology), and bone interfaces of the temporal bone are an ideal place to apply such a filter function, which in turn can take spatial resolution to its lowest possible limits (about 0.375 to 0.5 mm at a pixel size of 0.25 mm). For this increase in spatial resolution one trades contrast resolution. Fortunately raw data can be saved and one should never hesitate to reconstruct both standard soft tissue *and* bone algorithms if the clinical situation dictates. This situation arises most frequently in temporal bone–brain, sinonasal, and orbital studies. Frequently only selected images need to be reconstructed using both algorithms. The penalty again is time, and that the study becomes more physician intensive. Most extracranial head and neck CT already is detailed and physician intensive if done properly. Set protocols help but cannot substitute for active physician supervision.

Contrast Resolution

It is obvious from the previous discussion that the separation of contrast and spatial issues in a discussion of resolution is somewhat artificial. The separation is more useful in MRI, in which pulse sequence selection can affect more factors (T_1, T_2, proton density, and flow), than in CT, in which one is primarily dealing with electron density. The overriding principle in CT is that anything done to reduce pixel size reduces photon flux per voxel and may reduce tissue contrast. Currently this only seems important in the brain, where with sections of 3 mm or less one might want to increase dose (mainly by increased milliamperage but also by increased scan time) to compensate (Table 1.2). The inherent contrast based on electron density elsewhere in the head and neck region is good enough not to require increased technique. Generally kilovoltage is kept at 120 kV and not manipulated to alter contrast. Altering kilovoltage is much more important in abdominal work, in which more energy per photon may be necessary to get the photons to the detector. A typical adjustment in dose might include going from 170 to 200 mA for 5- versus 3-mm sections through the posterior fossa (Table 1.2). This is aimed at improving contrast resolution in the brain. One note of caution: Older systems or newer ones with less favorable tube-detector system design may require dramatic increase in dose to achieve adequate contrast (and spatial) resolution. This is usually accomplished by increasing both milliamperage and scan time. Increase in time has obvious disadvantages in marginally cooperative patients or in areas where motion artifacts are common, such as the upper aerodigestive tract.

Artifacts

There are machine-related and scan technique–related artifacts. Assume the machine is working perfectly (i.e., no rings, calibration and tube are good, etc.). The physician in charge can then have a profound effect on image quality by ensuring that technical, positioning, and other factors have been brought into proper focus for the problem at hand.

Gross motion artifacts can first be overcome by proper restraint of the head and *chin* in a comfortably extended position (Fig. 1.2). Motion due to swallowing and breathing is overcome by using 2-sec scan times and instructing the patient to "stop breathing and do not swallow" during each period of data acquisition (Fig. 1.1). Standardization of positioning and doing scans in suspended respiration will eliminate virtually all motion artifacts in patients who are able to cooperate. The disadvantage of breath holding comes only in the larynx, where additional sections through the true and false cords during quiet breathing may be required to look for subtle abnormalities. Since installation of modern CT equipment at the University of Florida, we have not had a head and neck study that was nondiagnostic because of motion artifact, and well over 90% of our studies are of excellent quality.

Streak artifacts through the shoulders are common, although much less apparent, on newer units as a result of more efficient tube-detector systems (i.e., improved sampling interval and frequency). Extending the neck slightly as a routine overcomes much of this because it "pulls" the structures of the visceral compartment up and out of the trouble spot. A simple trick in patients with thick, short necks is to put a blanket or sheet around the soles of the feet and have the patient grasp the free ends. Often some encouragement to relax the shoulders and gently pushing down on them will get the patient to relax the upper body and significantly drop the shoulders. Some patients are simply difficult and here the time, kilovoltage, and milliamperage can be increased if necessary to minimize the artifacts, especially if the low neck or thoracic inlet are sites of critical interest. All studies are done with manufacturer-supplied restraining and positioning hardware. Some custom devices are commercially available to help with more hyperextended neck positioning and as a substitute for the "blanket-around-the-feet" method of lowering the shoulders.

In the posterior fossa, the familiar artifacts between the petrous ridges remain an intermittent problem, although much less so on newer units. Immobilization is essential. Scanning parallel to the IOML is probably the most critical factor in reducing this artifact. These done, one can also decrease section thickness to 3 mm or less, increase time (sampling frequency), and increase milliamperage (improve tissue contrast in brain). Practically, this is becoming a less important issue since MRI has become the predominant imaging tool in the posterior fossa. However, at the University of Florida 3-mm axial sections done parallel to the IOML are now used routinely from the roof of the orbit to the foramen magnum in studies of the brain to help minimize these artifacts.

Intravenous Contrast

Iodinated contrast is an extremely valuable tool when used properly in conjunction with intra- and extracranial studies of the head and neck. Its use involves risk. Because of this a risks/benefits decision must be made about its use in every patient. Sometimes it is difficult to anticipate whether a study done with contrast will yield a more informative set of images. Perhaps the most difficult decisions must be made in considering the use of contrast in diseases of the paranasal sinuses, nasal cavity, and orbits. Specific indications are discussed in appropriate chapters. The nonionic/lower osmolarity products will make the risk/benefit decisions easier but at increased cost.

The aims of contrast infusion in extracranial head and neck radiology are *(a)* to determine the vascularity of a lesion, *(b)* to see the margins of a lesion with greater clarity, *(c)* to distinguish normal vessels from pathology (primary tumor and lymph nodes) and study the effects of pathology on these same vessels, and *(d)* to aid in differential diagnosis. These goals require that iodine be in the "vascular" phase throughout image acquisition. Over the years the best strategy to accomplish these goals has resulted in two approaches. These differ based on whether or not a power injector is used:

1. Without a power injector:
   a. Start I.V. to keep open (TKO) (D_5W or 300 ml of 25% low-viscosity contrast) with 19- or 20-gauge intracath. Three-way stopcock facilitates use of I.V. fluid rather than contrast during TKO (planning) phase.
   b. Plan study—obtain "scout" projection radiograph and first axial slice to assess CT plan.
   c. Inject 40- to 60-ml bolus of 60% contrast over *1 to 2 min* (to avoid nausea and vomiting).
   d. At completion of bolus, open I.V. to maximum flow rate and begin scanning.
2. With a power injector:
   a. Start I.V. with 19- or 20-gauge intracath TKO (see above).
   b. Plan study—obtain a "scout" projection radiograph and first slice to assess CT plan.
   c. Load injector with 60% contrast—infuse at 0.5 ml/sec. Start scanning after approximately 60-sec delay.
   c. (Alternate method) Start scanning after 90-sec delay and give intermittent 15- to 25-ml boluses depending on intravascular enhancement observed as images become available. This assumes that on-line viewing by physicians/technologists is occurring during study.

The bolus-drip method delivers about 50 g of iodine to the patient. The power injector method delivers about 42 g. The bolus-drip method is easy to perform and runs less of a risk of serious extravasation of contrast. It also may allow a slightly longer period of time during which the contrast is at maximal "intravascular" concentration; this is probably due to the approximately 20% increase in iodine load delivered. Both techniques will allow about a 10- to 12-min window for acquisition of images during which vessels are heavily opacified, mucosa is enhancing, and tumor margins are best visualized. These two techniques are equally efficacious and reasonably safe. A power injector is not necessary and it does raise the risk of a large-volume extravasation with potential soft tissue sloughing.

Dynamic studies are occasionally a useful adjunct to the more routine technique just described. These were first popularized in the head and neck region for studies of the posterior fossa, but their use in identifying hypervascular masses was probably simultaneously appreciated. The studies may be done either by hand or with a power injector. This can, at least in selected cases, be used to improve differential diagnosis and, rarely, obviate conventional or digital angiography under the proper clinical circumstances (Fig. 1.3). Dynamic studies can be used as a routine; however, the techniques usually involve reduced milliamperage per second and potentially diminished contrast resolution; the potential trade-offs here are machine dependent. Most importantly, the images are batch reconstructed after acquisition, which makes on-line physician supervision less convenient. Such supervision is the cornerstone of good head and neck imaging in our practice.

The technique of dynamic scanning for the purposes of differential diagnosis is quite simple. The lesion in question is scanned in one plane during rapid bolus injection of contrast. The accumulation and washout of contrast is plotted over time and compared to that of surrounding control structures (i.e., artery, vein, and muscle) on the same section. The computer-generated curves can show a clear separation between lesions with rapid flow (washin/washout) and those with other patterns (Fig. 1.3). This taken with clinical data, gross morphology, and location can usually lead to a highly accurate differential diagnosis and help determine the need for angiography. Although this technique has been popularized by some groups, these authors use it infrequently in clinical practice, preferring to select the patient needing angiography based on a high-quality bolus-drip study and clinical data.

CT-Guided Biopsy

The overwhelming majority of biopsies in head and neck patients are done in the clinic or during endoscopy. In highly selected circumstances, however, CT-guided biopsy can obviate a significant and sometimes difficult operation. This happens most frequently in those lesions that are discovered on CT or MRI studies and are not palpable or visible clinically.

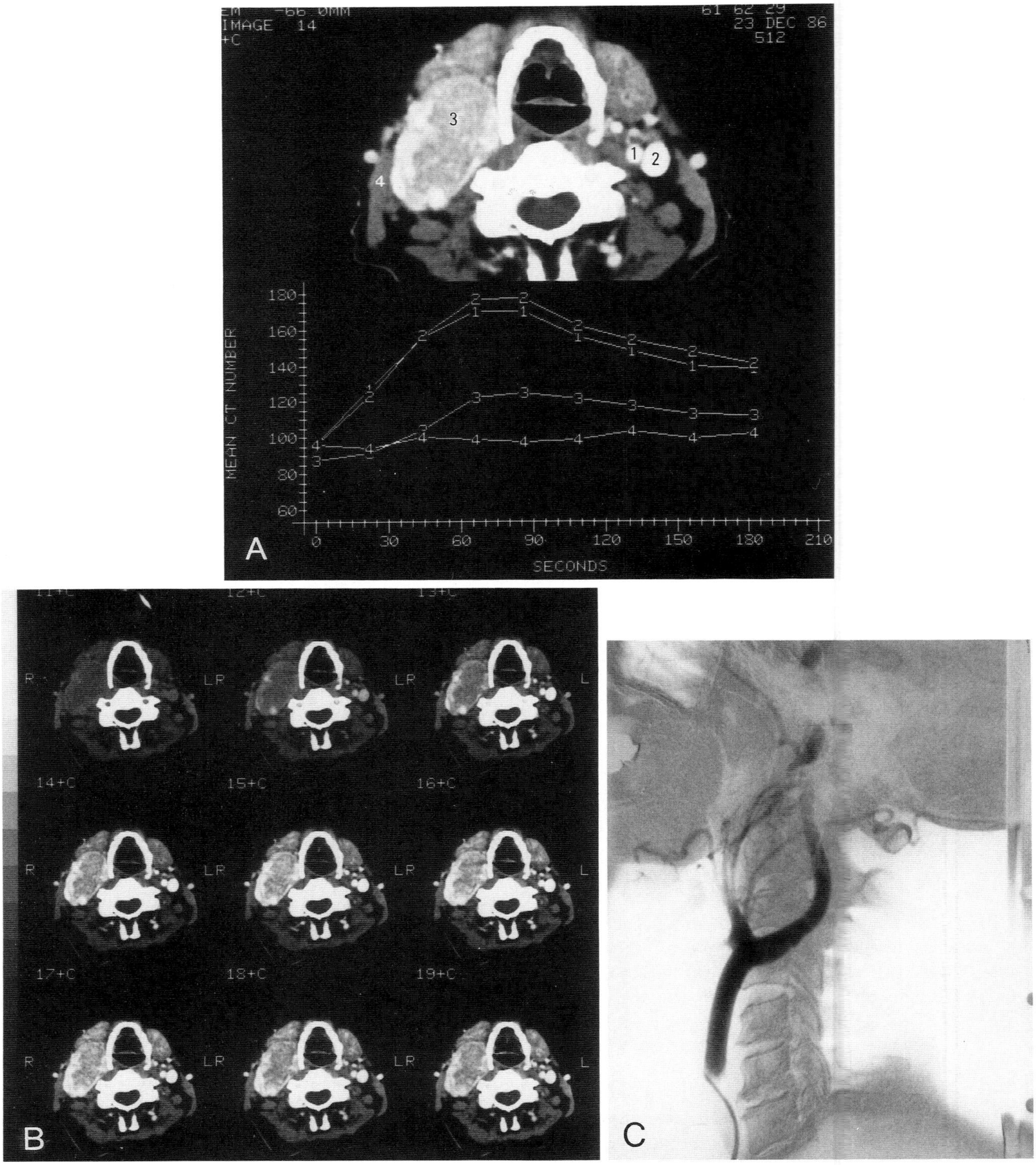

Figure 1.3*A–C*

Figure 1.3. Example of a "semiquantitive" dynamic CT study. *A,* Areas of interest are selected, including: 1. carotid artery; 2. jugular vein; 3. tumor; and 4. muscle. Contrast bolus is given and mean CT numbers are recorded as a function of time. *B,* individual scans at about 25-sec increments. *C,* arteriogram correlates well with the dynamic CT study, showing a relatively hypovascular mass.

Comment: From its position this mass should be a paraganglioma (carotid body type). Since it was hypovascular on both angiography and dynamic CT, neuroma was suggested as the preferred preoperative diagnosis. Pathologically this was a predominantly fibrotic carotid body tumor (paraganglioma).

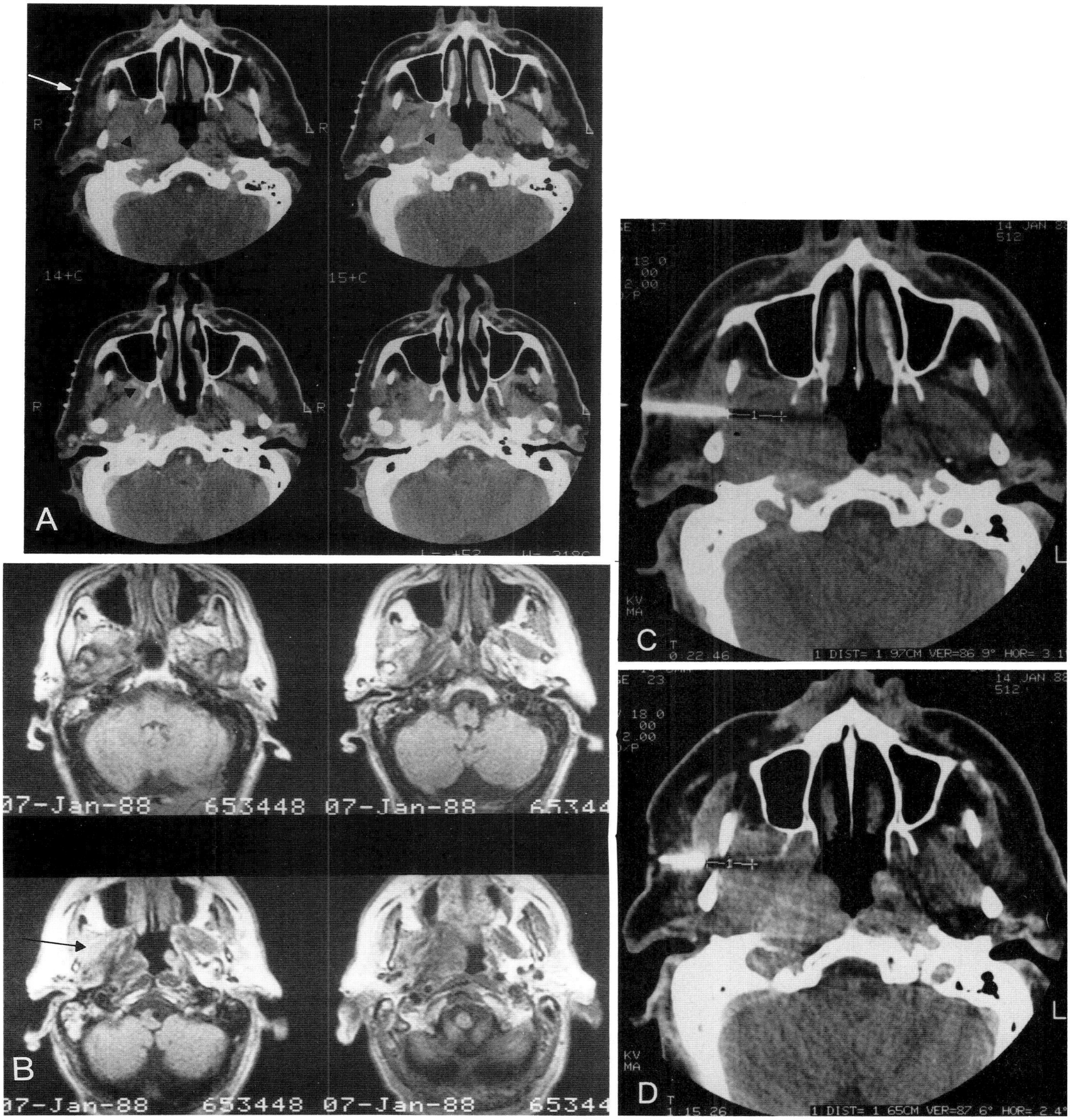

Figure 1.4*A–D*

Figure 1.4. General procedure for CT-guided biopsy. *A,* four views with localizing catheters *(arrows)* in place. Dynamic study with contrast infusion localizes the maxillary artery *(arrowheads)*. *B,* correlation with four views from MRI study shows target area of tumor *(arrow)* distinctly different in signal than surrounding muscle; this aids site selection and cuts down on false sampling of muscle. *C,* 19-gauge guide needle in place. Having established optimal angle and access, excursion of 22-gauge aspiration is planned; this will be done coaxially. Aspiration did not yield positive diagnosis. *D,* 18-gauge ABC needle positioned so that cutting action begins deep to facial nerve (note tip of needle in masseter muscle). Excursion of needle directed inferior to course of maxillary artery; depth was controlled as further safeguard *(dashed line)*. Core specimen was hand carried to surgical pathology. Diagnosis was poorly differentiated carcinoma.

Biopsies may be done with fine needles (20 gauge or smaller) or large needles with or without cutting action. Cutting needles have been used only in cases in which the lesion is shown to be hypovascular, relatively superficial, and large enough so that the likelihood of lacerating the pterygoid venous plexus, major vessels, or facial nerve is remote.

A lesion may be sampled in one of the following ways depending on its location:

1. *Infratemporal fossa*—Just under the zygomatic arch via the notch between the condyle and coronoid processes of the mandible. Cutting needle can be used with proper precautions (Fig. 1.4).
2. *Deep parotid space, parapharyngeal space; deep to angle of mandible*—Posterolateral approach between the mastoid tip and mandible; level varies with site and lesion. Cutting needle has never been used by us with this approach.
3. *Poststyloid parapharyngeal space (carotid sheath), deep posterior upper neck*—Suboccipital approach or posterior approach. Cutting needle may be used in the posterior upper neck with proper precautions in larger, more superficial lesions if hypovascular. The cutting needle is *never* used in the vicinity of the carotid sheath.
4. *Neck*—Any direction that will avoid damage to major vessels or chance of airway obstruction.
5. *Transnasal*—Rarely used; should be done with ear, nose, and throat surgeon and following cocainization.

The policy at the University of Florida is to have a cytotechnologist present with a microscope and equipment for basic slide making. Samples are obtained and viewed by that person and the diagnostic radiologist. After just a few cases the diagnostic radiologist can become quite proficient at judging the adequacy of a sample, although specific diagnosis requires a very experienced cytopathologist. The procedures are done at a time when pathologists are available for immediate consultation. When core specimens are obtained, these are sometimes hand carried to pathology for frozen section confirmation before the patient is released. Recently core needle and cytologic specimens have been used for flow cytometry, which can be useful in identifying and typing lymphoma.

Over the years these infrequent procedures have proven highly efficacious. They often lead to definitive management without the need for major surgery. They have confirmed recurrent tumor earlier than possible in previous times and have led to more prompt triage of patients to either palliative treatment or salvage-for-cure categories when combined with the overall clinical and imaging findings.

Summary

Modern CT is an extraordinarily powerful imaging tool when used and interpreted properly. By following the steps outlined in Table 1.1 and discussed in detail in the preceding sections anyone can produce high-quality CT studies capable of providing a large amount of information relevant to patient care.

MAGNETIC RESONANCE IMAGING

It is essential to understand basic MRI physics in order to use this imaging tool to its fullest advantage, and there are many excellent sources of this information (see Suggested Readings). This discussion assumes a basic fund of MRI knowledge and centers on clinically applied physical principles, much as was done in the CT section.

Images of maximum quality and information content are the goal. The importance of field strength toward these ends has been overemphasized for various reasons. For a while there was great confusion regarding was the "optimal" field strength for proton imaging. Excellent head and neck imaging can be done at fields of 0.15 T and greater (Fig. 1.5). It is important not to become unduly biased on this matter. It is simply an issue of signal to noise. This is no different than any other imaging technique. One can increase the signal, decrease the noise, and preferably do both to improve the image quality. Signal may be increased by raising the field strength, by capturing more signal (e.g., optimized receiver coil, quadrature detection), or by using varied techniques (e.g., three-dimensional Fourier transform, improved radiofrequency (Rf) slice-selective pulse profile). Noise can be reduced by improving system electronics (e.g., properly located preamp, narrowing receiver bandwidth) or by decreasing body-related noise (e.g., with a closely coupled small-volume receiver coil). The difficulties in exercising these options vary with field strength and individual system design. The bottom line is that practical diagnostic information will prove roughly equivalent at all fields in *optimized* systems operating from 0.15 to 1.5 T, with the possible exception of information resulting from magnetic susceptibility differences such as that induced by iron stores or deposition, which is easier to recognize with higher field (0.5- to 1.5-T) units. Magnetic susceptibility effects are *routinely* visible on 0.15- to 0.35-T instruments, so that only relative sensitivities are at issue (Fig. 1.6). High-field systems (1.0 T and above), on the other hand, suffer significant losses as a result of physiologic motion, tuning difficulties, and coil loading effects that are expressed most acutely in body imaging but are present in head and neck imaging as soon as one goes beyond the brain. No system is without its faults.

A more important issue is what constitutes reasonably acceptable technique for studying the areas of interest presented subsequently. Based on 4 years of experience and over 7000 cases at the University of Florida with an *optimized* 0.15-T resistive unit, we have set certain minimum guidelines for ourselves in head and neck imaging. These have proven fully capable of providing very sophisticated data in intra- and extracranial pathology, and there has been no need to supplement studies from this system with studies done on another unit. These routine techniques include:

1. SLT: 4 to 5 mm on T_1-weighted sequences and 6 to 8 mm on T_2-weighted sequences
2. FOV: 21 to 28 cm (14 cm for temporomandibular joint)
3. Acquisition matrix: 192 × 256 or 128 × 256 (in multiecho mode)
4. Acquisition time: 6 to 14 min/sequence (total exam time 45 to 60 min)

Spatial Resolution

The basic concepts of the voxel, and the relative impact of image contrast, spatial resolution, and SNR on resolution, were introduced at the beginning of this chapter (see "Resolution—General Considerations"). The interrelationships of those factors are fundamental to understanding the following discussion. They should be reviewed now if necessary.

The need for some finite amount of spatial resolution determines in part the lower limits of acceptable SNR in any imaging system. In MRI, when voxel size is decreased the number of protons per voxel decreases. When SLT is narrowed the effect is linear, that is, one-half the SLT results in one-half the protons and one-half the original signal. When pixel size is reduced (FOV decreased), the situation is more serious. Since the reduction is in two dimensions, reduction of the pixel width by a factor of 2 diminishes the SNR by a factor of 2.8. One can immediately begin to realize the trade-off in balancing the needs of spatial resolution and image contrast when deciding which pulse sequences are necessary to study the brain. With spin echo techniques adequate contrast between normal brain and intra-axial pathology implies the use of pulse sequences with long pulse repetition times (TRs) (therefore limiting the amount of signal averaging possible) and pulse-echo intervals (TEs) in the 70- to 90-msec range. The longer TEs are inherently lower signal situations because of the position of most tissues on the decay curve at these relatively late echo delay times. Five-millimeter sections with a 21- to 28-cm FOV are fairly well tolerated at any field strength for short TR/TE (e.g., 500 to 700/20 to 30

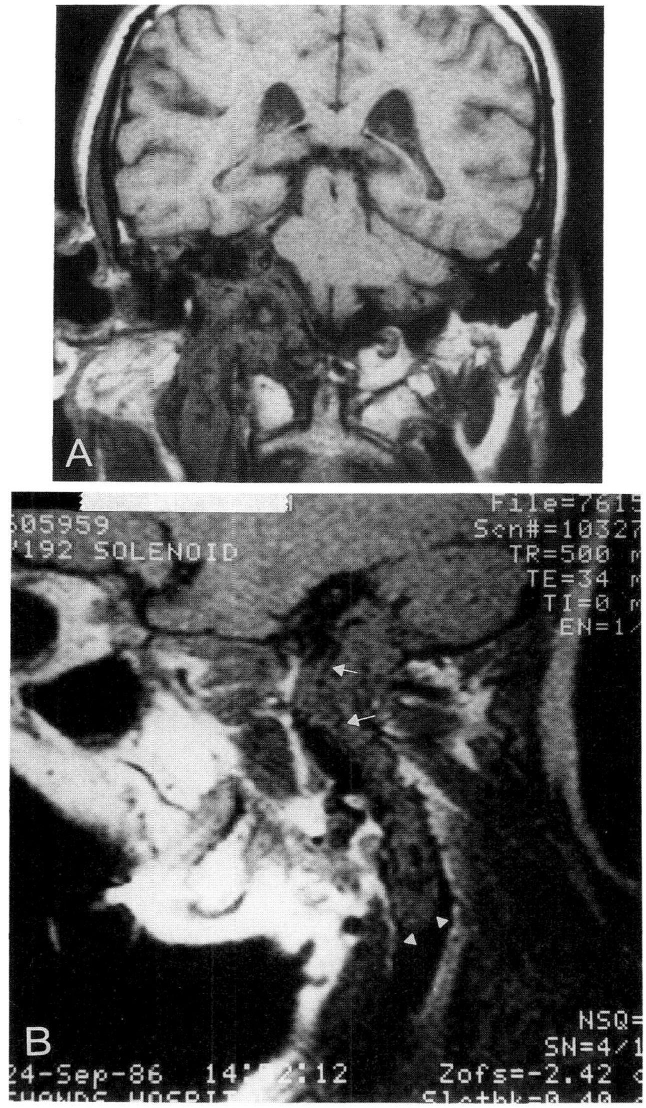

Figure 1.5*A* and *B*

Figure 1.5. Two different patients each with a paraganglioma (glomus jugulare type). *A,* MRI image done on a 1.5-T GE unit, routine head coil, with 3-mm section, partial saturation 500/20-msec pulse sequence, and about 8 min acquisition time. *B,* image done on a 0.15-T resistive Technicare unit, our own custom volume head coil, 4-mm section, spin echo 500/34-msec pulse sequence, and about 8 min acquisition time.

Comment: Although the higher field image is clearly aesthetically more pleasing, the low-field image contains all necessary diagnostic information [i.e., flow void in serpiginous vascular structures *(arrows),* obvious intraluminal pattern in jugular vein *(arrowheads)*] and is reasonably aesthetic as well.

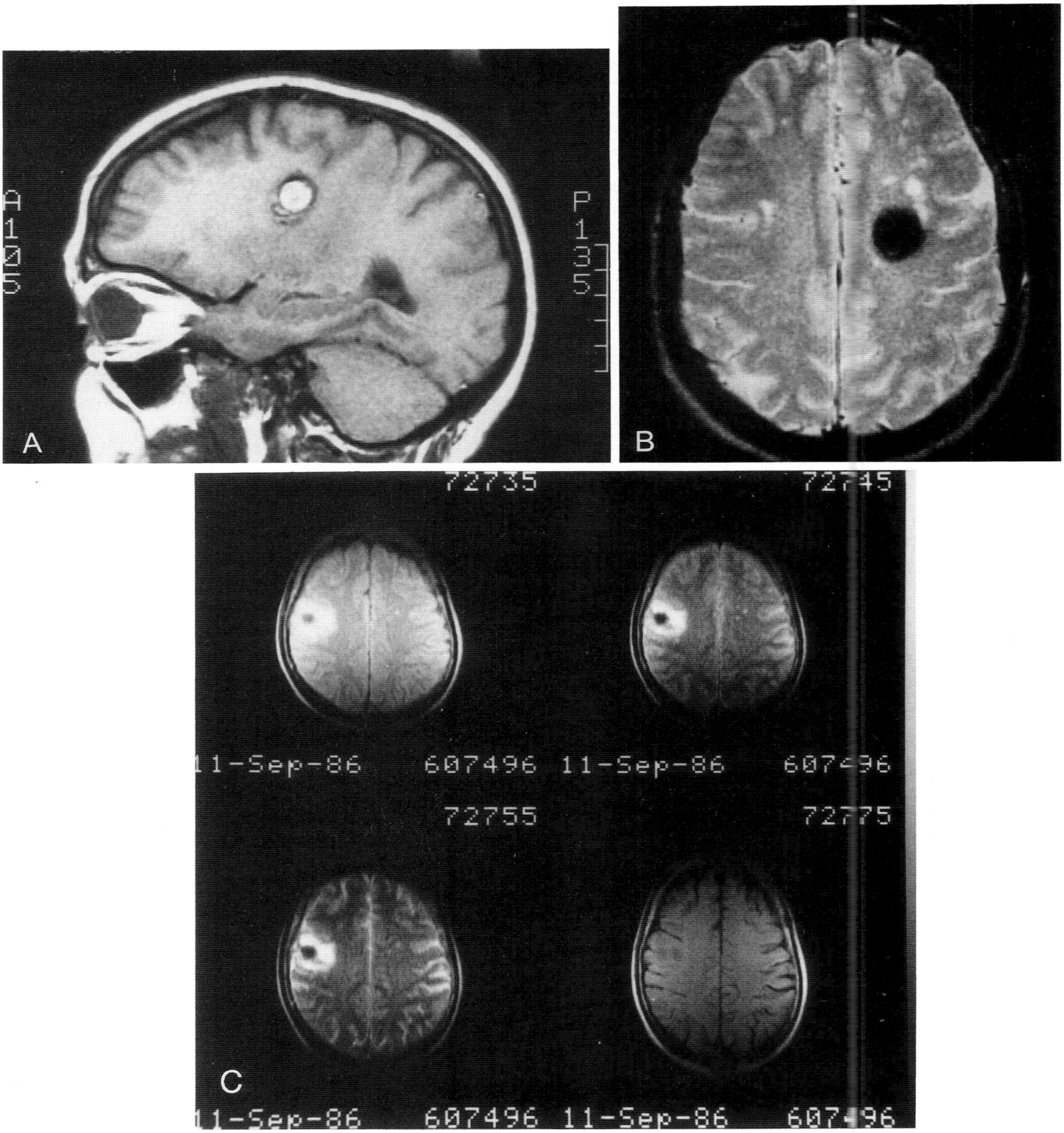

Figure 1.6*A–C*

Figure 1.6. Two patients with intracranial hemorrhagic lesions. *A* and *B*, T_1- and T_2-weighted, respectively, images from study done on a 1.5-T unit. *C*, four images—single echo (SE) 2000/45-, 90-, and 135-msec pulse sequence and 500/30-msec pulse sequence from a study done on a 0.15-T resistive unit. *A* and *B* show findings typical of a chronic hemorrhagic lesion believed to be related to a vascular malformation. In *C* only preferential T_2 shortening in seen in the surgically proven recently hemorrhagic metastasis.

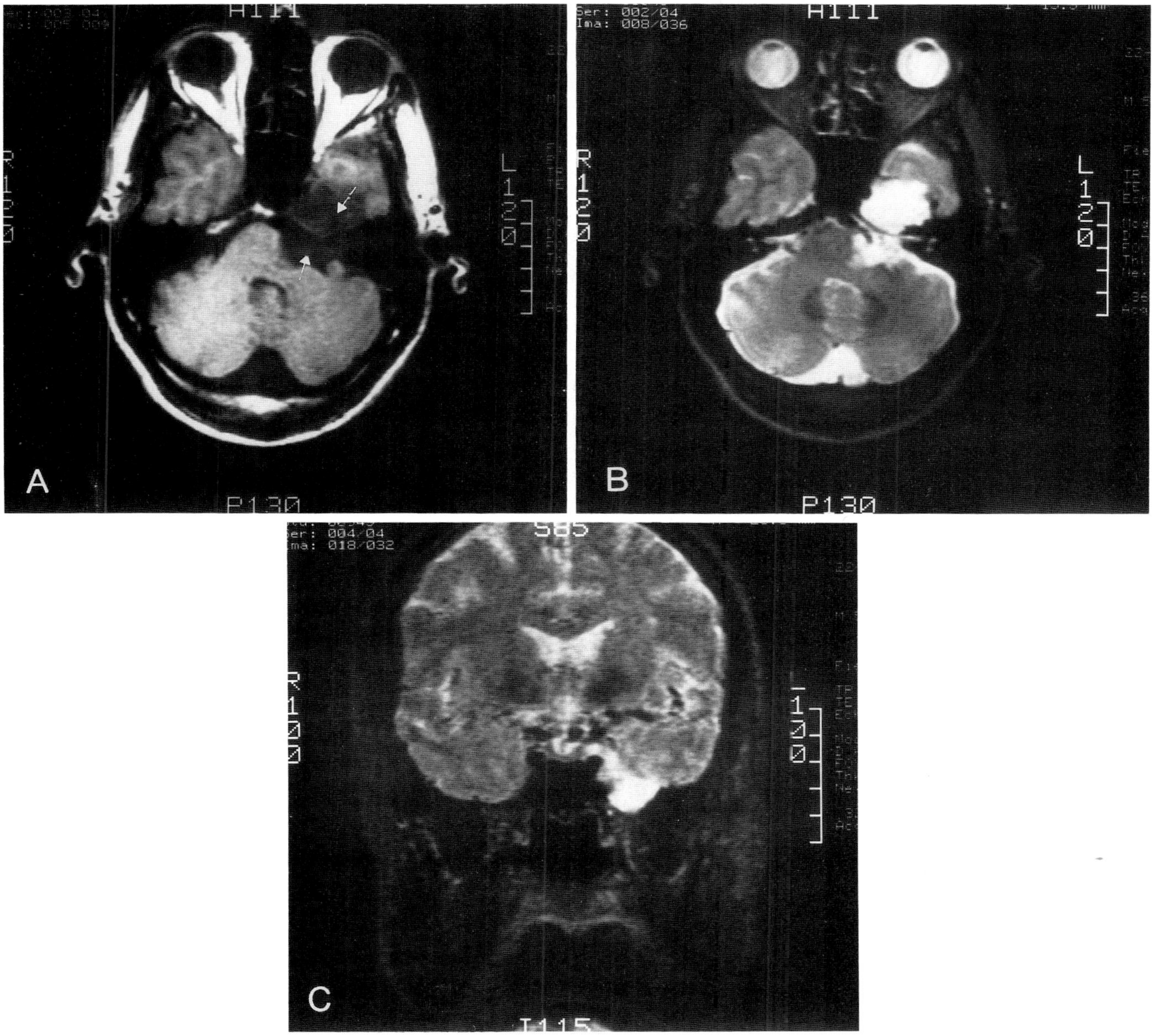

Figure 1.7*A–C*

Figure 1.7. Patient with typical appearing, surgically proven epidermoid tumor studied on a 1.5-T system. *A*, with partial saturation 600/25-msec pulse sequence, lesion shows low intensity *(arrows)*. *B*, SE 2000/80-msec pulse sequence, 5-mm section with FOV 24 cm. *C*. SE 2000/30-msec pulse, 3-mm section with FOV 20 cm.

Comment: Note that even in the excellent SNR environment of a high-field system pushing the spatial resolution of a moderately T_2-weighted image can result in significant degradation. The image in *C* is obviously more grainy and less aesthetically pleasing than that in *B* at least in part because of the markedly reduced voxel volume.

msec). The combination of a 3- to 5-mm section and a 12- to 14-cm FOV with even these moderately T_1-weighted pulse sequences will push to the SNR limits of most units when standard head coils are used (Fig. 1.7). Fortunately, in the extracranial head and neck, skull base, internal auditory canals (IACs), and cerebellopontine (CP) angles one is often dealing with anatomic structures of relatively high inherent (object) contrast on T_1-weighted images, that is, bone with relatively immobile protons, surrounding fat, cerebrospinal fluid (CSF), and nervous tissue. The key questions to ask in MRI are "What am I trying to contrast?" and "What is the relative importance of image contrast and spatial resolution?" If the structures have high inherent contrast, relatively short TR/TE pulse sequences (e.g., bone of IAC, CSF, cranial nerves VII and VIII) then spatial resolution can be emphasized by using short TR/TE (T_1-weighted)

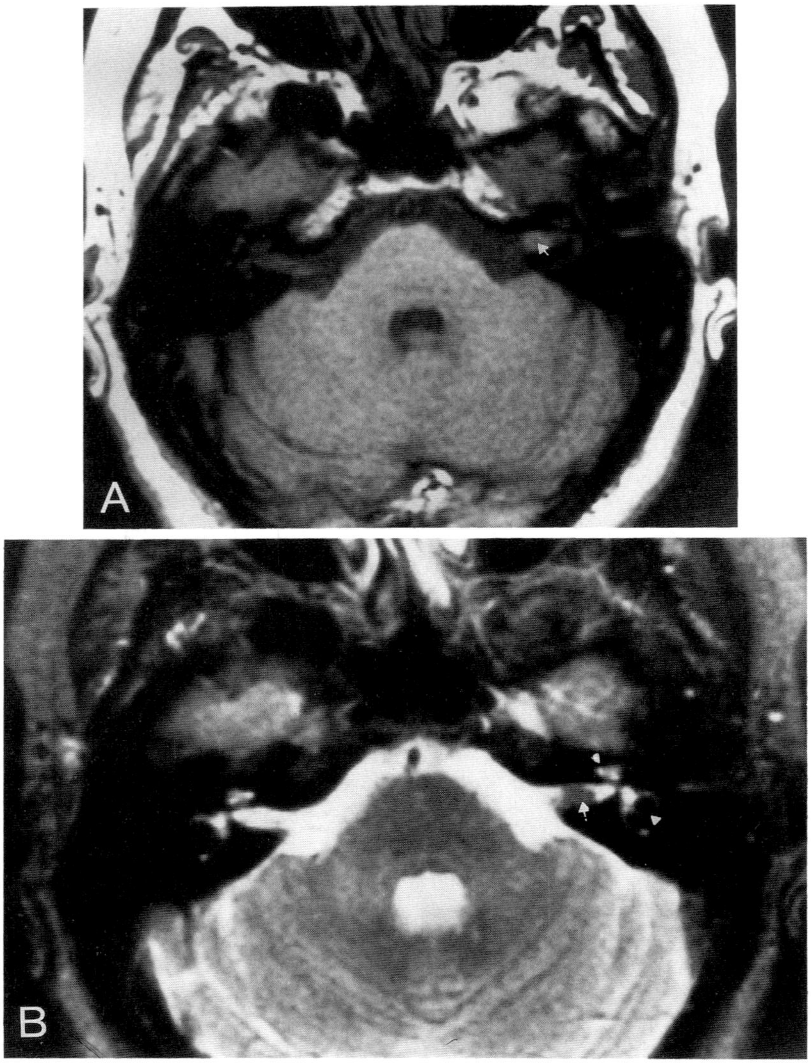

Figure 1.8A and B

Figure 1.8. Patient with intracanalicular acoustic neuroma. *A*, inherent contrast between CSF, bone, and tumor *(arrow)* make a highly spatially resolved image the most obvious choice for identifying such a tumor. This 3-mm section was done with a FOV of 24 cm and a 256 × 256 matrix. *B*, ordinarily an acoustic neuroma would be much brighter than brain on this T_2-weighted pulse sequence, and one might expect to decrease conspicuity by causing it to blend with the signal of CSF on less spatially resolved intermediate or T_2-weighted images. This happens not to be the case in this patient *(arrow)*. This also illustrates that at mid and high fields it is possible to produce highly spatially resolved T_2-weighted images. Note how well the cochlea, vestibule, and semicircular canals are seen *(arrowheads)*.

pulse sequences that allow for signal averaging (increasing SNR) (Fig. 1.8). A three-dimensional (3DFT) rather than two-dimensional (2DFT) Fourier transform technique can also be used in this situation, the former having SNR advantages as well as the ability to produce truly contiguous sections (Fig. 1.9). However, if one must detect a subtle intra-axial brainstem lesion, the study will require a significantly T_2-weighted pulse sequence and/or a paramagnetic contrast agent. High-resolution, thin section, relatively T_1-weighted MRI work suffices for areas such as the cavernous sinus–skull base, orbit, IAC/CP angle for acoustic neuroma, and craniovertebral junction. The trade-off between image contrast, spatial resolution, and SNR to produce a certain resolving power for a given object in this region is beautifully described in an article by Enzman and O'Donohue concerning optimized techniques for detecting intracanalicular acoustic neuromas (see Suggested Readings). This type of consideration must be applied for each region and indication for MRI studies. At first glance the larynx, tongue base, and other areas seem amenable to a totally "T_1-weighted" (i.e., short TR/TE) approach, but a closer look at image contrast issues in the next section reveals that such a simplistic approach has potentially serious limitations. For now the discussion concentrates on the areas amenable to high-resolution thin section images and the techniques used to produce them.

Slice Thickness

The shape of the slice-selective Rf pulse used with 2DFT techniques creates an interesting problem when trying to do contiguous thin (3- to 5-mm) sections. Since the Rf pulse is actually a curved function if the sections lie too close together, they "bang into" one another in multislice acquisitions (Fig. 1.9). This is often called "crosstalk" and is most noticeable in long TR/TE acquisitions. The partial saturation that occurs

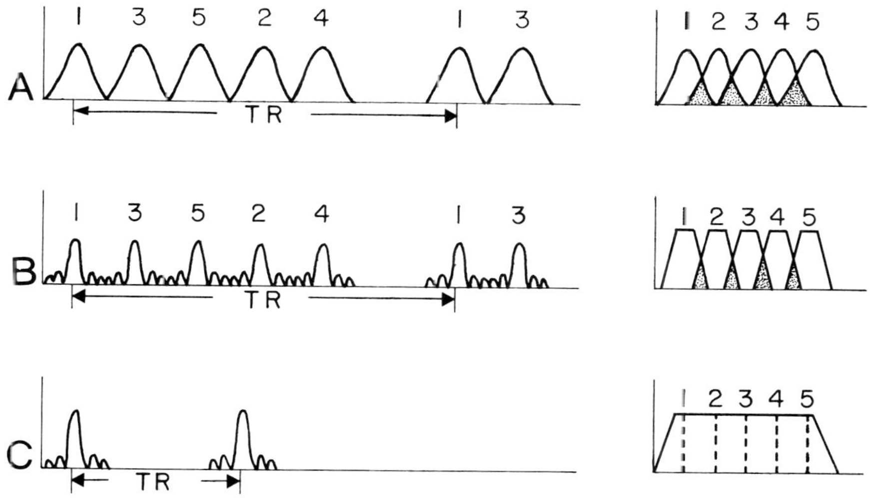

Figure 1.9*A–C*

Figure 1.9. Comparison of 2DFT and 3DFT modes of slice selection. *A*, gaussian slice selection in time domain *(left)* done such that slices will be contiguous (no gap). Gaussian shape of slice profile *(right)* results in considerable "partial saturation" (crosstalk) in adjacent slices, indicated by shaded areas. Note that in time spatially adjacent slices are typically perturbed out of sequence within a given TR interval as indicated by numbering. *B*, sin C pulses in time domain result in a more square, trapezoidal slice profile than the gaussian; this reduces but does not eliminate crosstalk; note the difference in the shaded area. *C*, 3DFT spin echo typically has TR of one-half or less of T_1-weighted 2DFT spin echo. Each pulse perturbs a slab. Slices are then selected by a second phase-encoding gradient (number of steps being equal to number of slices desired). This effectively produces gapless imaging without crosstalk. Note that slices on outer edges will have less optimal profile and SNR. This would have been worse if a gaussian profile had been used to select the slab.

because of this overlap is undesirable in a situation in which much of the SNR per voxel reserves have been spent for thin sections and a relatively small FOV. Solutions to this vary with manufacturers. Some leave a full SLT gap, offset, and then fill in the gaps with a second acquisition (interleaving). Others leave a small gap stated to be 15 to 20% of the SLT and accept "noncontiguity," but this really is not an ideal solution when sections of 5 mm or less are required. Three-dimensional Fourier transform techniques can produce excellent-quality 2- to 3-mm, truly contiguous sections; time constraints dictate that these be used with TR less than 500 msec (probably around 250 msec) and short TE (15 to 30 msec) to be practical (Fig. 1.9). As discussed before, in areas of high inherent contrast this relatively T_1-weighted technique is perfectly acceptable and, combined with gradient echo pulse sequences, may provide more options for varying tissue contrast in high-resolution thin section images. The capacity to do 5-mm sections has existed on virtually all systems since 1984. The 3- to 5-mm sections necessary for detailed work in the head, neck, spine, and extremities have been available since late 1985. Improved localized receiver coils coupled with new techniques, such as 3DFT and improved slice-selective pulses, made 3- to 5-mm contiguous or nearly contiguous sections available on many systems during 1986. Continued improvement in all of these factors as well as new pulse sequences are likely to lead to even more refinement over the next several years.

As with CT, one must be aware of the cephalocaudal extent of a study when using thin sections. With MRI this is even more critical with standard spin echo techniques. The duty cycle of most units for an Rf-refocused spin echo sequence requires about 50 msec/section, so for a TR of 500 msec one can do 10 sections (somewhat more or less depending on the TE). If one is doing 2-mm sections with a TR of 500 msec or less then only 2 cm or less will be covered. This means that initial localization (i.e., a "quick" view) will usually be necessary. If the region of interest is larger than that covered, another acquisition must be done. Gradient-refocused echo techniques may well stand up to the thin section, small FOV requirements of high spatial resolution techniques but at present experience in this regard is limited. If so, rapid acquisition of contiguous single slices, as in CT, becomes possible. A marriage of gradient echo, reduced tip angle imaging techniques with 3DFT offers an alternative to covering more territory per acquisition. With good receivers and further refinements, however, 2DFT multislice, spin echo techniques still remain the mainstay of thin section imaging at this time.

Pixel Size

Acquisition matrix size is a more critical issue in MRI than in CT because it has a direct impact on imaging time. The acquisition matrix in the readout (frequency encoding) gradient is usually 256; this number can be increased to 512 rather simply by increasing the computer's sampling rate without a penalty in imaging time. The matrix size in the phase-encoding direction, however, depends on the number of gradient steps used during the acquisition. The number of phase-encoding gradient steps is directly proportional to imaging time. A 256 × 256 matrix produces a symmetrical pixel. A 128 × 256 or 192 × 256 matrix image may be obtained in one-half or three-quarters of the time, respectively, but the pixel will be asymmetric. At 192 × 256 this does not produce any visually disturbing artifacts. A 128 × 256 matrix results in a "truncation" artifact seen as parallel bands that are especially noticeable at borders of markedly different signal intensity (e.g., fat-muscle interface) and that "ring through" the image. Time savings must be weighed against image quality. A 192 × 256 or 256 × 256 matrix should be used whenever spatial resolution is an overriding concern. Lesser numbers of phase-encoding steps may be possible without significant truncation artifacts. A 512 × 512 acquisition matrix is even practical if the number of signal averages can be cut to two for a T_1-weighted and one for a typical T_2-weighted pulse sequence. A 512 × 512 matrix can also be used in a reasonable time frame with more signal averages if the phase-encoding steps are made only over the portion of the FOV containing the anatomy in question (i.e., not over the air to each side of the head). This is called a "selective" FOV. The time savings here is again directly proportional to the number of phase-encoding steps that can be eliminated without ignoring the more useful data within the anatomic limits of the structure being studied.

The basic trade-offs in SNR caused by decreasing FOV were discussed in the CT section. When the voxel is reduced in two dimensions, the cost in SNR is considerable. It is very helpful to have more field strength (i.e., over 0.15 T) when one wishes to have a FOV less than 21 to 28 cm, if standard head coils are being used.

There is another problem in MRI if the FOV becomes small. If the receiver coil "sees" a signal from anatomy outside the FOV the reconstruction processes will place those data in the display. This is sometimes referred to as an aliasing or "foldover" or "wrap-around" artifact. This can be avoided by choosing a larger FOV or by matching the volume of tissue "seen" by the receiver coil (sensitive volume) more closely to the FOV chosen. The latter is accomplished by using smaller localized receiver coils or sometimes just centering the anatomy better in the existing coil. An additional benefit of a smaller coil is that it will usually be more closely coupled to the area of interest and suffer less losses (noise) from body-related loading. The merging of a closely coupled small-volume receiver coil and small FOV are then a logical combination for high-resolution thin section imaging of a relatively small area of interest (e.g., temporomandibular joint, orbit, sella, knee) (Fig. 1.10).

Contrast Resolution

Electron density alone influences contrast in CT. In the case of MRI, proton density, relaxation times (T_1 and T_2), and flow are the determinants of image contrast. No matter how the MRI experiment is done, T_1, T_2, and proton density and flow (motion) will influence tissue contrast. The experiment can be biased by varying TR, TE, and TI (inversion-recovery interval), but one must understand the reasons for wanting more T_1 or more T_2 weighting in the images. The reasons vary with the clinical questions at hand, need for spatial resolution versus image contrast, and region of anatomy versus pathology under study. With gradient echo techniques flip angle may also be varied to affect contrast. Gradient echo images are also very flow sensitive and can be used to dramatically alter contrast due to flow.

In the intracranial compartment the choices are relatively simple. The detection of intra-axial pathology requires a relatively T_2-weighted image with TR between 1500 and 3000 msec and TE between about 60 and 120 msec. If the TE can be kept between 60 and 90 msec, relatively thin section (5 to 8 mm) high-

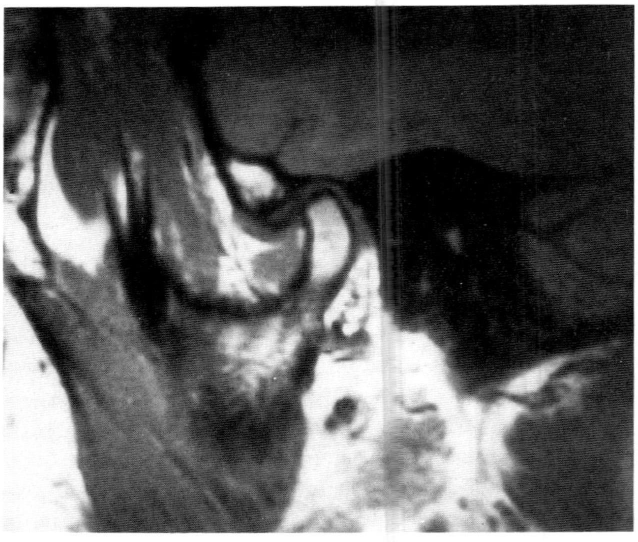

Figure 1.10

Figure 1.10. Temporomandibular joint study in the closed mouth position. This is a partial saturation 600/20-msec pulse sequence, 16-cm FOV, 3-mm section with 256 × 256 matrix. Such a small voxel volume is possible in large part because of the use of a small, closely coupled received coil.

resolution images can be made at fields of 0.15 T or more. The selection of a specific TR in this range (1500 to 3000 msec) is often related more to the imaging time than to anything else. The choice of a specific T_2-weighted pulse sequence within these TR and TE ranges seems to be a highly individualized matter, which means that most of those chosen probably work well for detecting intra-axial pathology. Most imagers choose to use a dual-echo acquisition with a TR of 2000 to 2500 msec and TEs of 20 to 90 msec. This produces a "spin density image" (first echo) and moderately T_2-weighted image (second echo) in the same acquisition.

In the extracranial compartment there are tissue contrast issues that differ considerably from those of the brain. The general principle that tissue contrast improves with more T_2 weighting holds to some degree (as it does for the brain), but the differentiation of pathologic and normal tissues is somewhat more complex depending on the pathology and surrounding anatomy. In tumor imaging below the skull base one seeks to contrast tumor with fat, muscle, and lymphoid tissue while maintaining a highly spatially resolved image (Fig. 1.11). It has been our experience and that of others that one should not expect to differentiate tumor (e.g., squamous cell carcinoma or lymphoma) from normal lymphoid tissue at most of the pulse sequences in standard use. Some workers suggest that long TR (greater than 3 sec) pulse sequences with early (<30 msec) echo delay times can produce an image that potentially "discriminates" normal lymphoid tissue from tumor (R. N. Bryan, personal communication). This spin density approach certainly merits some further investigation, since it might have application in staging lymph nodes if it is correct. Thus far this has not come into widespread usage. Reduced tip angle, spin density, gradient echo images may be capable of the same thing. At present our working assumption is that tumor and normal lymphoid tissue (e.g., adenoid, faucial tonsils, lingual tonsils) cannot be distinguished reliably by manipulating pulse sequence techniques. One must rely on observing deep infiltration of surrounding fat and muscles as the feature that differentiates aggressive pathology from the ubiquitous lymphoid tissue seen as a normal variant in the upper aerodigestive tract (Fig. 1.11). Of course imaging is not a substitute for biopsy, and superficial cancer coexists with normal lymphoid tissue frequently. With MRI as with CT, imaging remains an excellent compliment to endoscopy and biopsy; no imaging test other than tissue under the microscope yet "diagnoses" cancer.

Tumors of the upper aerodigestive tract must also can be difficult and usually requires a combination of T_1- and T_2-weighted images. Some combination of T_1- and T_2-weighted images is usually required in the initial study of tumors and other lesions affecting the extracranial head and neck. Deep infiltration remains the best sign of an aggressive lesion versus a normal variation in the upper aerodigestive tract.

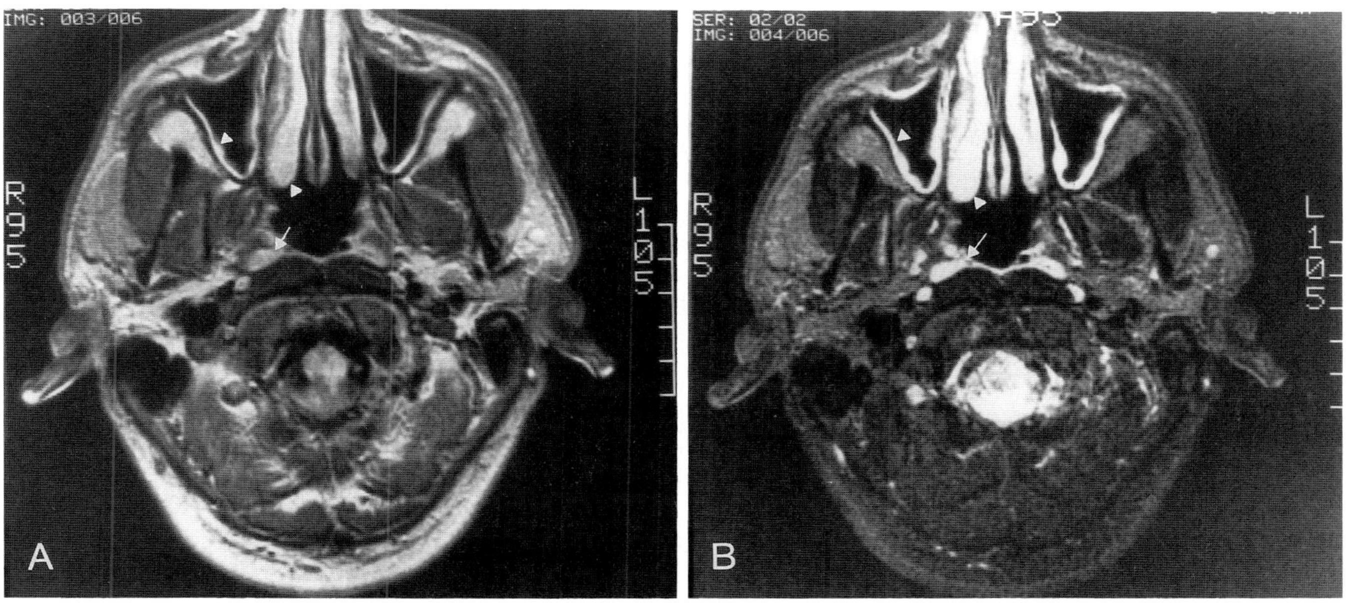

Figure 1.11*A* and *B*

Figure 1.11. Dual-echo 2000/40-msec *(A)* and 2000/80-msec *(B)* pulse sequence shows range of tissue contrast that must be differentiated from extracranial head and neck pathology. Lymphoid tissue *(arrow)* is relatively easy to differentiate from muscle. Mucosal disease and well-hydrated turbinates *(arrowheads)* usually are much brighter than tumors. Contrast between tumor, lymphoid tissue, and fat, however,

be contrasted with muscle and fat, most conveniently with both on the same image. Tumor-fat contrast, however, is best on relatively T_1-weighted pulse sequences (e.g., 500 to 700/20 to 30 msec), whereas contrast between tumor and muscle is optimized on more T_2-weighted pulse sequences. When using thin sections with high spatial resolution, it is best to retain a relatively short TR so that signal averaging can be used to retain the SNR lost to thin sections and small FOV. At the University of Florida a basic pulse sequence of 600/45 msec has been chosen (Fig. 1.12). The 45-msec TE provides enough T_2 weighting to differentiate most tumors and muscle but does not introduce enough T_2 weighting to cause most tumors to become isointense with surrounding fat. If more tumor-muscle contrast is required, a spin echo (SE) 2000/60 to 70 msec–type pulse sequence is used. Moderate to heavily T_2-weighted (2000/90 msec) pulse sequences are most effective for differentiating tumor from inflammatory/obstructive changes in the sinuses (Fig. 1.13). Both T_1- and T_2-weighted images are usually necessary when trying to differentiate fibrosis from residual tumor, although good-quality T_2-weighted images are most important in answering this question (Fig. 1.14). Here again, imaging data *never* equal biopsy; viable (clonogenic) tumor cells may exist in a "bed" of dense fibrosis. In this circumstance even biopsy may fail to provide an answer. Sometimes careful clinical and imaging follow-up is the only hope for finding recurrent or residual tumor while salvage therapy is still possible. Unfortunately, sometimes the best one can offer is confirmation that recurrence is beyond the limits of salvage for cure (Fig. 1.15). Specific uses of various pulse sequences are discussed in appropriate chapters; however, a simplistic view that "one pulse sequence fits all" should never be adopted. Each pulse sequence should be thought out for each particular diagnostic problem in each anatomic region of interest.

Paramagnetic Contrast Agents

Gadolinium-DTPA is the first of what will undoubtedly be a long line of contrast agents developed for use with MRI. FDA approval for intracranial indications was given as of July 1, 1988. Many more compounds are in various phases of development and testing but none are anywhere near FDA approval, and Gd-DTPA is likely to be the only agent generally available in the United States from 1988 to 1991 or 1992. All of this family of compounds depend on the presence of a strongly paramagnetic element (e.g., gadolinium) that can form a stable chelate. This compound is injected in very small concentrations (e.g., 0.1 to 0.2 mmol/kg). The contrast accumulates in areas of blood-brain barrier breakdown or other extracellular spaces much as do iodinated compounds. At the doses used this compound produces a preferential, dramatic T_1 shortening of tissues where it localizes. Actual contrast ratios will depend on: *(a)* the relative concentrations of gadolinium in the lesion versus that in the surrounding normal extracellular volume, *(b)* the time course of its accumulation and clearance from the compartments, and *(c)* the inherent contrast in these areas, which is dependent on the T_1, T_2, and proton density of the tissue versus

Figure 1.12. Patient with squamous cell carcinoma of the nasopharynx. SE 600/45-msec pulse sequence produced excellent tumor-muscle contrast; note the infiltration of the lateral pterygoid *(arrow)*. Tumor *(T)*–fat *(F)* contrast is reasonably good. Tumor–lymphoid tissue *(L)* contrast is marginal.

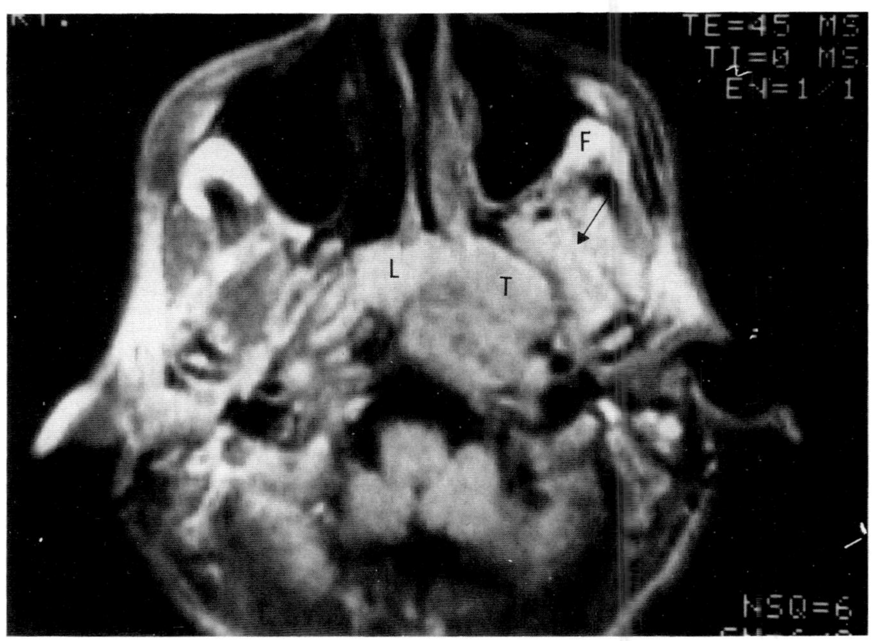

Figure 1.12

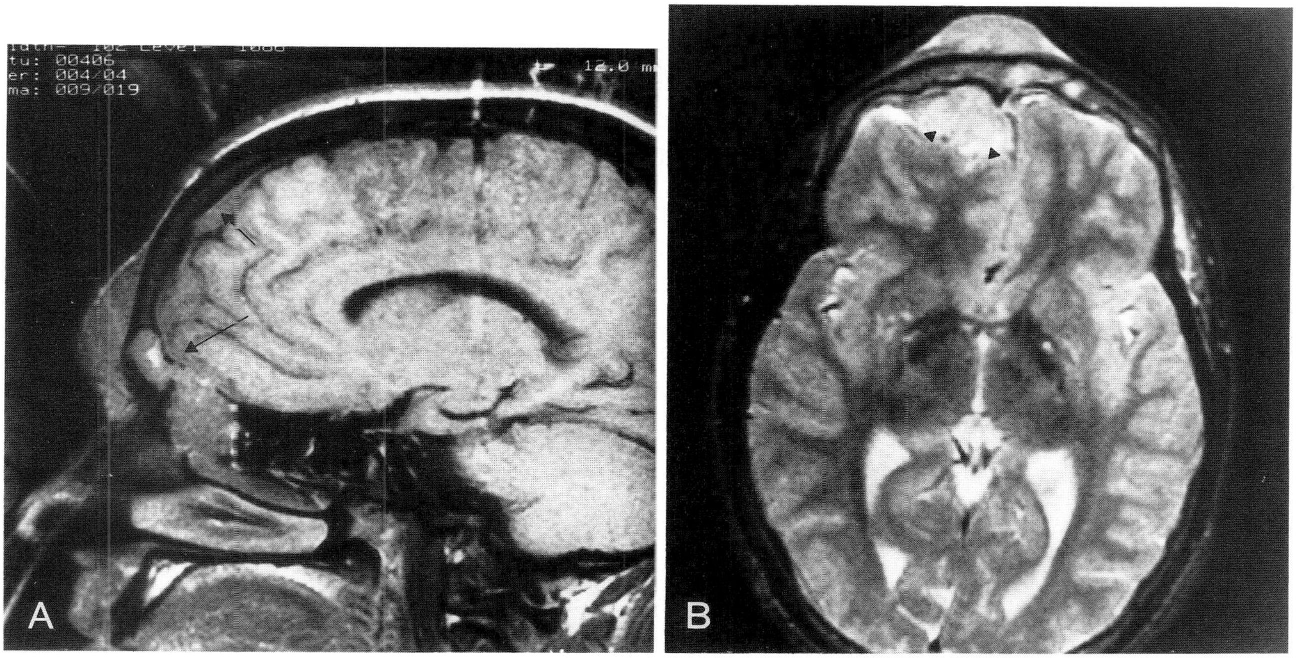

Figure 1.13A and B

Figure 1.13. Several examples of how MRI may help improve diagnosis if its contrast resolution properties are exploited properly. *A* and *B*, T_1- and T_2-weighted images, respectively, in a patient believed to have pyomucocele of the frontal sinus. MRI shows this to be an infiltrating lymphomatous mass with dural spread *(arrows)* and brain invasion *(arrowheads)* manifest by edema. Pyomucocele would have been much brighter on the T_2 image and would not have shown such an infiltrating spread pattern. *C* and *D,* CT and MRI of patient with expansile mass in the ethmoid. *D,* MRI clearly shows that this is a mococele *(arrow)*. Density was indeterminate on CT. *E,* Patient with nasopharyngeal carcinoma. Tumor *(T)* is clearly differentiated from secondary, obstructive sinus disease *(arrow)* on this spin echo 2000/80-msec pulse sequence. (Parts *C–E* are on page 20.)

pathology and the pulse sequence(s) selected for study. One can see that such compounds are not useful for intravascular opacification, so that a major benefit gained with iodinated contrast and CT in combination is not available with MRI and paramagnetics (Fig. 1.16). However, gradient echo or other flow-sensitive techniques can be used to evaluate flow qualitatively when necessary.

Paramagnetic contrast agents such as Gd-DTPA may then be used to artifically produce contrast between intra- and extra-axial pathology and the brain and other surrounding structures; this allows the use of T_1-weighted, highly spatially resolved images that retain sensitivity to pathologic changes. Gadolinium-DPTA can be used very effectively with gradient echo techniques. Paramagnetic contrast is likely to prove useful in detecting small acoustic neuromas, meningiomas, and basilar-meningitic-type processes (Figs. 1.17 and 1.18). It is also likely to help with the separation of chronic inactive foci of brain disease and edema from active areas of blood-brain barrier breakdown (Fig. 1.19). The exact uses and efficacy of the paramagnetics are yet to be determined, but they will have a role to play.

It is unlikely that MRI and paramagnetics such as Gd-DPTA will add to the sensitivity or specificity of MRI in the *extracranial* head and neck; in fact, it might actually be expected to reduce tumor-fat contrast on T_1-weighted pulse sequences (Fig. 1.20). Mucosal and cavernous sinus enhancement is frequently seen, and this might prove useful in selected cases (Fig. 1.16). It may show a lesion to be "enhancing" but this is unlikely to add specificity over the history, physical exam, and plain MRI, flow-sensitive MRI, or enhanced CT findings. The rate of accumulation and washout of the contrast in a lesion can be plotted, but this probably will not prove specific enough to eliminate angiography in paragangliomas, juvenile angiofibromas, and other highly vascular masses. Applications in the extracranial head and neck (excluding the spinal cord) are therefore likely to be limited. It is possible that such contrast combined with fast scan techniques could help characterize the aggressive tumor margins and possibly the internal morphology of cervical nodes as iodinated contrast does in CT, so one should keep an open mind about this subject, which is still in its developmental phase (Fig. 1.20).

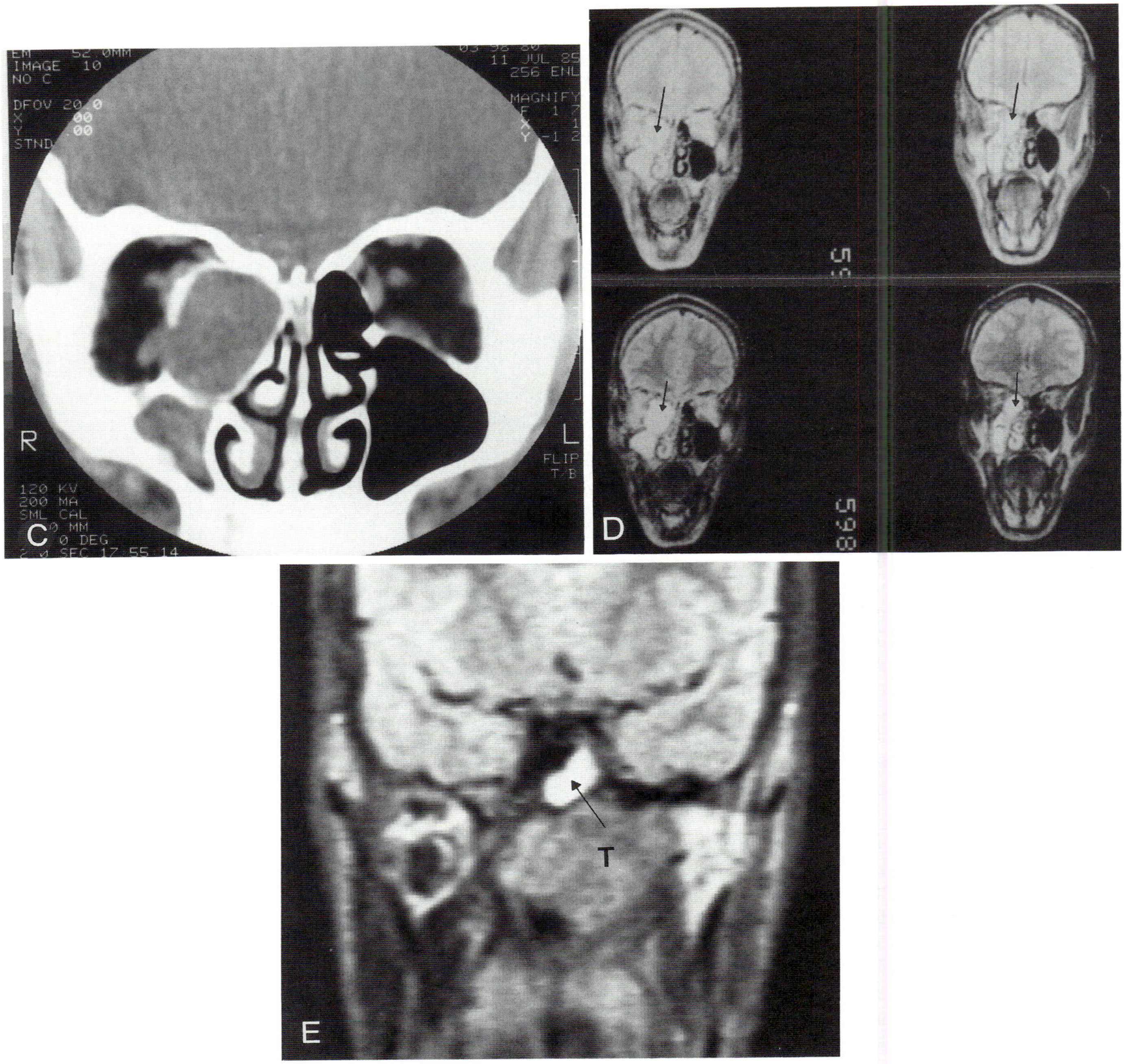

Figure 1.13*C–E*

RELATIVE ADVANTAGES AND DISADVANTAGES OF CT AND MRI

The following chapters deal very specifically with the relative usefulness of CT and MRI in lesions of the head and neck. Here the advantages and disadvantages are considered in a more general way. This discussion does not consider MRI field strength because it has not proven significant at 0.15 T at the University of Florida and is almost certainly not significant at fields from 0.3 to 1.5 T. Excellent images are available on *optimized* systems working at 0.15 T and higher.

Cost

The cost of acquiring and maintaining a superconducting MRI system is currently far greater than that for CT. In order to prevent MRI from becoming a loss center, cost per exam for the average superconducting system is kept high compared to CT. Charges for studies on resistive, permanent, and per-

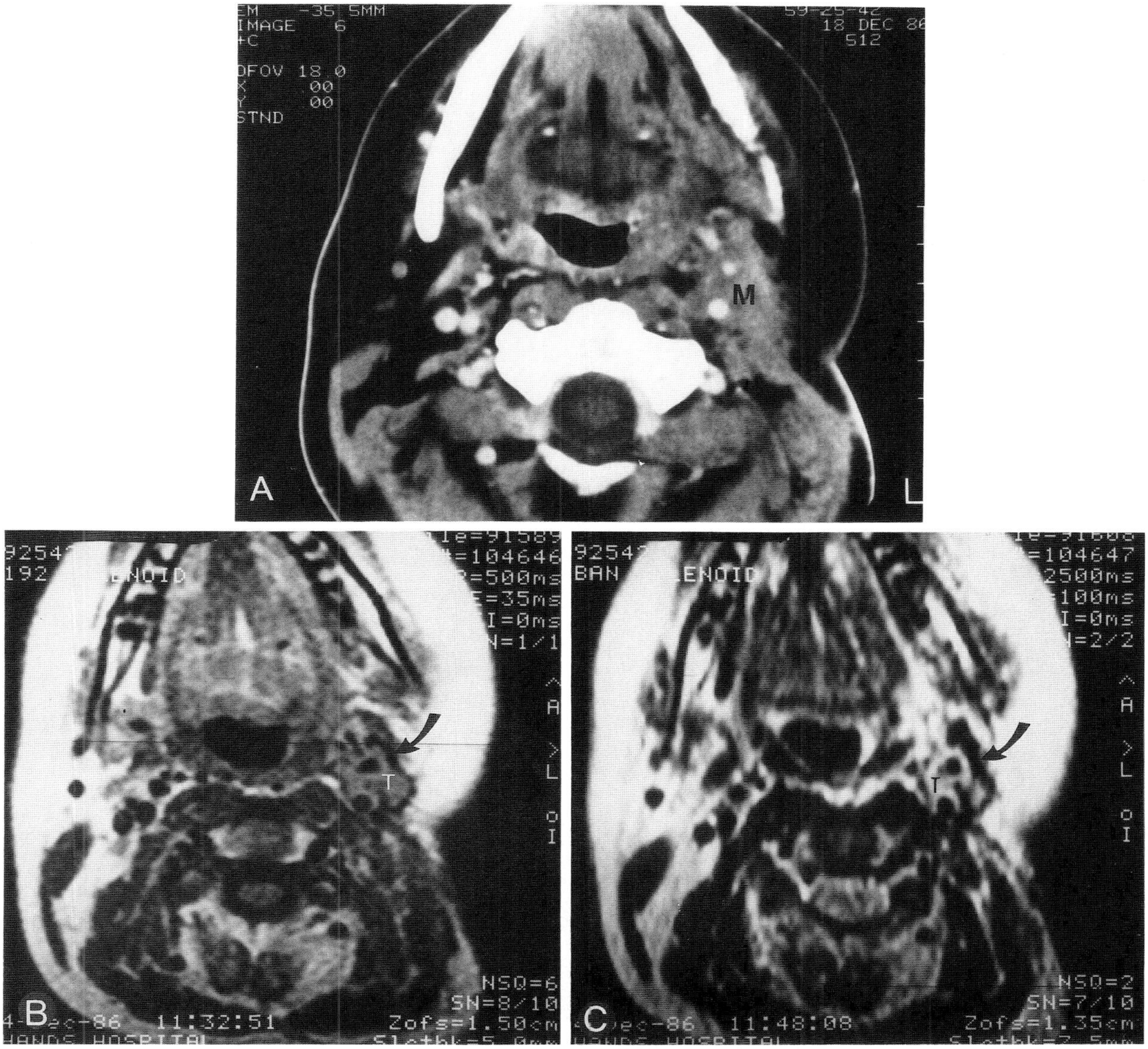

Figure 1.14*A–C*

Figure 1.14. Eighteen-year-old male who had very aggressive but localized non-Hodgkins lymphoma of the left neck. Patient had undergone chemotherapy followed by radiotherapy and then surgery for this locally aggressive lesion. *A,* CT 6 months after surgery showed residual mass *(M)* around internal and external carotid arteries. It was uncertain whether this was postoperative scarring or tumor. *B* and *C,* SE 500/35 and 2500/200-msec pulse sequence images, respectively, done 1 week after CT in *A*. Combination of tumor *(T)* and scar *(arrow)* are present. CT-guided biopsy was offered for confirmation but patient was treated with chemotherapy on basis of these imaging findings. Follow-up MRI showed prompt response of tumor to therapy.

Comment: MRI resulted in reduction of delay in diagnosis of this patient. If biopsy had been done the needle would have been positioned in tumor rather than one of the areas of scarring noted on MRI.

haps lower end superconducting systems can be kept at the same or lower levels than comparable contrast-enhanced CT studies. There is likely to be some downward pressure on MRI charges as a result of reimbursement policies and competition; however, it will be difficult to break even at a reasonable price per exam if the extraordinary costs of purchase, maintenance, and upgrades that come with some systems persist. The industry seems to be coming around to the notion that excellent proton imaging can be done on a cost-efficient unit; perhaps they will be more sensitive to the issue after recovery of their

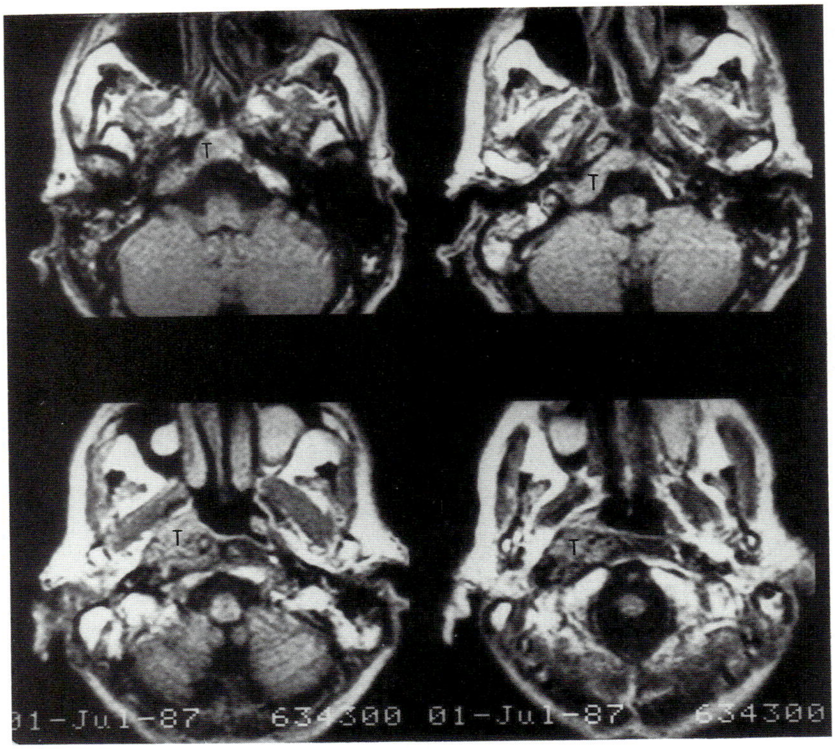

Figure 1.15

Figure 1.15. Sixty-five-year-old male 3 years following radiotherapy for soft palate cancer; his only complaint was dysphagia. Myotomy for cricopharyngeal achalasia was being considered. No masses were visible on clinical exam. This series of MRI scans show extensive recurrent tumor mass *(T)* involving the nasopharynx and prevertebral muscles and extensive invasion of the skull base. All disease was submucosal. Patient was offered palliative chemotherapy.

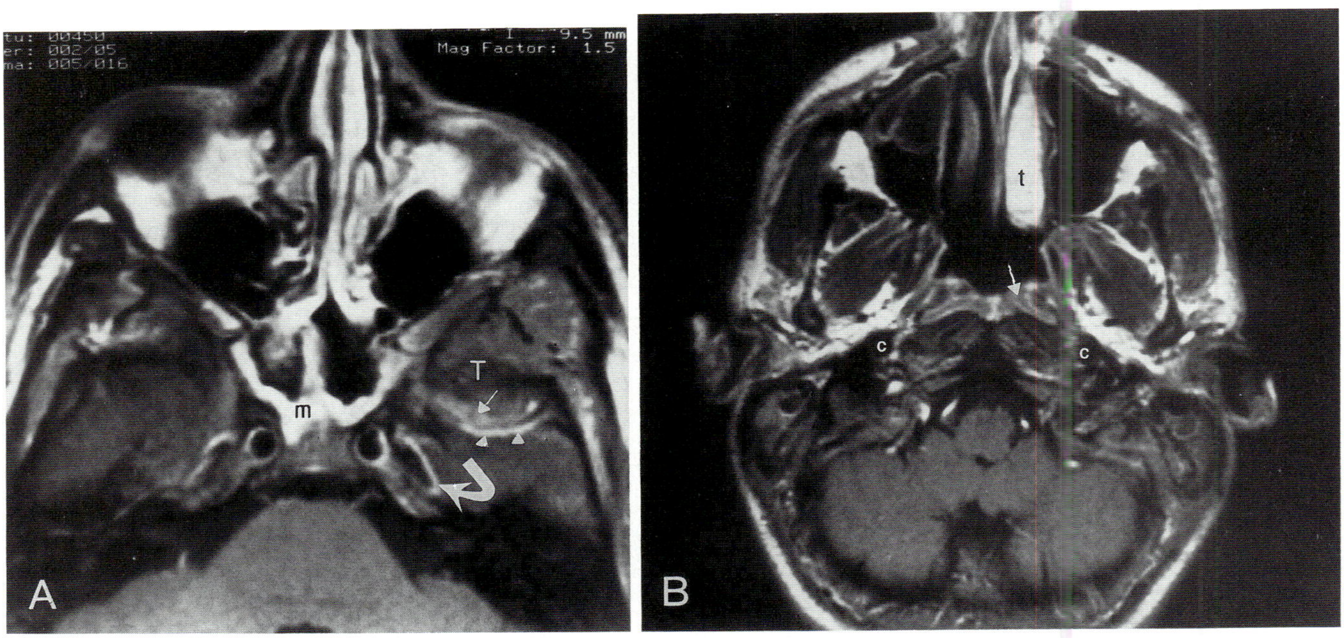

Figure 1.16*A* and *B*

Figure 1.16. Patient with lymphoma involving the skull. Gadolinium-DTPA was given. *A*, part of tumor *(T)* enhances slightly *(arrow)*. Dura is displaced and enhancing where tumor is pushing intracranially *(arrowheads)*. Note enhancement of the cavernous sinus *(curved arrow)* and sphenoid sinus mucosa *(m)*. *B*, section somewhat lower shows the typical enhancement of a turbinate *(t)*. Also note enhancement of the lymphoid tissue in the nasopharynx *(arrow)*. The carotid arteries *(c)* show no enhancement.

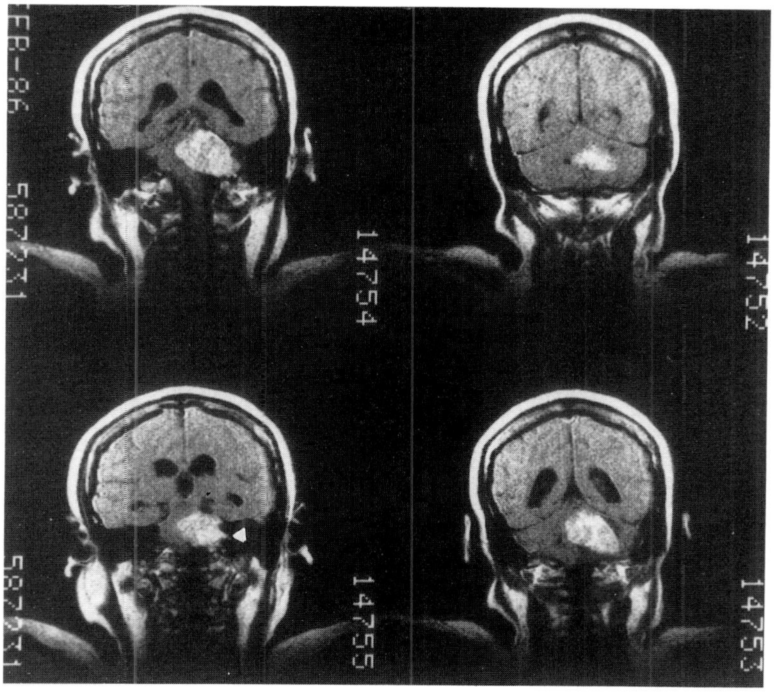

Figure 1.17. Patient with large acoustic neuroma. T_1-weighted image 3 min after injection of Gd-DTPA. Note tumor extending into internal auditory canal *(arrowhead)*.

Figure 1.17

Figure 1.18. Patient with sarcoidosis presenting as multiple cranial nerve deficits. *A–C,* SE 2000/45-, 90-, and 135-msec pulse sequence images done before Gd-DTPA infusion. *D,* SE 500/30-msec pulse sequence image started 3 min following Gd-DTPA shows extensive leptomeningeal involvement due to sarcoidosis.

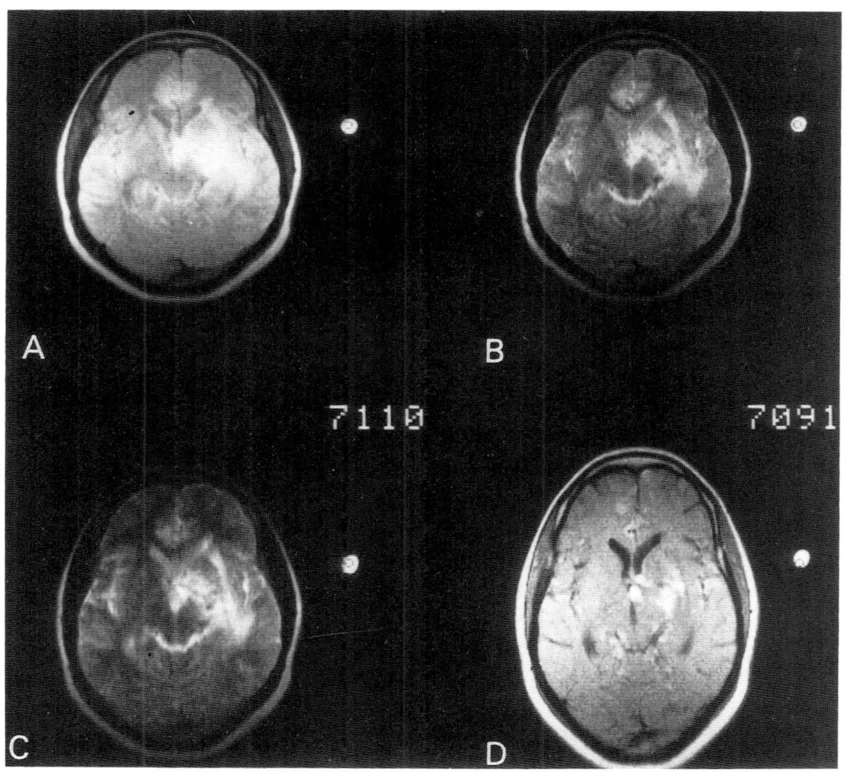

Figure 1.18*A–D*

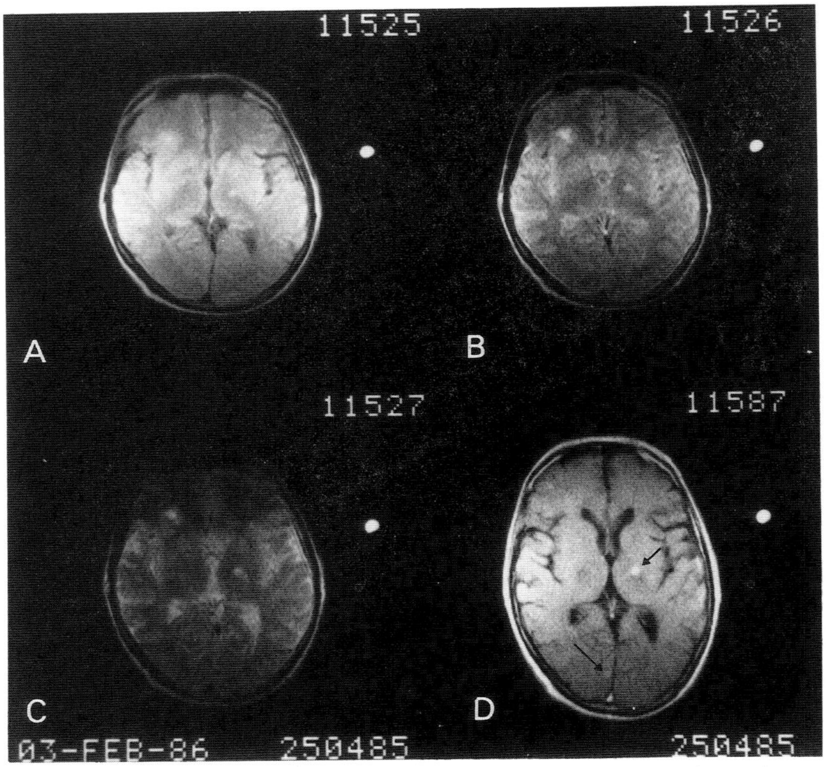

Figure 1.19A–D

Figure 1.19. Elderly patient suspected of having cerebral metastatic disease. *A–C,* SE 2000/45-, 90- and 135-msec pulse sequence images on which it is difficult to be certain whether areas of increased signal intensity were due to chronic ischemic disease or metastases. *D,* SE 500/30-msec pulse sequence image following Gd-DTPA enhancement shows two metastatic foci *(arrows)*. Right frontal lesion showed no evidence of blood-brain barrier breakdown and is believed to represent a coexistant focus of abnormality related to chronic ischemic disease.

initial investment and under pressure from foreign products. Until MRI prices come down (or CT goes up) price per examination will remain a significant advantage of CT in most institutions.

Contraindicated and Failed MRI Studies

Magnetic resonance imaging exams are contraindicated in patients for a wide variety of well-known reasons. All MRI facilities have strict intake interviews to avoid potentially lethal situations (e.g., cerebral aneurysm clips). Cochlear implants and stapes prostheses may be found with more frequency in a situation in which a large number of referrals are coming from otolaryngologists. About 5% of patients will be too claustrophobic to study; the incidence of claustrophobia may be as much as doubled in the smoking and drinking population that tend to have head and neck cancer. Sedation and optical devices can improve this failure rate but not reduce it to zero.

Critically ill patients can be studied, but the logistics of patient monitoring and maintenance of vital functions are much more difficult, and at times impossible, for MRI studies. Critically ill patients are routinely studied with CT.

Failed MRI studies due to excessive motion artifact are common. In the pediatric age group sedation is over 90% effective at relieving this problem. In adults sedation usually does not help except in the mildly claustrophobic group. Rapid single-slice techniques using I.V. paramagnetic contrast may reduce this failure rate in patients who are unable to fully cooperate. Overall CT retains a distinct advantage over MRI in the rate of failed studies due to all of the circumstances outlined above, and this represents a distinct advantage especially in a primarily hospital-based practice.

Efficiency of Examination

An average CT study takes 30 min of table time, whereas an average MRI exam takes 45 to 60 min of table time. There is little reason to believe this will change for the next several years. This assumes that studies are being *actively* supervised by a physician. The time advantage is important economically (increased throughput) as well as for patients. Many patients will become fatigued or "fidgety" after two or three acquisitions and the rate of failed or suboptimal acquisitions clearly rises as the time of exam lengthens (Fig. 1.21).

The potential complexity of MRI exam (e.g., T_1- and T_2-weighted images, multiplanar) that results in many of its advantages may actually impede throughput in a survey situation. The entire upper aerodigestive tract and neck can be studied in 20 to 30 min on CT in a patient with a neck node from an occult primary tumor. Such an "unfocused" MRI study might take two to three times longer to produce the same information. In general, MRI is in its best and most efficient mode when its considerable advan-

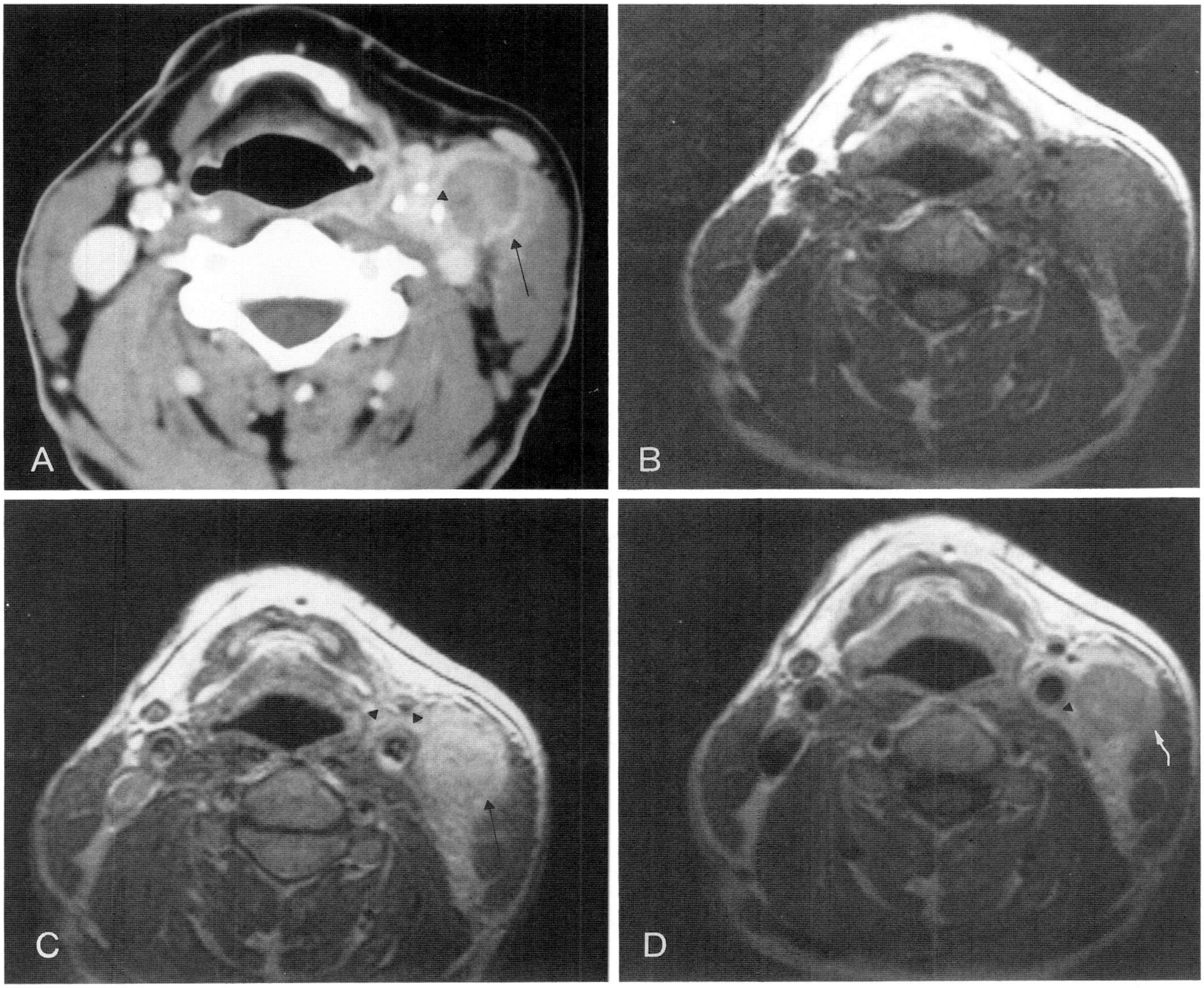

Figure 1.20*A–D*

Figure 1.20. Patient with metastatic cervical adenopathy from primary tumor of unknown origin. *A,* CT shows nodal mass with capsular involvement and penetration *(arrow)* with fixation to sternocleidomastoid muscle. Tumor is likely to be focally adherent or fixed to carotid at this point *(arrowhead)* but carotid is *not* encased. *B,* T_1-weighted MRI without Gd-DTPA at same level shows nodal mass but little discrimination of extranodal extent of tumor. *C,* spin echo 2000/30-msec pulse sequence MRI without Gd-DTPA shows muscle involvement *(arrow)* and abnormal tissue around carotid *(arrowheads)*. *D,* spin echo 500/20-msec pulse sequence *with* Gd-DTPA produces an image similar to the CT in *A*. Muscle involvement is noted *(arrow)*. Small strands of tissue, perhaps tumor, seem to be extending to carotid *(arrowheads)*.

Comment: At present, for MRI to approach the overall utility of CT in evaluating nodal disease T_1- and T_2-weighted images of high quality must be available or Gd-DTPA must be used. Still at issue is the ability of MRI to show focal metastases in normal-size nodes with the same clarity as CT.

tages in tissue contrast and multiplanar display are focused on a confined region of anatomic interest. There are exceptions to this, and the relative advantages of CT and MRI with respect to efficiency of examination must be decided on a case-by-case basis since so many competing factors are operational.

Artifacts

All imaging systems produce artifacts, but those of MRI are more numerous and more likely to be interpreted as pathologic change by inexperienced observers. Gross motion artifacts were discussed pre-

Figure 1.21. Patient with pyriform sinus carcinoma. All sections of the CT study were same quality as that seen in *A*. *B*, excellent-quality MRI images were obtained on the first acquisition, which took 9 min on a 0.15-T resistive unit. *C*, second acquisition showed considerable motion artifact. Additional acquisitions were nondiagnostic and the study was terminated.

Comment: In *B* note the potential advantages of MRI for showing relationship of primary tumor *(T)* to infrahyoid strap muscles and musculature of the posterior pharyngeal wall. *N*, metastatic lymph node.

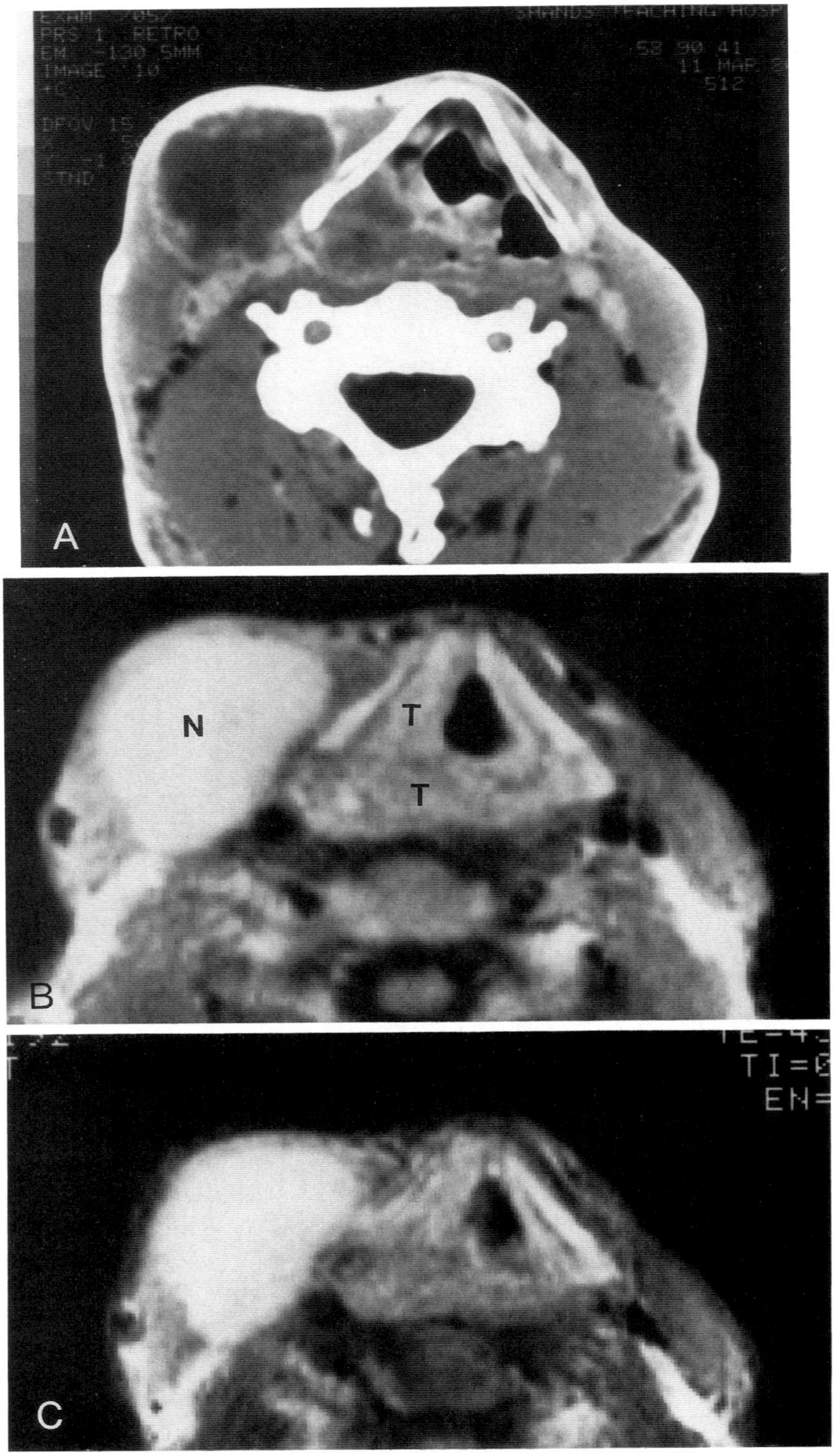

Figure 1.21*A–C*

viously and pose a far more significant problem for MRI compared to CT. Gross motion is mainly a problem outside of the brain. Eye movements degrade orbital images. Jaw motion frequently obscures important detail in the oropharynx and oral cavity (Fig. 1.22). Swallowing and labored breathing routinely degrade laryngeal and hypopharyngeal studies, and this may be compounded in patients with cancers in the region which often aggravate airway problems (partial obstruction) and swallowing and coughing (as a result of increased secretions or chronic inflammation). The rate of technically inadequate studies approaches 20% in patients with oropharyngeal and laryngopharyngeal cancer because of these factors, and marginally diagnostic studies occur about 20 to 30% of the time. CT failure rates under the same situations are near zero at the University of Florida. In the nasopharynx motion is not a problem and MRI is the preferred exam because of its superior contrast resolution and multiplanar capabilities.

Flow-related MRI artifacts (both blood and CSF) may degrade images, hide pathology, and lead to misinterpretation (Fig. 1.23). Dealing with flow-related artifacts increases the complexity of performing and interpreting MRI studies, a potential disadvantage. However, these same "artifacts" may be the source of important and unique diagnostic information (Fig. 1.5). One must be totally familiar with these phenomena so as not to make critical errors in reading MRI studies of the head and neck and other regions. These factors will come into play even more as gradient echo pulse sequences are used (Fig. 1.24). Excellent discussions of flow-related artifacts are available in a number of sources (see Suggested Readings).

Artifacts due to dental hardware and fillings can be avoided on CT in almost all cases by proper positioning of the head and gantry angulation. Local field distortions caused by these materials may have little or no effect on images or may produce serious degradation (Fig. 1.22); the latter are unavoidable when present but can frequently be overcome, in part, by altering the plane of section.

The streak artifacts in posterior fossa CT have been largely overcome by improved tube-detector systems and thin sections; beyond this a well-tuned CT system runs relatively artifact free nowadays. Magnetic resonance imaging is still subject to many more technical artifacts than those just discussed. These include:

1. *Aliasing (Foldover)*—caused by a mismatch of the volume of tissue under study and the chosen FOV.
2. *Chemical Shift*—caused by separation of fat and water resonance. A problem mainly in high field systems and imaging outside of the brain. These can be overcome by using steep imaging gradients (i.e., at least 0.5 to 1.0 gauss/cm).

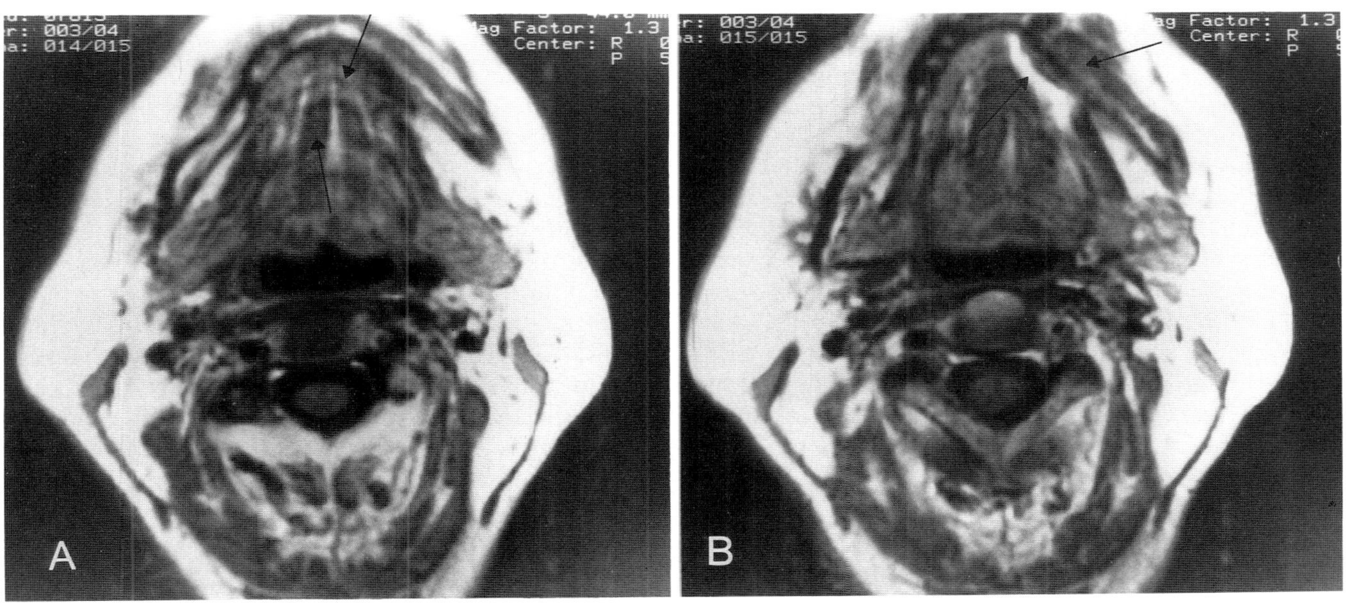

Figure 1.22*A* and *B*

Figure 1.22. Patient with oropharyngeal tumor (not shown) studied on a 1.5-T system. *A*, typical artifacts due to jaw motion *(arrows)*. These are the mild variety visible on a large number of cases; they decrease image quality but do not usually impede diagnosis. *B*, same patient with field distortion artifacts due to dental work *(arrows)*. These are very common, frequently completely distorting detail in the oral cavity, floor of the mouth, and even nasal cavity, sinus, and oropharynx if severe enough. These become worse with gradient echo techniques.

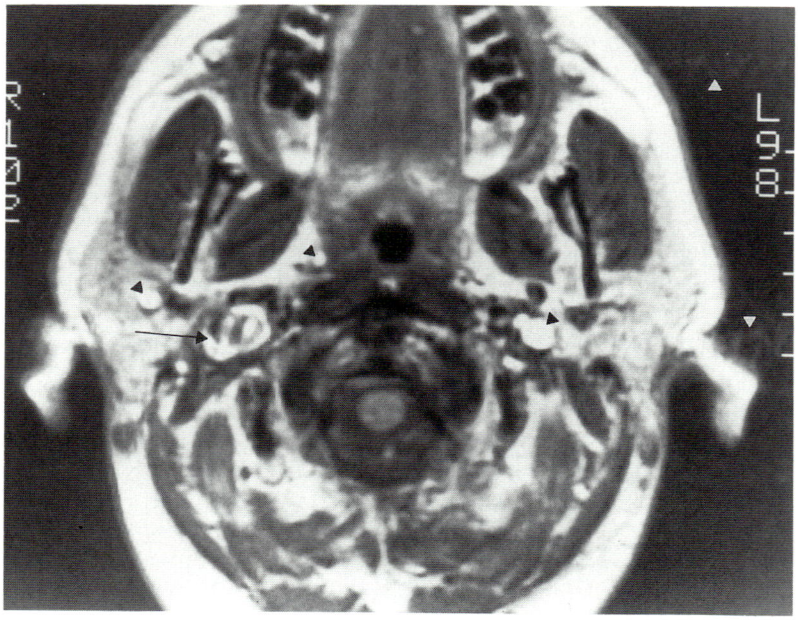

Figure 1.23

Figure 1.23. This section illustrates the potential complexity of flow-related phenomena as seen on spin echo pulse sequences. Right jugular vein has a very complex appearance (*arrow*) probably as a result of turbulent flow. Such findings can be mistaken for pathology, especially in the jugular fossa region. Left jugular vein, pharyngeal vessels, and retromandibular vein *(black arrowheads)* show flow-related enhancement. External carotid and internal carotid show familiar "flow void." Pulsatile motion artifacts from various artifacts ring through the image *(white arrowheads)*; these sometimes cause significant degradation.

3. *Inhomogeneous Rf Reception*—caused by improper tip angles or poorly shimmed fields.
4. *Truncation Artifacts (Edge Effects)*—occur at high-contrast interfaces (e.g., fat-muscle); can be reduced by expanding matrix while holding FOV constant (i.e., going from 128 × 256 to 192 × 256 acquisition matrix).
5. *Crosstalk (Cross-excitation)*—partial saturation of adjacent slices due to overlapping of slice-selective pulses. Can be improved by creative Rf pulse shaping (e.g., sin C pulses), leaving gaps (with or without interleaving), 3DFT.
6. *Distortions of Aspect Ratio*—caused by mismatches in phase and frequency encoding gradients that, when severe, cause the image to appear warped. These can cause serious problems in MRI-guided stereotactic procedures. To avoid make sure pulse programs are properly "tuned," especially in new software upgrades.
7. *Rf Interference*—causes a variety of artifacts; may come from the system, patients, or external sources and all may interact.

This is by no means a complete discussion of MRI or CT artifacts, but it should be clear that CT is a mature, relatively artifact-free technique. Magnetic resonance imaging, on the other hand, is still immature in some regards but as systems become "tighter" many of the troublesome system-related artifacts will disappear. Some of the flow-related "artifacts" are being put to good diagnostic use. At present, however, CT retains a distinct advantage for producing rapid, high-quality images in virtually all patients. This still remains a goal for MRI.

Unique Capabilities

There are certain things that MRI does better than CT and vice versa. This must be taken into account when one is developing imaging algorithms to deal with the very complex anatomy and pathology of the head and neck region.

Bone (and Cartilage) Detail

Computed tomography is clearly better than MRI at showing bone detail. However, MRI is remarkably good at demonstrating bony structures such as the skull base when they contain fatty marrow and their cortical surfaces are surrounded by tissue or fluid (Figs. 1.5, 1.13*E*, and 1.15). Magnetic resonance imaging in fact is probably more sensitive than CT and radionuclide bone scans for demonstrating processes spreading *primarily* within the marrow-containing space of bones (Fig. 1.25). This is high and deserved praise for MRI, but do not be fooled. Serious interpretive errors can be made by assuming that bone is not destroyed because a destructive pattern is not visible on MRI. A mistaken false-positive diagnosis of bone invasion is a less common fault. Bone and cartilage destruction and invasion are such key diagnostic and prognostic issues in head and neck disorders that the diagnostic imager must assume full responsibility for demonstrating their presence or absence with a very high degree of certainty. This is one reason why CT is chosen first in the paranasal sinuses, oral cavity, oropharynx, and larynx in the University of Florida protocols and diagnostic imaging algorithms in the following chapters.

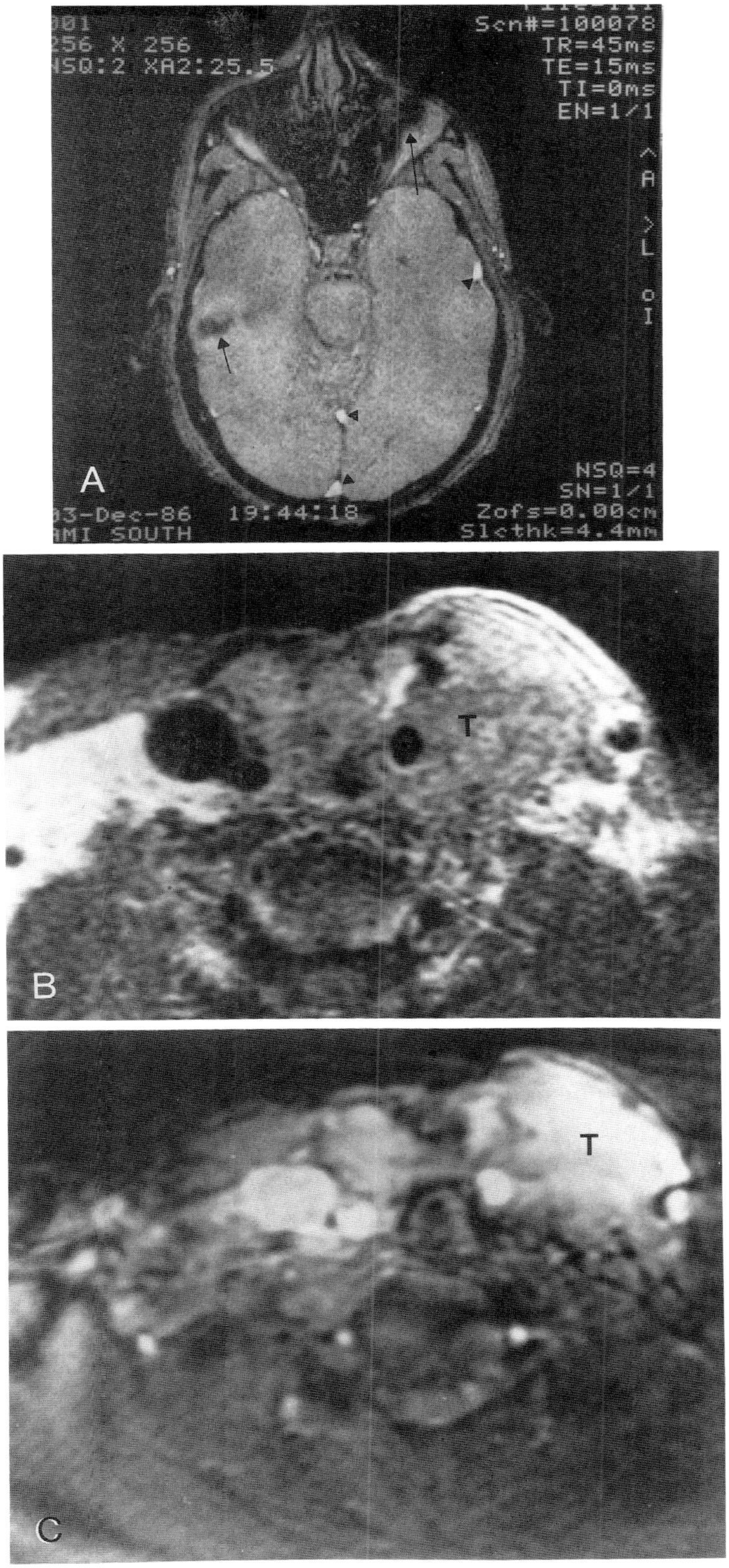

Figure 1.24A–C

Figure 1.24. *A*, gradient echo image, TR/TE = 45/15 msec with tip angle of approximately 30° at 0.6 T. Areas of flow-related enhancement are obvious *(arrowheads)*. Note mild field distortion artifacts at brain-bone and air-bone interfaces *(arrows)*. *B*, spin echo 500/20-msec pulse sequence image done at 1.5 T on patient with stomal recurrence of squamous cell carcinoma *(T)*. *C*, gradient echo image of same patient showing flow-related enhancement in vessels, but mass also becomes quite bright. This is obviously not a vascular mass. This points out the potential pitfall in gradient echo imaging of reducing contrast between vessels and pathology depending on sequence chosen. Gradient echo imaging combined with Gd-DTPA creates another variable that may prove confusing until optimal parameters for use of these techniques are established.

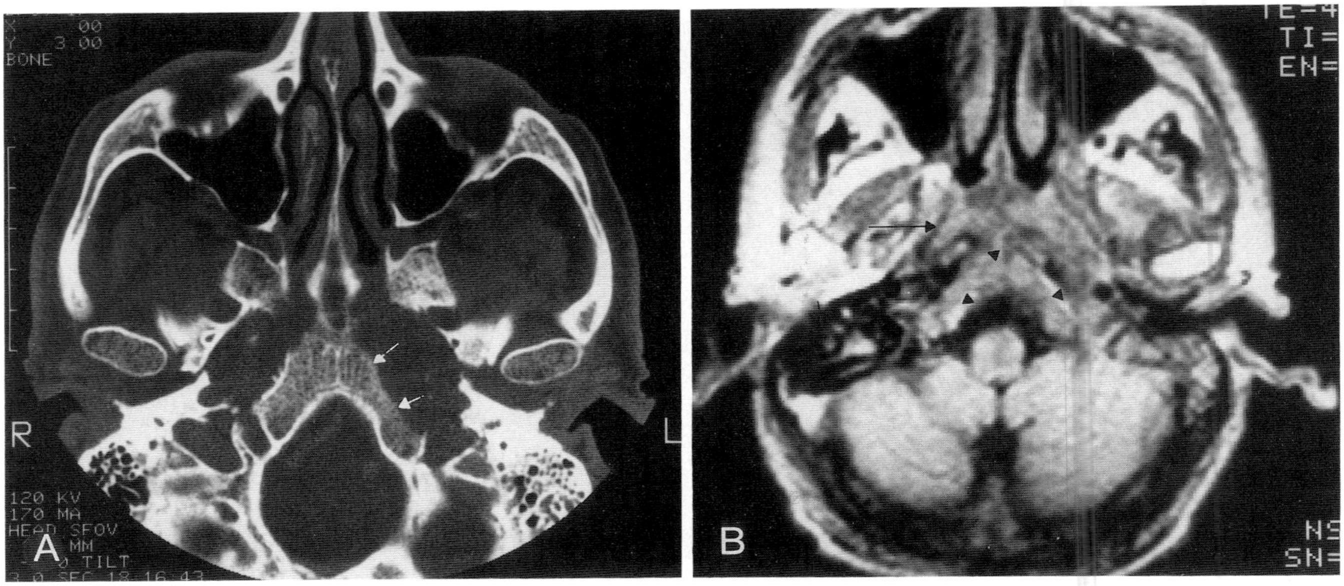

Figure 1.25*A* and *B*

Figure 1.25. Patient with carcinoma invading the skull base. CT and MRI were done 1 day apart. *A,* CT exam shows erosion of the cortical margin of the clivus *(arrows)* but bony trabeculae appear relatively normal. *B,* SE 600/45-msec pulse sequence, 5-mm section done on a 0.15-T resistive unit shows widespread infiltration of the clivus *(arrowheads)* in addition to deeply infiltrating spread to the prestyloid parapharyngeal space with obliteration of the pharyngobasilar fascia on the left compared to the right side *(arrow)*.

Calcification

Detection of calcifications in a lesion may aid in differential diagnosis and can potentially lead to altered treatment plans. MRI is poor at showing calcifications, but these may be recognized on occasion (Fig. 1.26). This is a supportive reason for our choosing CT as the initial tool for evaluating paranasal sinus pathology and whenever there is a hint of an inflammatory history in a parotid or submandibular region mass. The implications of this situation in intracranial pathology have been discussed extensively in the neuroradiologic literature.

Multiplanar Imaging

Although reformations and direct coronal CT offer some flexibility for multiplanar display, MRI is extraordinary in its rendering of coronal, sagittal, and off-axis views of anatomy and pathology in the head and neck and elsewhere. The impact of the multiplanar capability of MRI is felt in both diagnosis and treatment planning. Combining these data with three-dimensional display systems should further enhance the rapidly developing fields of skull-base surgery and high-precision radiotherapy. Although this is one of the most "simple-minded" benefits of MRI it turns out to be an extraordinarily important one and it clearly overcomes some of the weaknesses of MRI relative to CT. For example, even though CT is better at showing bone detail, both CT and MRI prove to be equivalent for showing skull base erosion in nasopharyngeal cancer (Fig. 1.13*E*). Magnetic resonance imaging becomes equivalent mainly on the strength of the ease of sagittal (for the clivus) and coronal (for the petroclival junction) display of the areas at major risk. The relative benefits of multiplanar display vary with the region and possible pathologies under study and are but one of a number of things considered in our protocols and problem-solving algorithms (Fig. 1.27). Magnetic resonance imaging is frequently used as an adjunct to CT because of its multiplanar capability, especially when anatomic issues remain unresolved (e.g., the relationship of tumor to the cribriform plate–olfactory bulb region) (Fig. 1.13*A*, *C*).

Contrast Resolution

T_1, T_2, and proton density all may be manipulated by varying MRI pulse sequences to produce contrast between pathology and normal tissue. This is a major advantage of MRI over CT and its effects are felt in detecting intra-axial pathology as well as showing tumor-muscle interfaces with a clarity that far exceeds CT in many cases (Figs. 1.11 to 1.13). Magnetic resonance imaging can clearly separate obstructed, fluid-filled sinuses from those grossly invaded by tumor and can even sometimes *suggest* that a pathologic diagnosis may be in error (i.e., suggest inflammatory rather than neoplastic etiology) (Fig. 1.28). It can also *suggest* that a mass is end-stage fibrosis rather than residual tumor (Figs. 1.14 and 1.28). It is, how-

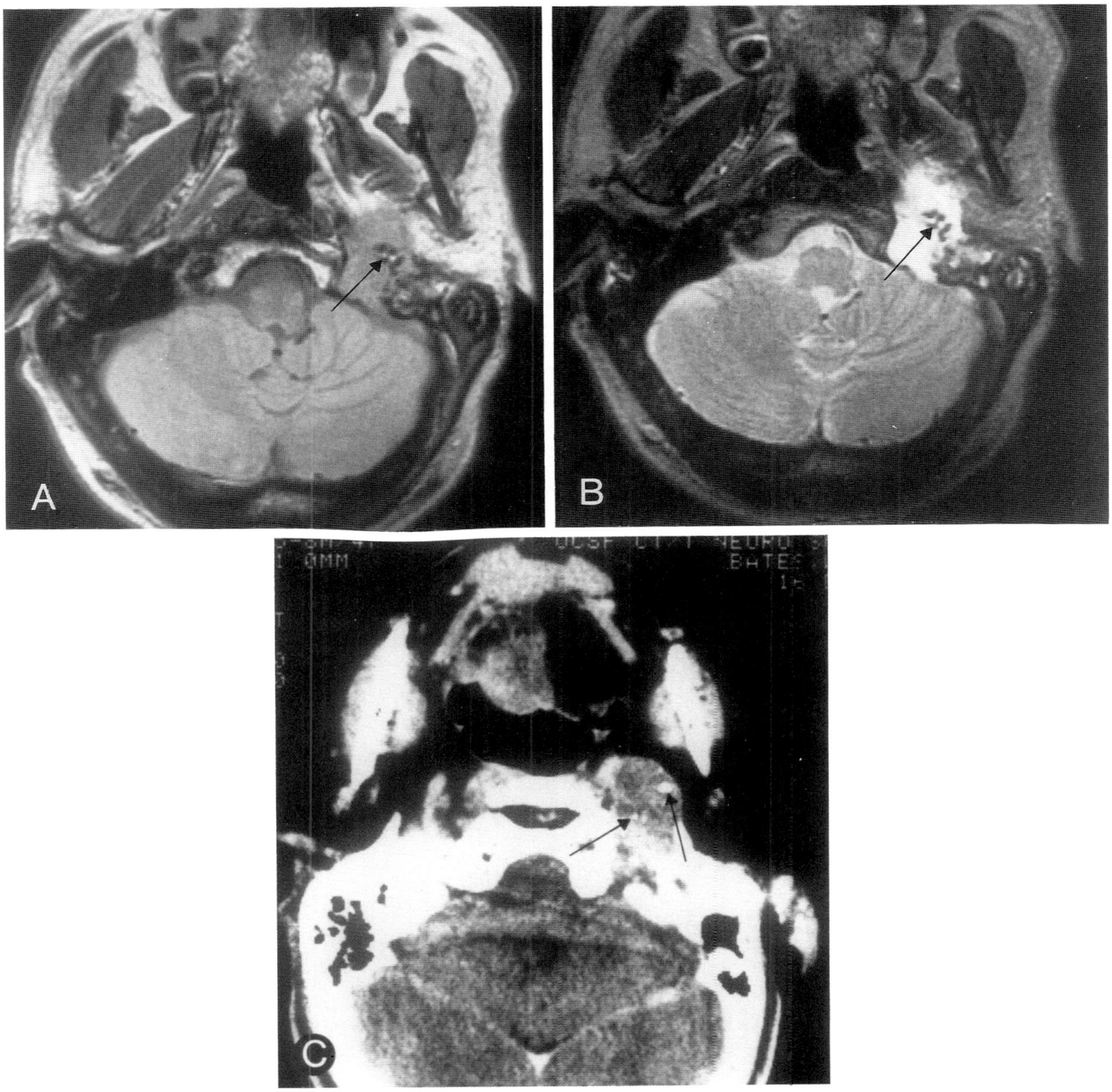

Figure 1.26*A–C*

Figure 1.26. Patient with a chordoma. *A* and *B*, T_1- and T_2-weighted images that both show discreet areas of low signal intensity *(arrows)*. This could be due to flow or to calcification. *C*, CT shows obvious calcifications *(arrows)*. Also note atrophy of tongue as a result of XIIth nerve compression.

ever, *never* tissue specific (except maybe for lipomas). Clonogenic (viable) tumor cells can replicate in a bed of dense fibrosis and what appears to be a lipoma can be a low-grade liposarcoma. An obstructed sinus filled with fluid can have mucosal invasion by tumor, and even though a mass appears inflammatory (very long T_2) it may prove on biopsy to be malignant. Imaging findings are worth little without the total clinical picture; this is what gives them their meaning.

A potential disadvantage to the extraordinary ability of MRI to contrast normal and pathologic tissues is its tendency to make the interfaces between aggressive pathology and normal structures appear smooth (as opposed to infiltrative). This can lead to errors in differential diagnosis and underestimation and possible undertreatment of the disease process. However, it is the same rendering of sharp, clear interfaces between lymphoid tissue, the walls of the nasopharynx, and deeper musculature that makes MRI so sensitive to early infiltrating carcinoma in the nasopharynx. One needs only to be aware of the tendency so as not to be fooled by it. The ability to vary tissue contrast is a clear, major advantage of MRI compared to CT.

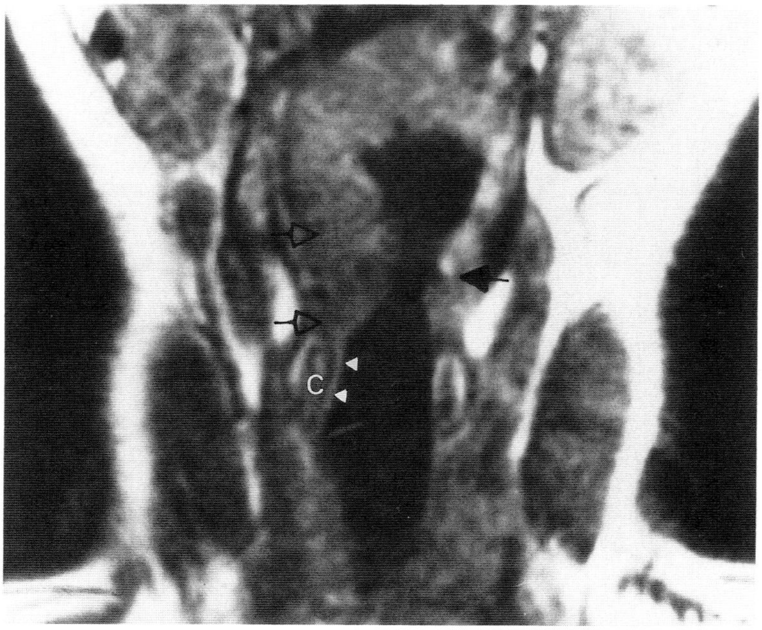

Figure 1.27

Figure 1.27. Patient with a primary supraglottic cancer. Coronal MRI clearly demonstrates tumor filling the paralaryngeal space and spreading across laryngeal ventricle to involve true and false cord level *(open arrows)*. Compare to normal paralaryngeal space and ventricular level *(closed arrow)*. There is also subglottic edema or tumor *(arrowheads)* manifest by soft tissue thickening medial to cricoid cartilage *(C)*.

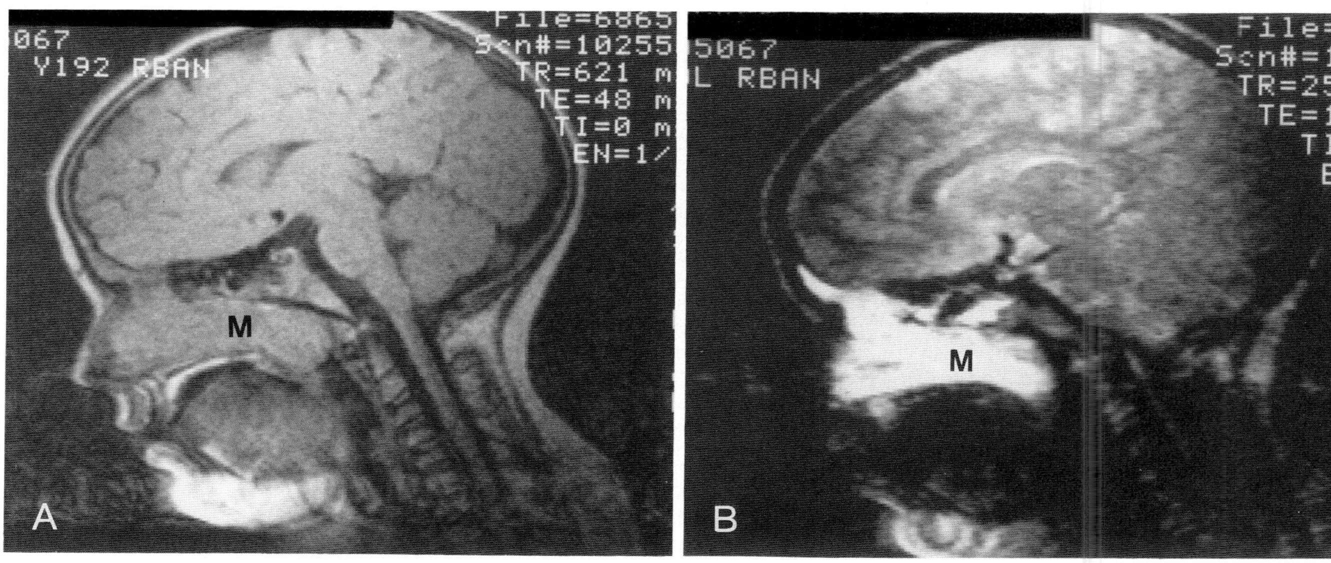

Figure 1.28*A* and *B*

Figure 1.28. Six-year-old with biopsy of nasal mass read as rhabdo- versus fibrosarcoma. *A* and *B*, T_1- and T_2-weighted images, respectively, show lobulated nasal cavity mass *(M)* bulging into nasopharynx. Very bright signal on heavily T_2-weighted image suggests inflammatory rather than neoplastic etiology but is not specific. Rebiopsy revealed fibroangiomatous, inflammatory polyp with "pseudosarcomatous" reactive changes.

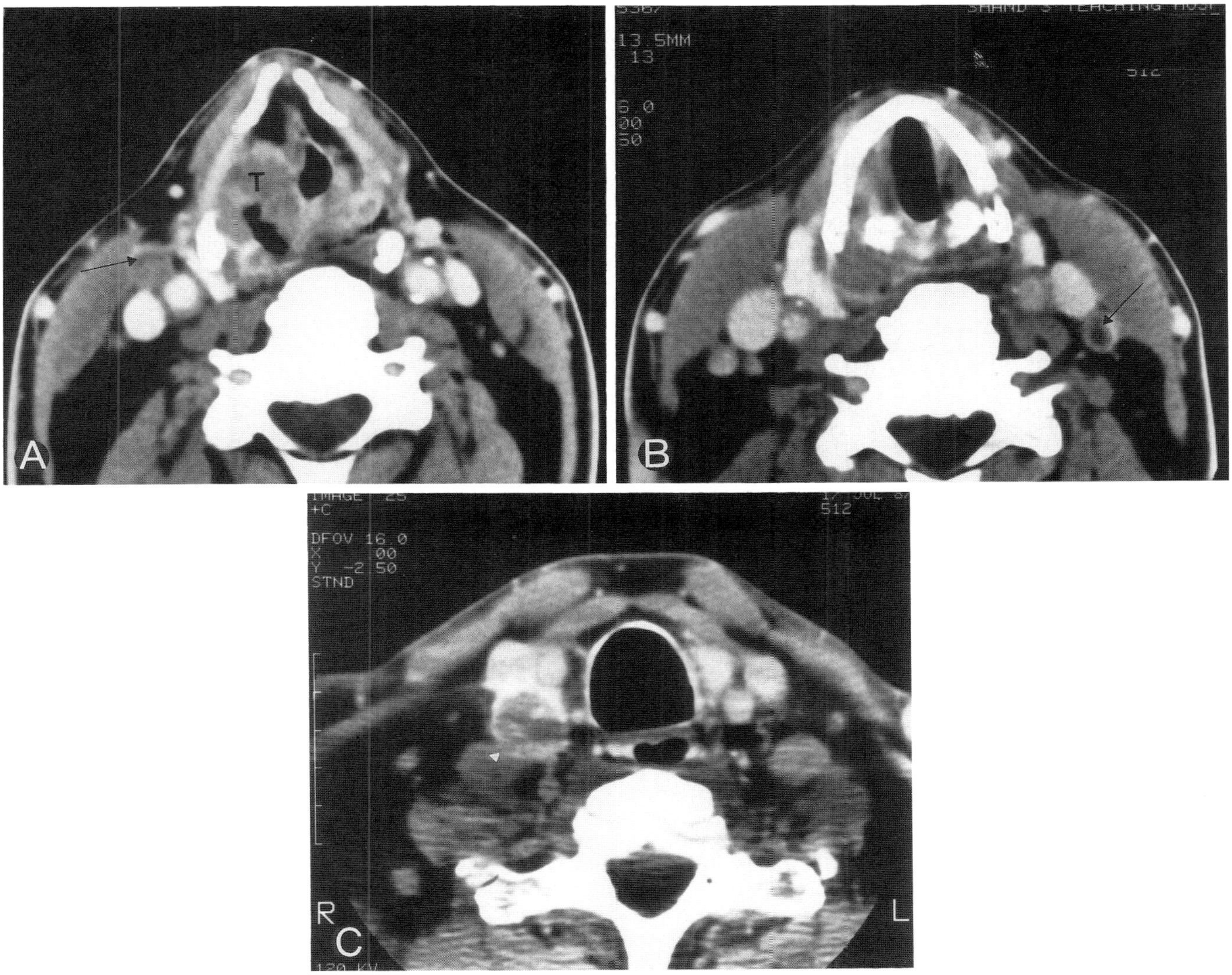

Figure 1.29A–C

Figure 1.29. Patient with pyriform sinus carcinoma. Neck was clinically *negative* on exam by numerous very experienced examiners. *A,* primary tumor *(T)* and positive 9-mm node on the basis of focal defect *(arrow)* *B,* positive 7- to 8-mm contralateral node with obvious focal defect *(arrow)*. *C,* positive 20-mm node deep in neck (scalene node) with evidence of capsular involvement and possible early capsular penetration *(arrowhead)*.

Comment: This neck is properly staged N3b rather than N0; individually the neck is N2b on right and N1 on the left. All findings were confirmed at surgery. This type of precision neck staging can be used to develop fully informed treatment plans for the neck. As yet such diagnostic capabilities for MRI have not been demonstrated either in preliminary or in detailed clinical trials.

The Posterior Fossa

The combination of contrast resolution, rendering of the basal cisterns free of interference from bone and artifacts, and reasonable depiction of the skull base make MRI a study ideally suited to the pathology arising in or affecting the posterior fossa. The use of Gd-DTPA can only enhance this dominance over CT, which is so clear at present. The addition of Gd-DTPA should aid in the detection of basilar-meningitic infiltrative processes as well as primary and recurrent acoustic neuroma, meningioma, and other lesions that can spread along the dura and within the meninges (Figs. 1.16 to 1.18).

Evaluation of Cervical Metastatic Disease

Evaluation of cervical metastatic disease is so critical to prognosis and management in patients with head and neck cancer that it deserves special men-

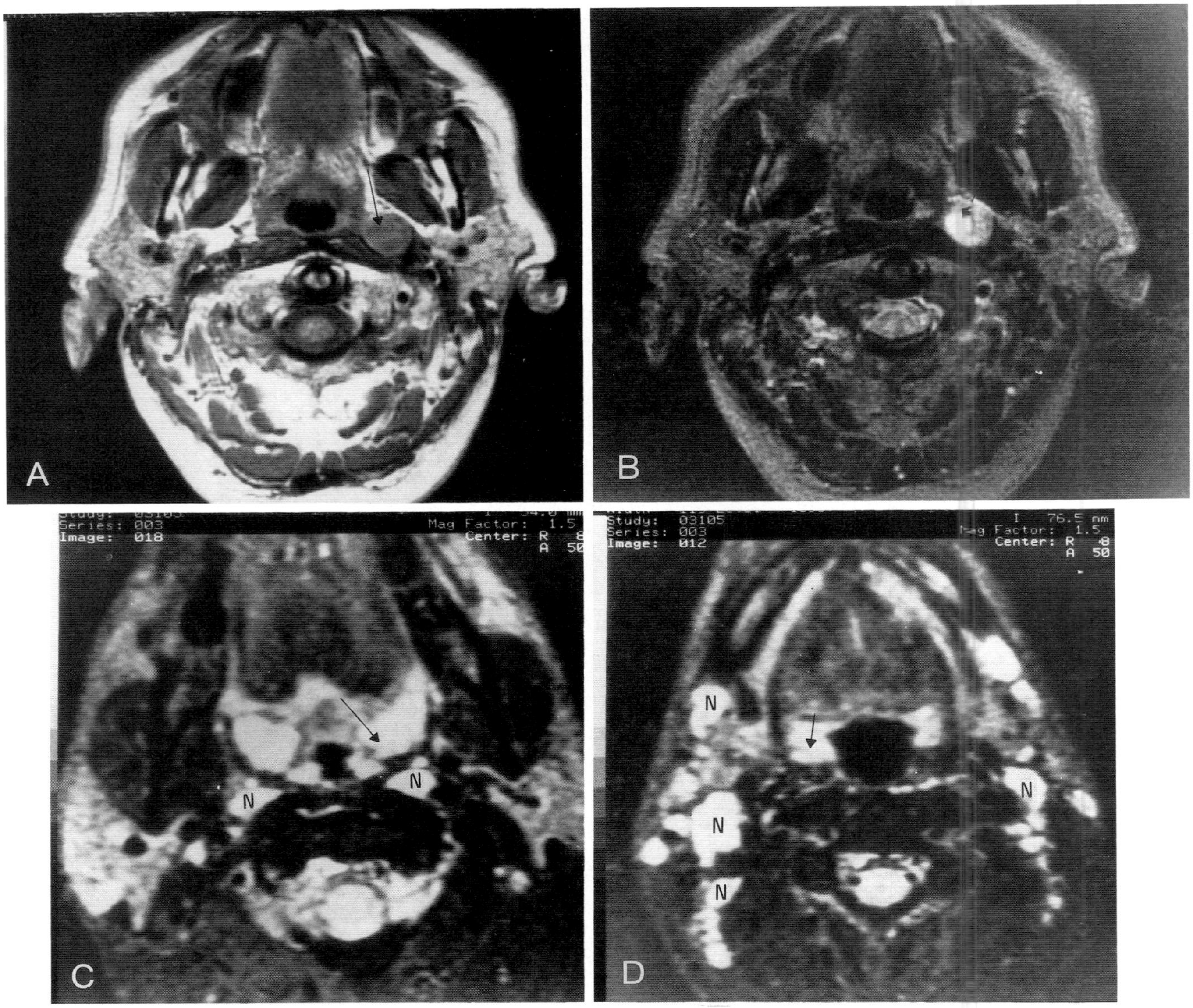

Figure 1.30*A–D*

Figure 1.30. Two different patients with adenopathy *(A)* and with squamous cell carcinoma of the nasopharynx *(B)*. *A*, partial saturation 500/20-msec pulse sequence image shows a positive (by size) retropharyngeal node *(arrow)*. *B*, discrete focal abnormality is only noted on SE 2000/70-msec pulse sequence *(arrow)*. *C* and *D*, SE 2000/70-msec pulse sequence images in patient with acquired immunodeficiency syndrome. Many nodes *(N)* are present and enlarged. All are same intensity of normal lymphoid tissue in tonsil *(arrow)*. Surgically sampled nodes showed reactive hyperplasia and no focal abnormalities.

Comment: From viewing the above cases it should be clear that at present definitive evaluation of primary site and nodes might require multiple pulse sequences as well as a coil change if entire neck is to be surveyed. These circumstances make MRI far more complex than CT for evaluation of upper aerodigestive tract malignancy at present.

tion here. Modern CT now routinely demonstrates metastatic foci in 5- to 8-mm nodes (Fig. 1.29). Magnetic resonance imaging is capable of this only with involved and time-consuming protocols when one considers that the primary site has to be studied in detail as well (Fig. 1.30). This does not even take into account the interpretive difficulties and often inferior image quality (on any system) that can arise on MRI images below the nasopharynx. Computed tomography shows the extent of early extranodal spread better than does MRI but MRI may prove a useful supplement in selected cases (Fig. 1 31). For

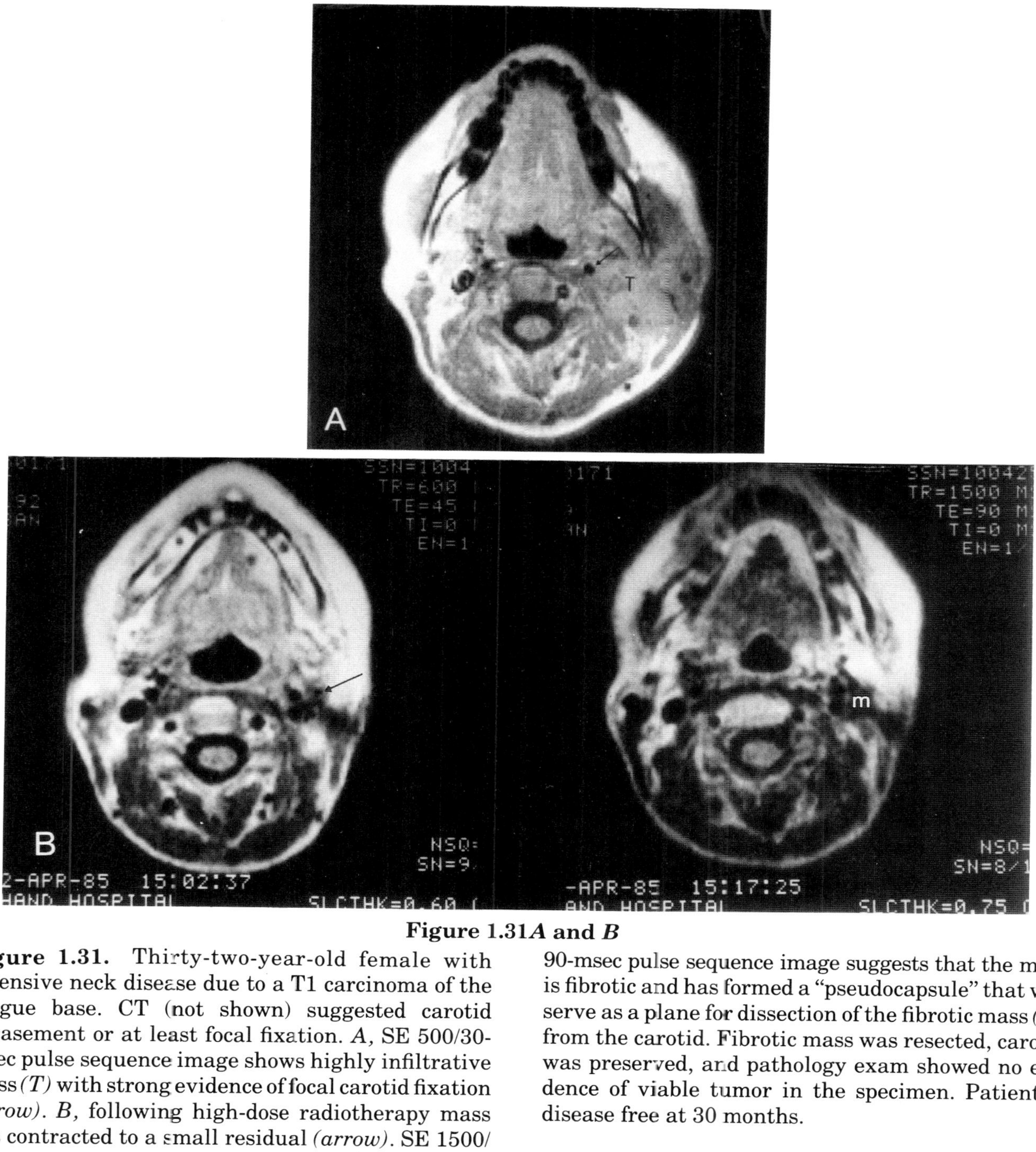

Figure 1.31*A* and *B*

Figure 1.31. Thirty-two-year-old female with extensive neck disease due to a T1 carcinoma of the tongue base. CT (not shown) suggested carotid encasement or at least focal fixation. *A,* SE 500/30-msec pulse sequence image shows highly infiltrative mass *(T)* with strong evidence of focal carotid fixation *(arrow)*. *B,* following high-dose radiotherapy mass has contracted to a small residual *(arrow)*. SE 1500/90-msec pulse sequence image suggests that the mass is fibrotic and has formed a "pseudocapsule" that will serve as a plane for dissection of the fibrotic mass *(m)* from the carotid. Fibrotic mass was resected, carotid was preserved, and pathology exam showed no evidence of viable tumor in the specimen. Patient is disease free at 30 months.

these reasons CT remains our primary tool for evaluating all primary tumors of the upper aerodigestive tract except those arising in the nasopharynx. This issue is developed more fully in subsequent chapters.

Intravenous Contrast Enhancement

Computed tomography with intravenous contrast enhancement frequently provides a more graphic depiction of inflammatory masses or the truly infiltrative margins of a malignant tumor. Markedly enhancing masses on CT may suggest a vascular lesion (e.g., paraganglioma, juvenile angiofibroma, arteriovenous malformation, aneurysm). There are, however, MRI findings that also lead one to suspect a highly vascular lesion, so that the advantage of CT here may be small and diminishing (with newer, more flow-sensitive pulse sequences and potentially Gd-DTPA dynamic studies (Fig. 1.32). The clinical

Normal Anatomy—Orbit
(use checklists in Appendix A as a study aid)

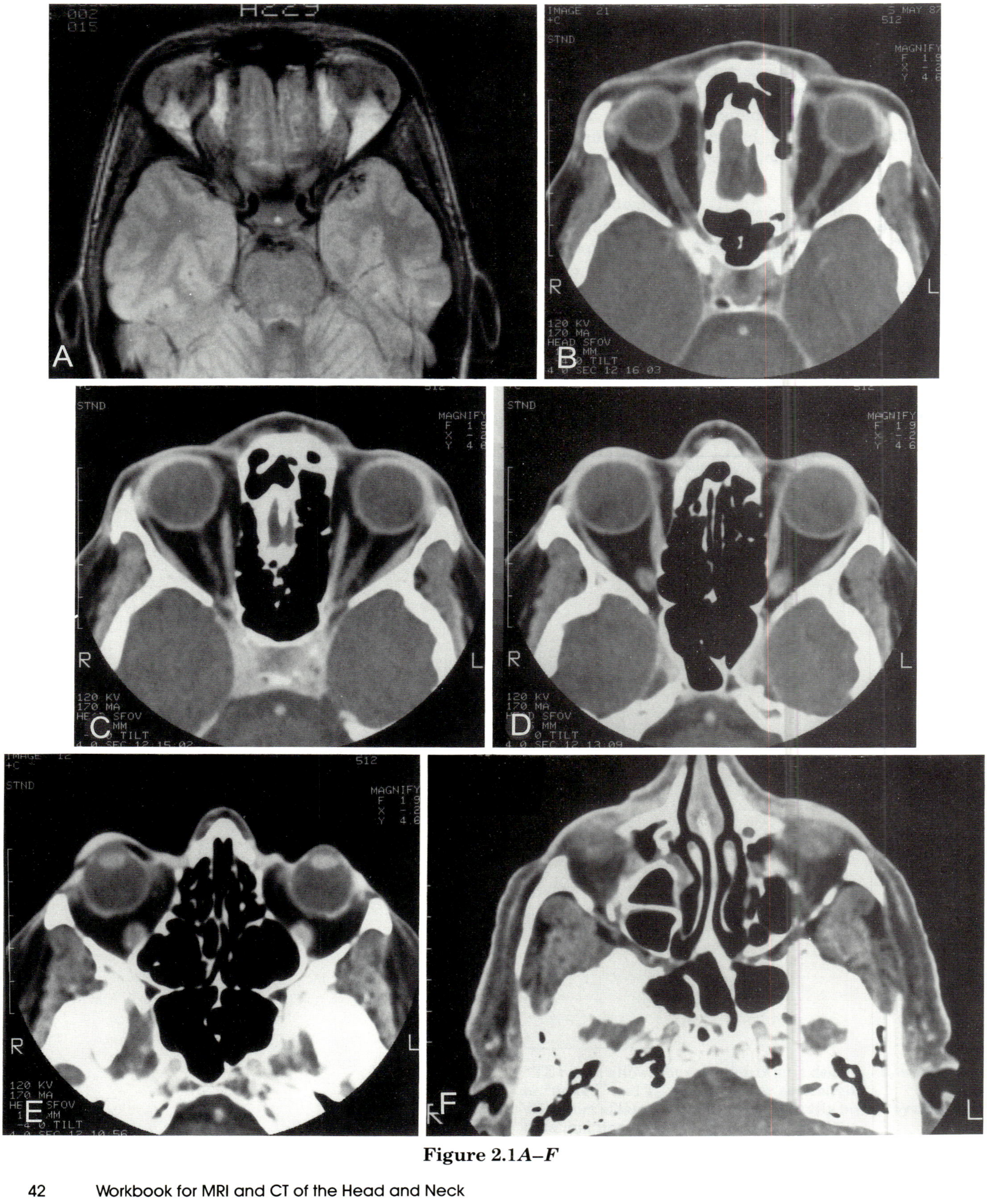

Figure 2.1*A–F*

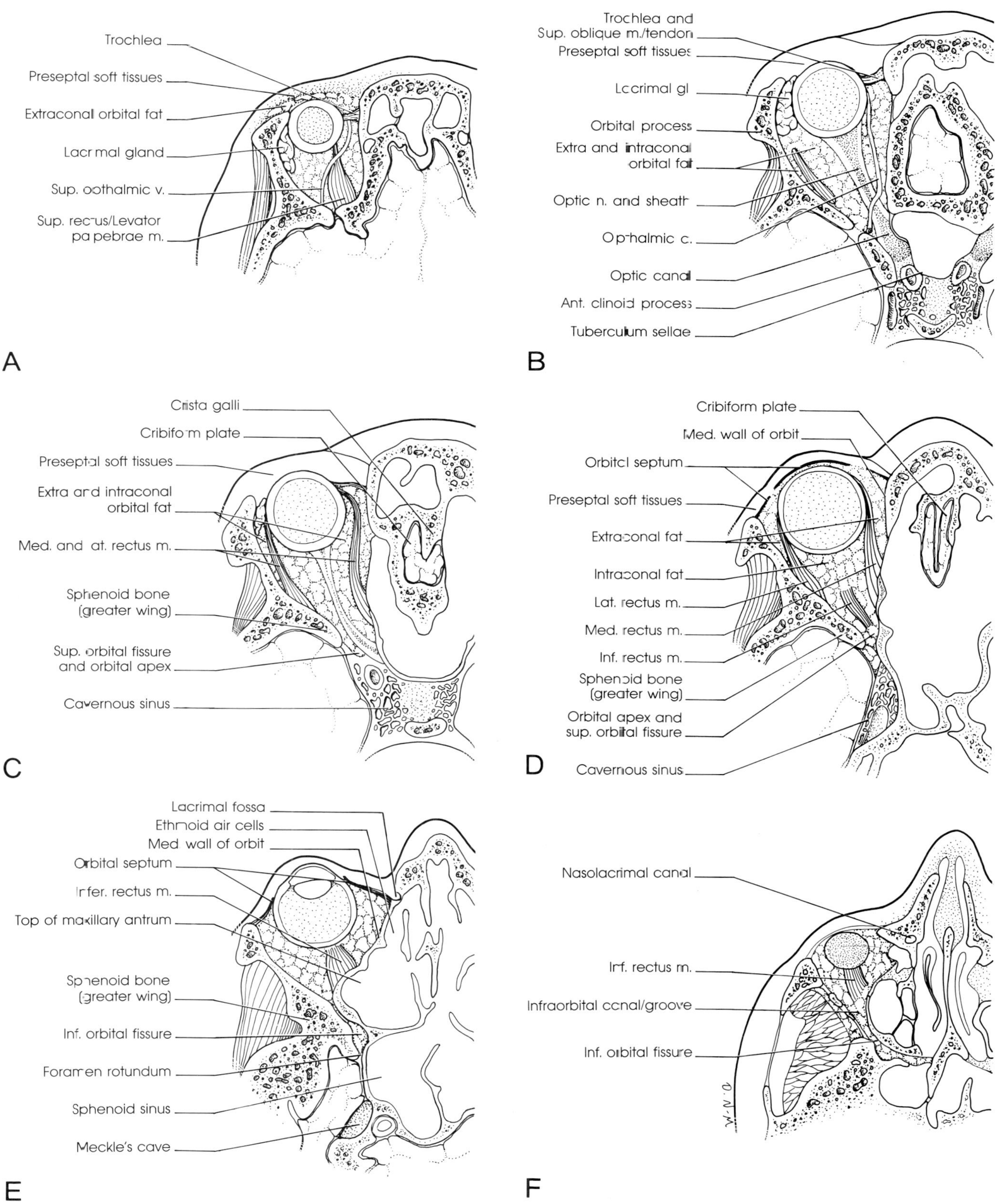

Trochlea
Preseptal soft tissues
Extraconal orbital fat
Lacrimal gland
Sup. ophthalmic v.
Sup. rectus/Levator palpebrae m.
A
Trochlea and Sup. oblique m./tendon
Preseptal soft tissues
Lacrimal gl
Orbital process
Extra and intraconal orbital fat
Optic n. and sheath
Ophthalmic a.
Optic canal
Ant. clinoid process
Tuberculum sellae
B
Crista galli
Cribiform plate
Preseptal soft tissues
Extra and intraconal orbital fat
Med. and lat. rectus m.
Sphenoid bone (greater wing)
Sup. orbital fissure and orbital apex
Cavernous sinus
C
Cribiform plate
Med. wall of orbit
Orbital septum
Preseptal soft tissues
Extraconal fat
Intraconal fat
Lat. rectus m.
Med. rectus m.
Inf. rectus m.
Sphenoid bone (greater wing)
Orbital apex and sup. orbital fissure
Cavernous sinus
D
Lacrimal fossa
Ethmoid air cells
Med wall of orbit
Orbital septum
Infer. rectus m.
Top of maxillary antrum
Sphenoid bone (greater wing)
Inf. orbital fissure
Foramen rotundum
Sphenoid sinus
Meckle's cave
E
Nasolacrimal canal
Inf. rectus m.
Infraorbital canal/groove
Inf. orbital fissure
F

Figure 2.2*A–F*

Normal Anatomy—Visual Pathways
(use checklists in Appendix A as a study aid)

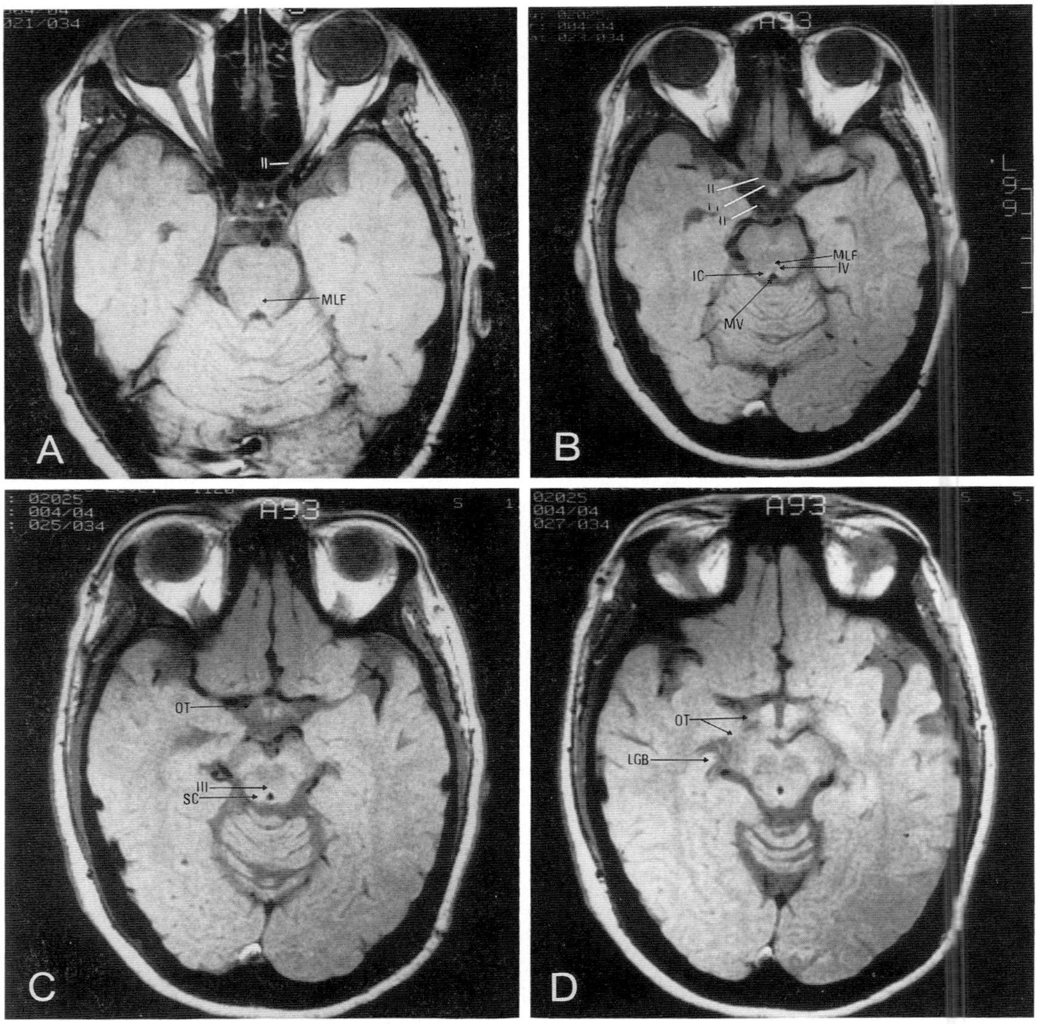

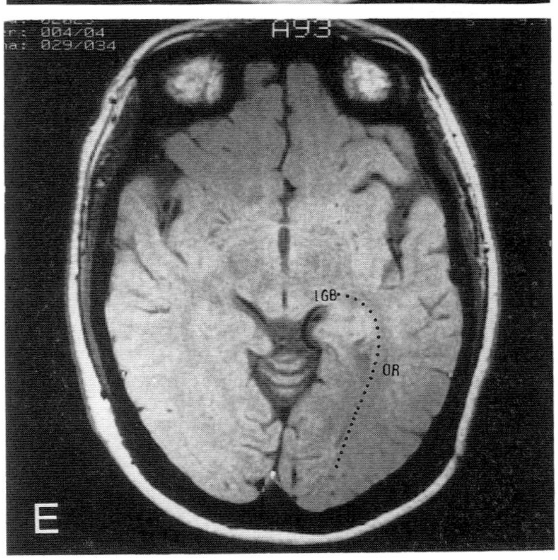

Figure 2.3*A–E*. Selected sections demonstrating major structures of the visual pathways from inferior to superior. Cranial nerves and their nuclei are numbered as follows: *II*, optic; *III*, oculomotor; *IV*, trochlear. Other structures labeled include: *MLF*, median longitudinal fasiculus; *OC*, optic chiasm; *IC*, inferior colliculus; *MV*, medullary vellum; *OT*, optic tract; *SC*, superior colliculus; *LGB*, lateral geniculate body; *OR*, optic radiation.

Figure 2.3*A–E*

Normal Anatomy—Cavernous Sinus (use checklists in Appendix A as a study aid)

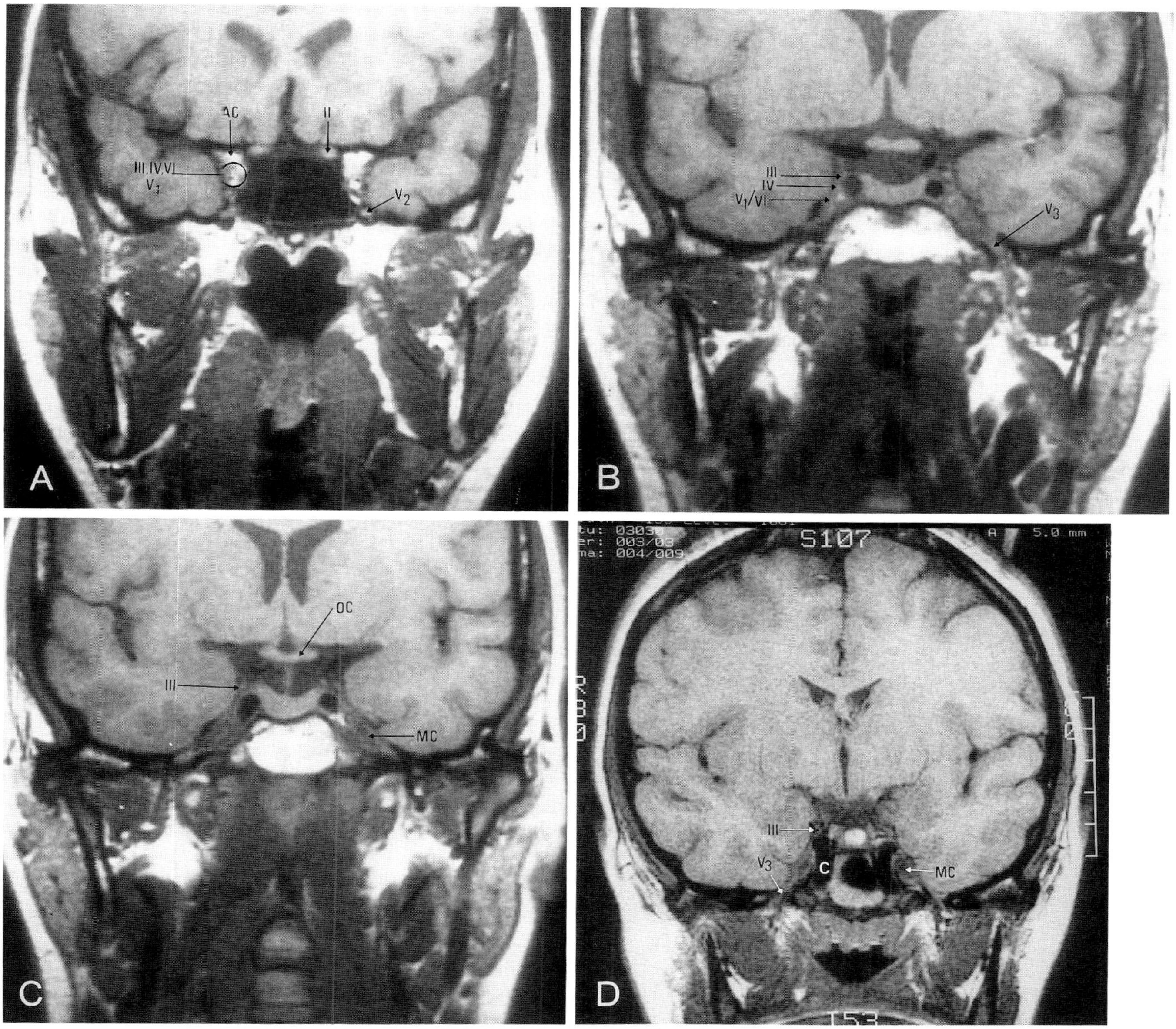

Figure 2.4*A–D*

Figure 2.4*A–D*. Selected coronal section from the orbital apex to the posterior cavernous sinus. Cranial nerves are numbered as follows: *II,* optic; *III,* oculomotor; *IV,* trochlear; *VI,* abducent; V_1, V_2, V_3, frontal, maxillary, and mandibular divisions of trigeminal nerve, respectively. Other labeled structures include: *AC,* fat in the anterior clinoid process; *OC,* optic chiasm; *MC,* Meckel's cave; *C,* internal carotid artery. On careful inspection one can see the trigeminal ganglion in Meckel's cave in part *C.*

CASES

Use checklists in Appendix A to analyze the following cases.

Problem I

Case 2.1A (Fig. 2.5)

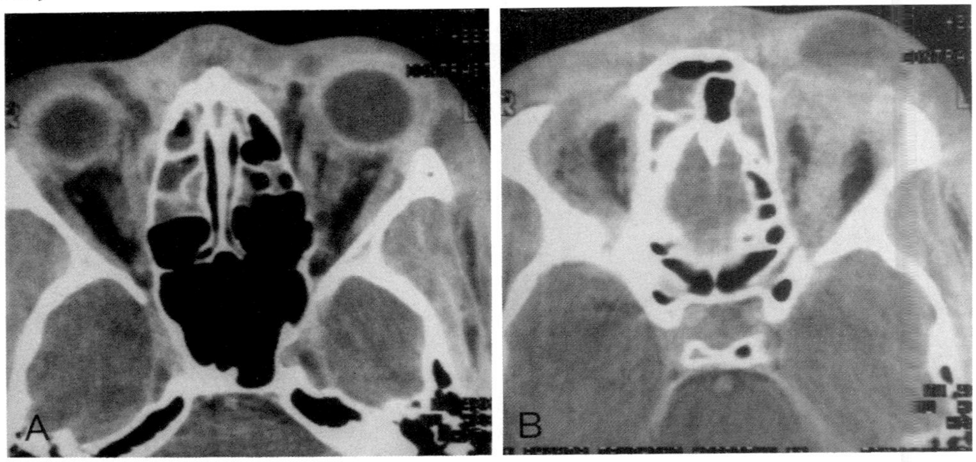

Figure 2.5*A* and *B*

Case 2.1B (Fig. 2.6)

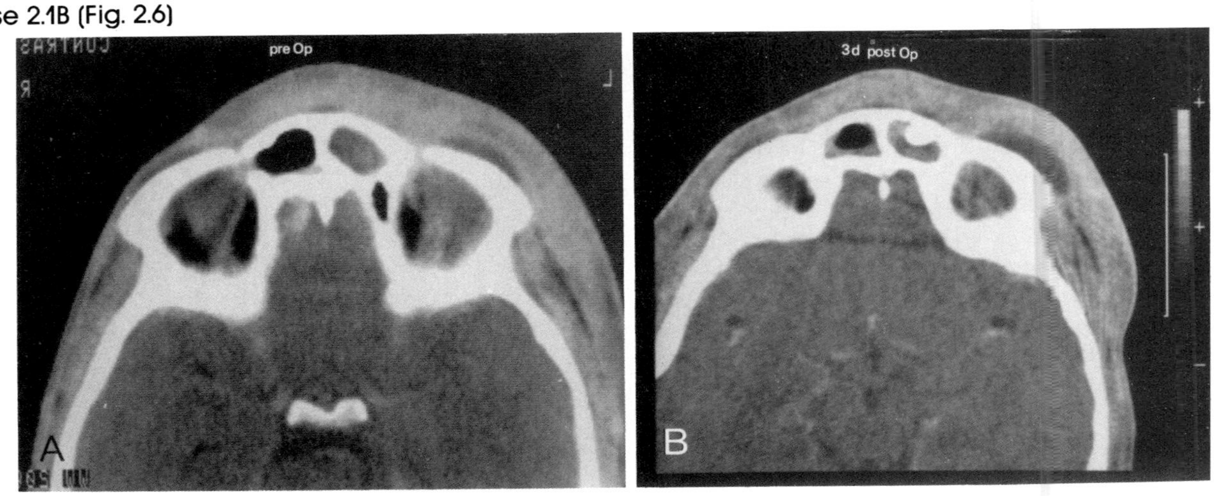

Figure 2.6*A* and *B*

Case 2.2 (Fig. 2.7)

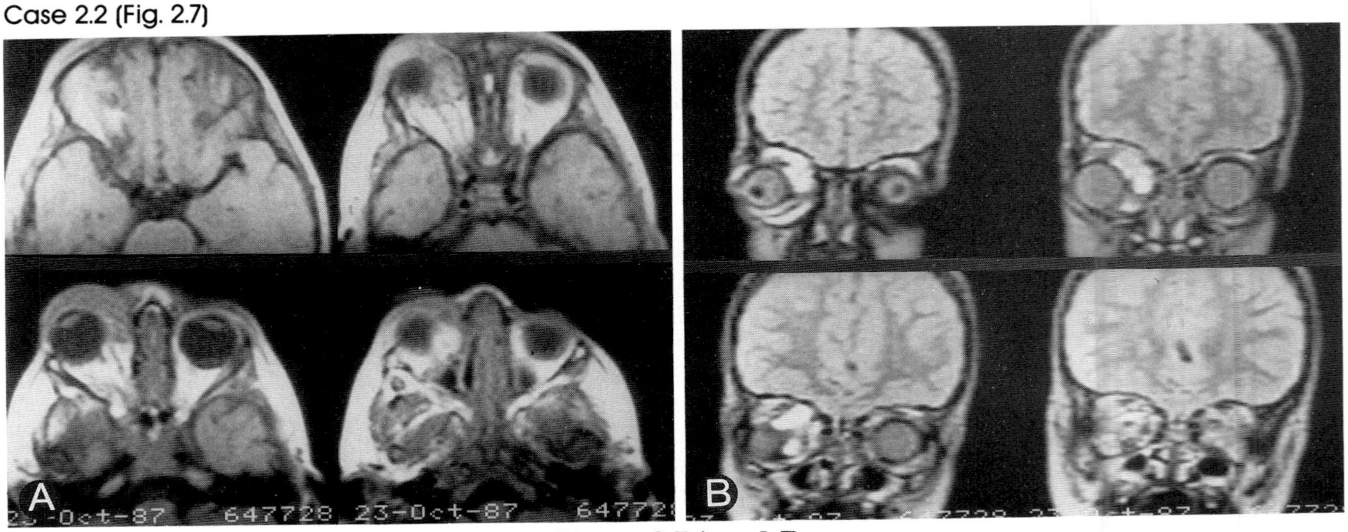

Figure 2.7*A* and *B*

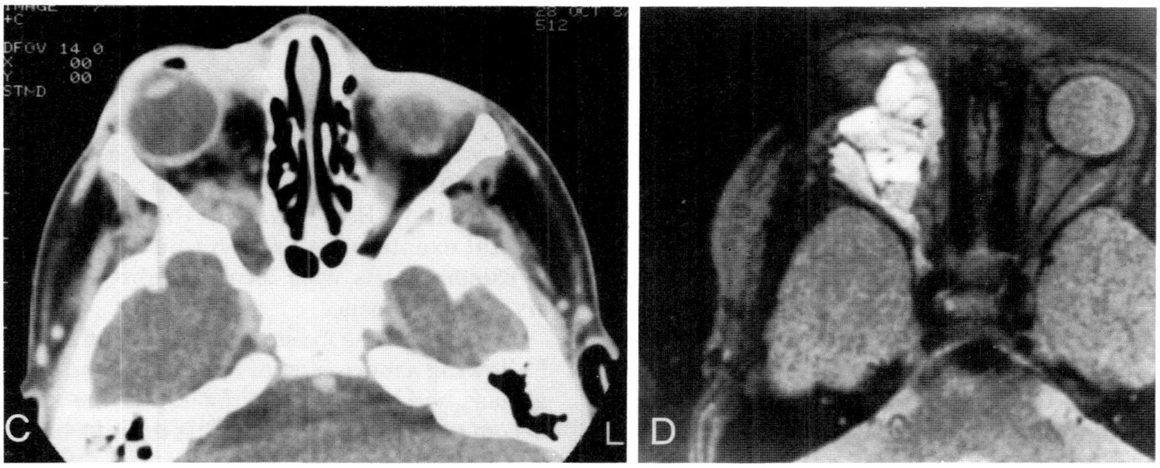

Figure 2.7*C* and *D*

Case Histories

Case 2.1A A 10-year-old male who presented with a temperature of 39°C and a swollen face.

Case 2.1B Eight-year-old male who did not respond to surgical drainage of ethmoids for orbital complications of sinus infection. *A*, initial study. *B*, 3 days after surgery and on antibiotics.

Case 2.2 An 8-year-old male with a 3-day history of fever and periorbital swelling not responding to oral antibiotics. *A*, SE 500/30. *B*, SE 2000/80. *C*, CT 5 days later. *D*, MRI of same lesion in a different patient (SE 2000/70).

Case 2.3 A 20-year-old nondiabetic male with prior history of orbital cellulitis secondary to aspergillosis. No history or lab findings indicative of immunosuppressive disease. He now has recurrent periorbital swelling. CT was done without contrast because of severe allergy. MRI was also done.

Questions

1. List your complete diagnosis for each case.
2. Is CT an accurate tool for distinguishing between preseptal orbital cellulitis and postseptal disease? Why did patient 1B not respond to surgery?
3. Is hemorrhage or cellulitis a frequent complication of the orbital pathology seen in Case 2.2?
4. Did MRI provide any additional benefit in Case 2.3?
5. List two reasons why CT might be better than MRI in evaluating orbital inflammatory disease.
6. Anatomic issue: What is the orbital septum?

Case 2.3 (Fig. 2.8)

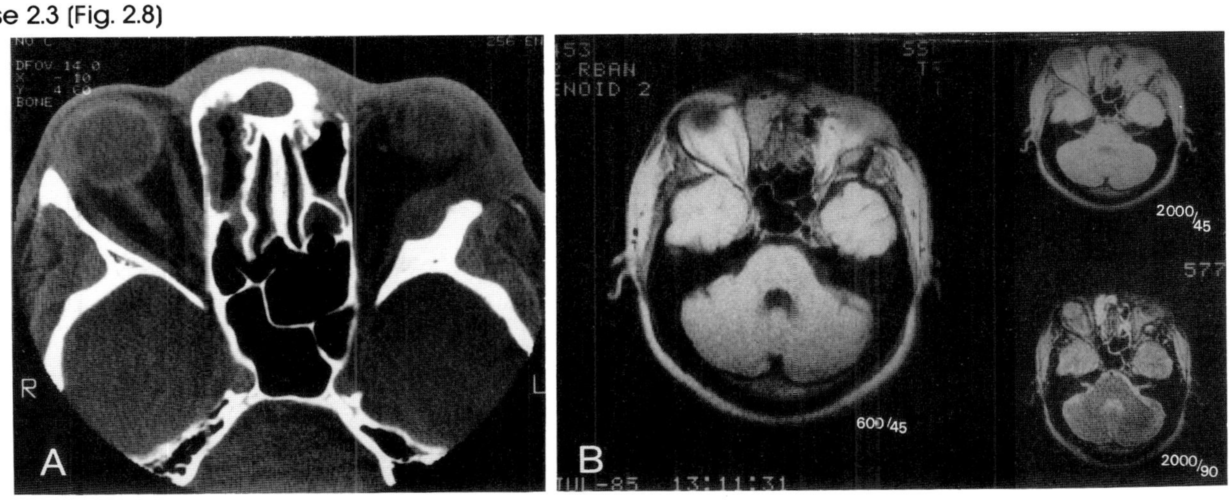

Figure 2.8*A* and *B*

Discussion

Problem I—Infiltrating, Possibly Inflammatory Orbital Masses Patient in Case 2.1A has bilateral preseptal orbital cellulitis complicated by a lid abscess on the left and postseptal subperiosteal orbital abscess

merely intensely inflamed tissues on MRI (Question 5). However, in Case 2.3, MRI data were quite helpful since they showed an area of discreet soft tissue swelling along the lateral wall to be a thick-walled, fluid-containing structure, in this instance strongly

Problem II

(Case histories and questions on page 52)

Case 2.4 (Fig. 2.9)

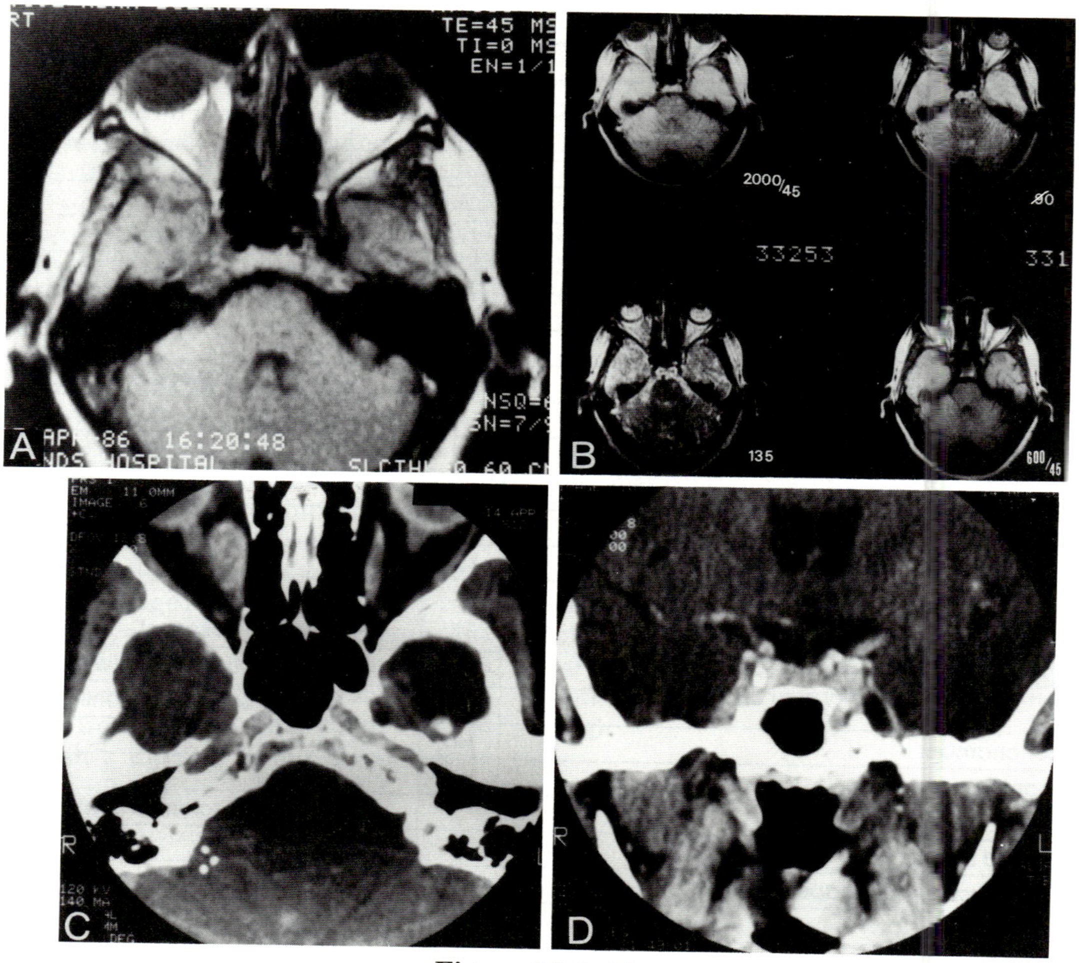

Figure 2.9*A–D*

Case 2.5 (Fig. 2.10)

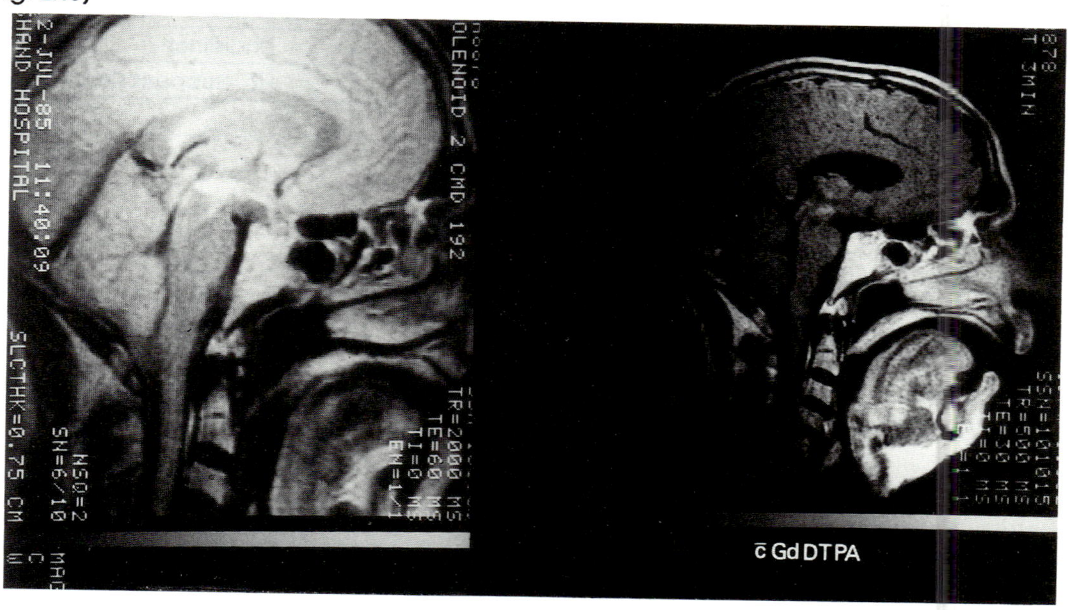

Figure 2.10

Case 2.6 (Fig. 2.11)

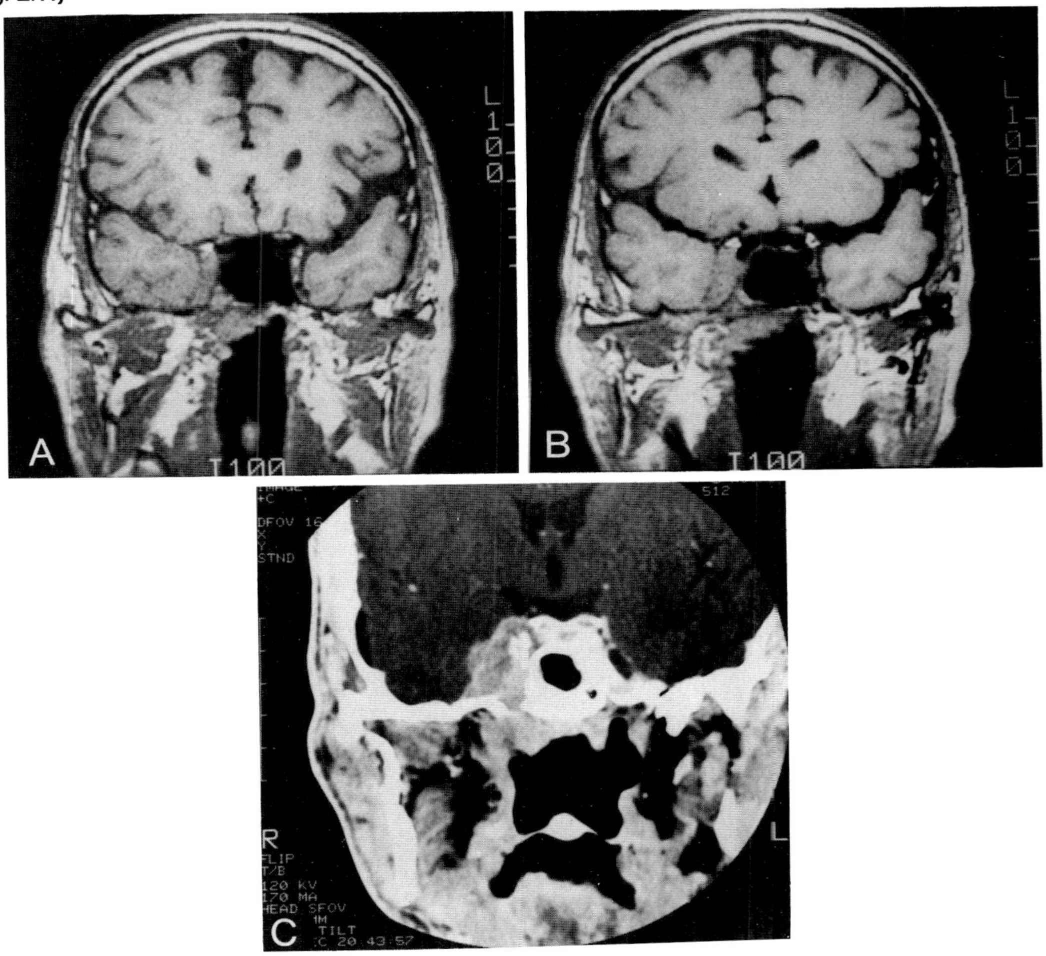

Figure 2.11*A–C*

Case Histories

Case 2.4 A 60-year-old female with a disorder of extraocular motility and right facial pain. Computed tomography and MRI were done.

Case 2.5 A 72-year-old male with intranuclear ophthalmoplegia. Spin echo 2000/60 and 500/30 (with Gd-DTPA) images in the midsagittal plane.

Case 2.6 A 50-year-old male with inability to abduct the right eye presented to our hospital with this MRI and a request for an angiogram to "evaluate meningioma of right cavernous sinus."

Questions

1. In two of these patients CT (Cases 2.4 and 2.5) preceded MRI imaging. Was this a reasonable course of action assuming equal access to CT and MRI?
2. If you had only one acquisition on each of these patients what would you do?
3. What is the most likely diagnosis in each case?
4. Give two reasons why MRI is better than CT for evaluating the optic pathways.
5. The chemical shift artifact makes evaluation of the optic sheath difficult at times. Would Gd-DTPA or a fat suppression pulse sequence be more helpful in solving this problem? Why?
6. Anatomic issue: Draw the approximate positions of the cranial nerves in the cavernous sinus as seen on a coronal section through its midportion.

Discussion

Problem II—Evaluation of the Visual Pathways The evaluation of the visual pathways falls clearly within the realm of MRI imaging. The CT studies done in two of these patients were informative and diagnostic but MRI could have been the first and only study for each (Question 1).

Question 2 brings up an interesting situation that one should always contemplate when doing MRI since there are times when patients, for one reason or another, will not cooperate for more than one acquisition. Its best to go for the most informative pulse sequence first. Case 2.4 is difficult because the lesion could be in the orbit, cavernous sinus, or brainstem. If Gd-DTPA were available the best choice might be a T_1-weighted pulse sequence with Gd-DTPA. This should be axial, high resolution, thin section, and encompass the orbit, cavernous sinus, midbrain, and pons. Without Gd-DTPA one must figure out a way to get both reasonable spatial resolution and enough T_2 weighting to see an intra-axial lesion. Any choice will be a compromise, but a dual echo spin density–T_2-weighted pair might be the best choice. The same reasoning could apply to Case 2.6. Case 2.5 is almost certainly due to an intra-axial lesion in the midbrain. A single echo moderately T_2-weighted, 5-mm axial section centered in the midbrain would be the best course of action.

Question 3 asks for specific diagnoses without much clinical data available. Perhaps this is unfair, but it is worth the exercise. Case 2.4 shows focal widening of the medial rectus muscle, obliteration of the cistern of the trigeminal ganglion–Meckel's cave, and infiltration of the petrous apex. The most likely etiology is metastatic disease. This patient was believed to have been disease free several years after treatment for ovarian cancer. With regard to Case 2.5, a 72-year-old man with intranuclear ophthalmoplegia is most likely to have had a brainstem ischemic event involving the medial longitudinal fasciculus. The patient's symptoms were of acute onset and this was the diagnosis. Note that the lesion enhances with Gd-DTPA. The patient in Case 2.6 had a VIth nerve palsy. Onset was subacute. Magnetic resonance imaging revealed a mass in the cavernous sinus but on initial interpretation the nasopharyngeal mass destroying the skull base was not noted, hence the referral to neurosurgery and request for angiography. Following review of the films at our institution, biopsy of the nasopharynx confirmed the diagnosis of carcinoma.

Question 4 is relatively straightforward, with sensitivity of MRI to intra-axial (especially brainstem) pathology as probably the leading reason for its superiority. Its multiplanar capability is very important for the evaluation of the optic nerve, chiasm, suprasellar cistern, and cavernous sinus. Question 5 highlights one limitation of MRI in the evaluation of the visual pathways: the chemical shift artifact that makes evaluation of the optic nerve/sheath precarious. On the surface Gd-DTPA would seem to be an answer, but realize that enhancement of a sheath lesion would tend to make it isointense with surrounding fat, potentially causing it to become less conspicuous. Fat suppression pulse techniques could eliminate the artifact and if used either alone or together with Gd-DTPA might produce excellent images of optic sheath pathology. Motion artifacts can further aggravate MRI imaging of subtle abnormalities of the nerve and orbit.

Anatomic Issue: Cavernous Sinus and Its Contents The coming of high-resolution CT brought with it the need for at least a rudimentary knowledge of the cavernous sinus anatomy. High-resolution MRI has made a detailed knowledge of this anatomy a requisite for those who wish to interpret these studies. To fully understand the cavernous sinus you should be able to draw it in the axial and coronal planes. Structures of main interest are the cistern of the trigeminal ganglion, the trigeminal ganglion itself, the three divisions of the trigeminal nerve and their exit foramina, and cranial nerves III, IV, and VI. The relationship of these structures to each other and the superior and inferior orbital fissures should be studied with checklists and MRI and CT images seen here and in Chapter 6. We are now far beyond the point where widening of the cavernous sinus is the only sure sign of involvement with pathology. Obliteration of the cistern of the trigeminal ganglion and even individual nerve enlargement can be signs of significant pathology. Recognition of such findings can make vast differences in patient management.

CHECKLIST—ORBIT (CASE 4)

	Seen	Nl	Abnl	Remarks
MID				
Orbital septum	√	√		
Preseptal soft tissues	√	√		
Globe	√	√		
Lens/anterior chamber	√	√		
Posterior chamber	√	√		
Intraconal fat	√	√		
Optic nerve and sheath	√	√		
Superior orbital fissure/orbital apex	√	√		
Cavernous sinus	√		√	Infiltrated
Sella and contents	√	√		
Medial rectus muscle	√		√	Focal thickening
Lateral rectus muscle	√	√		
Extraconal orbital fat	√	√		
Medial wall orbit/ethmoids	√	√		
Greater wing sphenoid	√	√		

CHECKLIST—VISUAL PATHWAYS BEYOND ORBITS (CASE 4)

	Seen	Nl	Abnl	Remarks
Optic nerve to optic canal	√	√		
Optic nerve in optic canal	No			
Optic chiasm	√	√		
Optic chiasm	No			
Optic tract	No			
Lateral geniculate body	No			
Optic radiations	No			
Visual cortex	No			
Cavernous sinus nerves (III, IV, VI)	√		√	Infiltrated
Quadrigeminal plate—tectum and pretectal regions	No			
Midbrain ventral to acqueduct	No			
Nucleus III	No			
Nucleus IV	No			
Median longitudinal fasiculus (MLF)	No			
Pontomedullary junction, floor 4th ventricle nucleus VI, lower MLF	√	√		

SUGGESTED READINGS

Books, Chapters, Reviews

Braffman BH, Zimmerman RA, Rabischong P: Cranial nerves III, IV, and VI: A clinical approach to the evaluation of their dysfunction. In Raymond HW, Zwiebel WJ (eds): *Seminars in Ultrasound, CT and MR*. New York, Grune & Stratton, 1987, vol 8, pp 185–213.

Bryan RN, Craig JA: CT of the orbit. In Bergeron RT, Osborn AG, Som PM: *Head and Neck Imaging—Excluding the Brain*. St. Louis, CV Mosby, 1984, Chap 14, Sect 1.

Daniels DL, Haughton VM: Magnetic resonance imaging of the sella and temporal bone. In Kressel HY (ed): *Magnetic Resonance Annual—1987*. New York, Raven Press, 1987, pp 1–47.

Hershey BL, Peyester RG: Imaging of the cranial nerve II. In Raymond HW, Zwiebel WJ (eds): *Seminars in Ultrasound, CT and MR*. New York, Grune & Stratton, 1987, vol 8, pp 164–184.

Mancuso AA, Hanafee WN: *Computed Tomography and Magnetic Resonance Imaging of the Head and Neck*. Baltimore, Williams & Wilkins, 1985.

Articles

Atlas SW, Bilaniuk LT, Zimmerman RA, et al: Orbit: initial experience with surface coil spin-echo MR imaging at 1.5 T. *Radiology* 164:501–509, 1987.

Atlas SW, Grossman RI, Axel L, et al: Orbital lesions: proton spectroscopic phase-dependent contrast MR imaging. *Radiology* 164:510–514, 1987.

Citrin CM: High resolution orbital computed tomography. *J Comput Assist Tomogr* 10(5):810–816, 1986.

Kwan ES, Laucella M, Hedges TR III, Wolpert SM: A cliniconeuroradiologic approach to third cranial nerve palsies. *AJNR* 8:459–468, 1987.

Mafee MF, Peyman GA, Grisolano JE, et al: Ocular MR imaging and spectroscopy: an ex vivo study. *Radiology* 160:201–205, 1986.

Sherman JL, Citrin CM, Barkovich, Bowen BJ: MR imaging of the mesencephalic tectum: normal and pathologic variations. *AJNR* 8:59–64, 1987.

Spires JR, Smith RJ: Bacterial infections of the orbital and periorbital soft tissues in children. *Laryngoscope* 96:763–767, 1986.

Towbin R, Han BK, Kaufman RA, et al: Postspetal cellulitis: CT in diagnosis and management. *Radiology* 158:735–737, 1986.

3

Paranasal Sinuses, Nasal Cavity, and Facial Bones

INDICATIONS

Tomographic study of the paranasal sinuses is probably the most common examination of the head and neck region done in a general radiology practice. Sinus disease is ubiquitous and the most difficult triage decision is when to move from standard plain films to the far more costly CT or MRI. Conventional pluridirectional tomography is still a reasonable alternative in benign disease if CT is not available; linear tomography really is not an alternative unless there is absolutely nothing else available within referral distance. The decision to go beyond plain films should be as rational as possible, but there is no question that some unnecessary CT, MRI, or pluridirectional tomographic studies will be done if one is to pick up more aggressive pathology when it is treatable with as little morbidity as possible. We do not believe that people should be "screened" with CT or MRI. Indications where one typically goes beyond plain films are listed in Table 3.1. More judgment is required in the following clinical situations:

1. Persistent pain in patient with chronic sinusitis.
2. Unilateral or otherwise isolated sinus disease unresponsive to medical therapy.
3. For planning endoscopic surgery on the ostiomeatal complex.
4. Any evidence of bone destruction or expansion on plain films or clinically (e.g., loose teeth without obvious dental disease).
5. Clinical signs/symptoms suggesting central nervous system (CNS) or orbital involvement.
6. Progressive atypical facial pain, especially if in the distribution of V_2.
7. Persistent headaches in patient with chronic allergy history, especially if headaches are retro-orbital or referred to the vertex (i.e., sphenoid sinus headache).

The multiplanar capability of MRI is very useful in the sinuses and nasal cavity, and its extraordinary capacity for contrast resolution frequently allows one to distinguish between obstructive/inflammatory opacification of a sinus and other pathologies. Modern I.V. contrast-enhanced CT, however, is quite good at the latter task and direct coronal sections often suffice for study in more than one plane. The lack of true bone detail, relative insensitivity to calcifications, and sometimes less obvious demonstration of a vascular mass on MRI lead us to choose CT as a starting point for most sinus disease. We have observed that MRI is more liable to error in both execution of the study and interpretation when used to evaluate general sinus disease. This is probably because of a combination of the complexity of the exam as well as inexperienced observers and may improve with time. Although this latter point is not a particularly objective criterion it has lent support to our policy of starting with CT under many circumstances Moreover, a low-cost, limited CT study done in the coronal plane may be used in selected patients. Magnetic resonance imaging is a highly valued adjunct in known cancer, selected benign-appearing masses, and when supplementary sagittal or coronal images are necessary. It is frequently useful after a diagnosis has been established; it can be used to follow known benign disease (e.g., fibrous dysplasia) or disease under therapy (e.g., cancer, juvenile angiofibroma). It is always used when the relationship of pathology to the orbit, intracranial structures, or skull base is uncertain on CT. Computed tomography is a clear first choice whenever bone detail is essential, for example, in trauma and craniofacial dysplasias.

Table 3.1
Indications for CT/MRI Facial and Sinonasal Region

Indication
Congenital malformations
Preoperative planning (CT, 3D if available)
Choanal atresia (CT)
Related meningoencephaloceles (MRI/CT)[a]
Fibrous and other dysplasias (CT/MRI)
Inflammatory disease
Preoperative planning endoscopic microsurgery (CT)
Local complications—polyps, mucocele/pyocele, impactions (CT)
Regional complications
orbital cellulitis abscesses (CT)
osteomyelitis (CT)
subdural/epidural empyema, venous sinus thrombosis (CT/MRI)
Rhinocerebral mucormycosis (CT)
Necrotizing granulomatoses (e.g., Wegener's) (CT)
Benign masses and neoplasms (CT/MRI)
Malignant tumors (CT/MRI)
Trauma (CT)
Acute—complex injury, ? inner table frontal sinus fracture, etc.
Preoperative planning of reconstructive surgery (3D selected cases)

[a]Where both studies may contribute unique data the usual beginning study is listed first.

TECHNIQUE

Specific CT protocols are presented by indication in Table 3.2. The study should be focused on a particular portion of the sinuses whenever possible. For example, complete study of the frontal sinus is often unnecessary, and supplemental coronals may often be done through a very limited region of interest. Three-millimeter-thick sections are standard, although in a "survey" situation they may be done at 5-mm increments and only in the coronal plane. Raw data will frequently be processed in bone and soft tissue algorithms; both bone and soft tissue window must always be recorded. Whether to use intravenous contrast is decided on a case-by-case basis. Since the value of contrast is not predictable in many cases we tend to avoid its use in potentially sensitive individuals. There is an increased tendency for patients with chronic sinus disease to have an "allergic" history, making sensitivity to iodinated contrast more likely. A sometimes useful strategy is to do axials without contrast and proceed to coronals with contrast if it seems that this would yield significant data. The only firm guidelines here are that contrast should be used in complex inflammatory disease and mass lesions (cancer and benign) but is not necessary in trauma and other circumstances when only study of the facial and other bones is required.

Magnetic resonance imaging studies of the paranasal sinuses and nasal cavity may be done with standard head coils or more localized volume receiver coils; the latter must allow for complete visualization of the sinuses, orbits, and nearby brain. Surface coils (i.e., flat receiver coils) are inappropriate in all except the most unique circumstances. Potentially interfering eye makeup and mobile dental work should be removed. The head should be positioned so that the IOML is perpendicular to the table top. A specific plane can be chosen following a preliminary "quick view" when necessary. Standard 2DFT, Rf-refocused, spin echo pulse sequences are used. Three-dimensional Fourier transform may be useful where 2- to 3-mm contiguous sections are desired, but these may be degraded by eye, jaw, and minor head motion. Gradient echo pulse sequences are likely to suffer degradation as a result of inhomogeneity at air-bone interfaces as well as dental fillings and hardware. Gadolinium-DTPA will probably only be used in highly selected cases (e.g., meningioma, early extradural versus intradural spread of tumor). Other basic technical factors are as follows:

FOV: 18 to 24 cm
SLT: 5 mm (occasionally 3 mm in selected region of interest)
Acquisition matrix: 160 to 192 × 256 or 256 × 256
General exam sinuses:
- Acquisition 1: Axial or coronal* single echo 500 to 700/20 to 30
- Acquisition 2: Axial or coronal* dual echo 2000/30 to 100†
- Acquisition 3: Opposite plane of section from 1 and 2 or sagittal, single echo, with most appropriate pulse sequence as judged from 1 and 2
- Acquisition 4: Optional—third plane, off-axis, concentrated 3-mm sections, gradient echo

---

*Choice of plane depends on clinical data and CT findings.
†TE range allows for selection of spin density—T_2-weighted or "mixed" and T_2-weighted pair as desired.

Case 3.4 (Fig. 3.8)

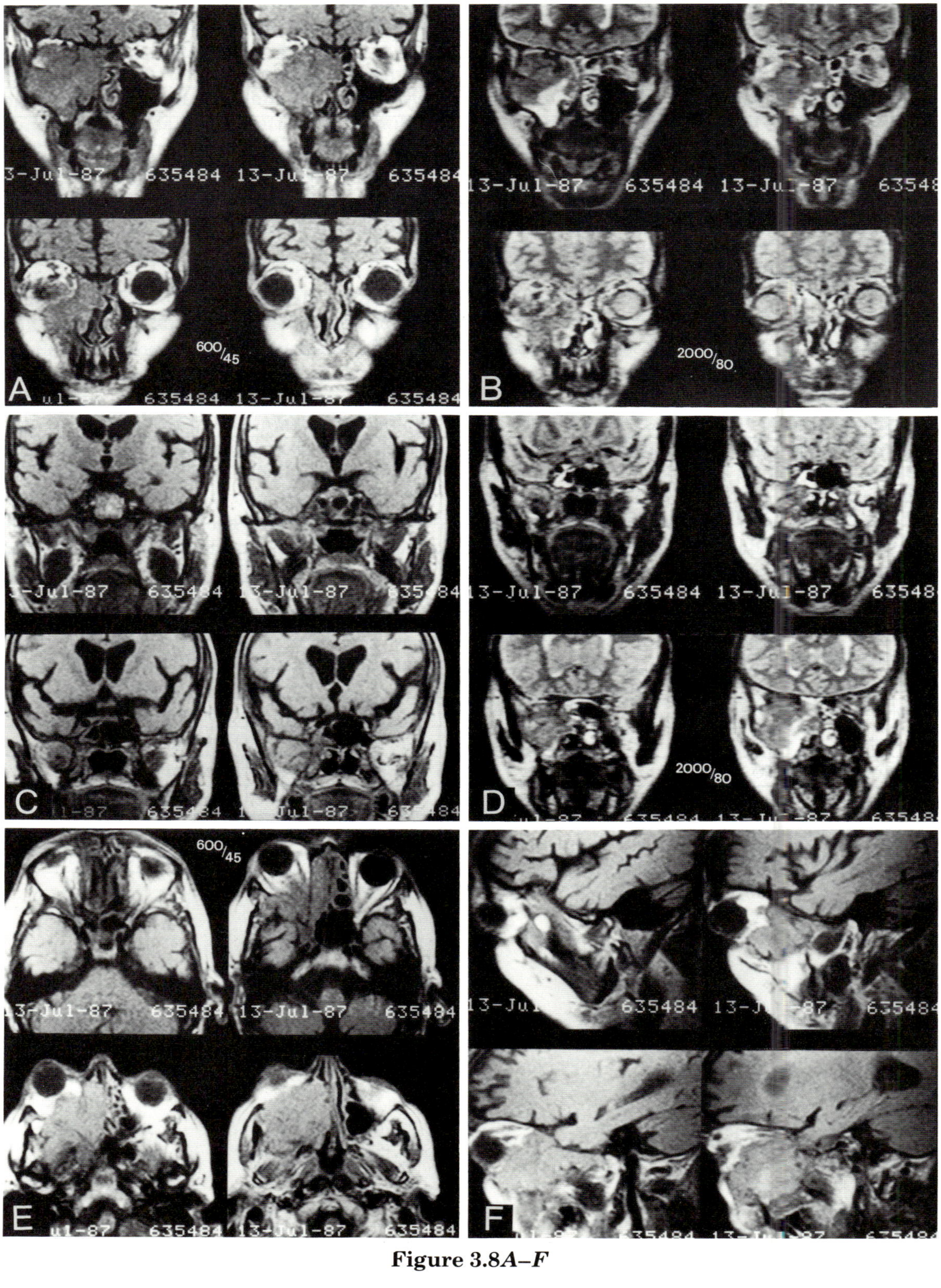

Figure 3.8*A–F*

Case 3.5 (Fig. 3.9)

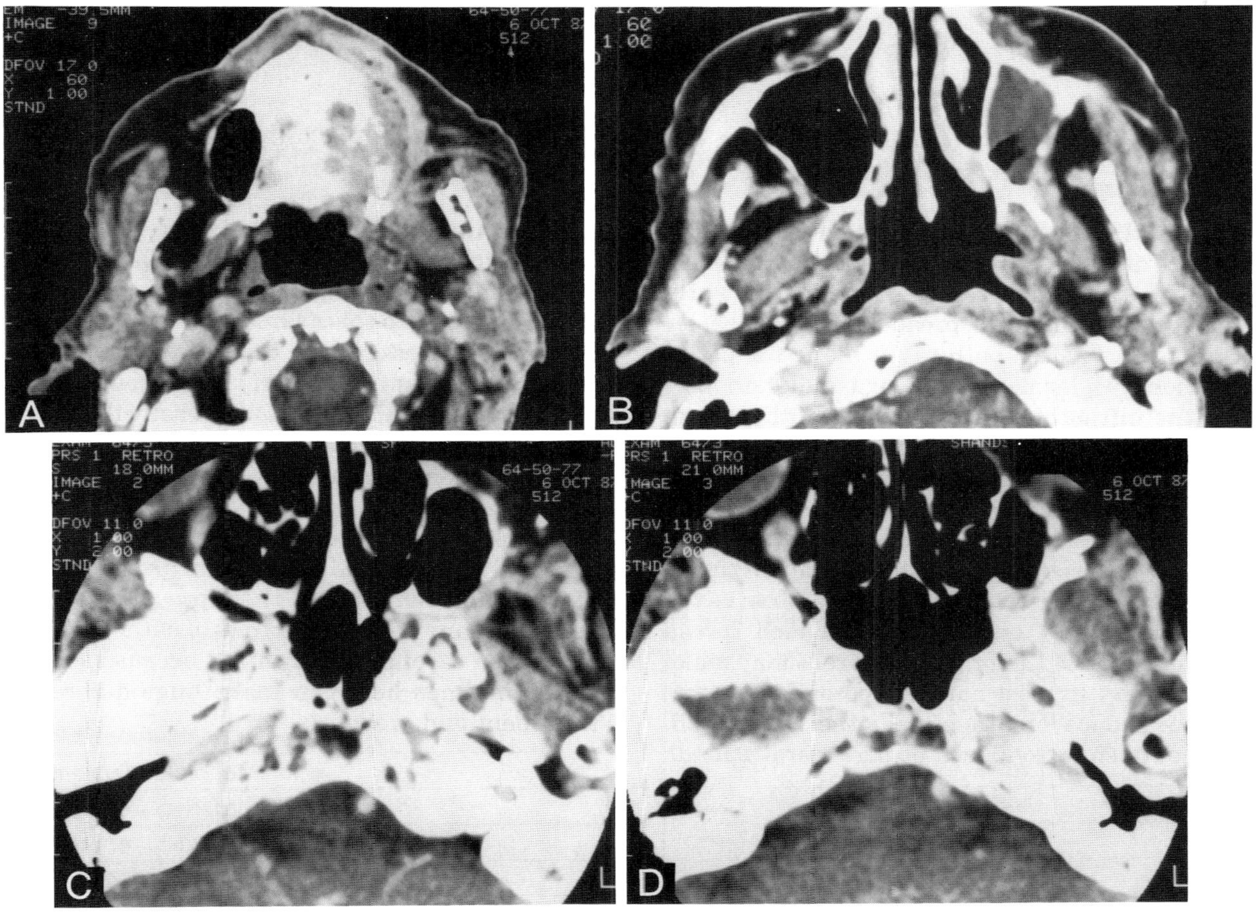

Figure 3.9*A–D*

Case Histories

Case 3.4 A 70-year-old male with carcinoma of the maxillary antrum.

Case 3.5 A 65-year-old female with carcinoma of the hard palate and inferior portion of the maxillary antrum.

Questions

1. Name four key regions of interest that must be evaluated in patients with sinonasal malignancy (i.e., those that are likely to alter treatment plan and related morbidity as well as prognosis).
2. Name two modes of intracranial spread that occur in sinonasal malignancies.
3. Does either of these patients have evidence of perineural spread of tumor? Name two neurovascular bundles along which sinonasal cancer spreads. What tumor often has perineural spread at initial presentation?
4. Anatomic issue: Describe the anatomy of the pterygopalatine fossa. What structures or spaces lead to it?

Discussion

Problem 2—Evaluation of Sinonasal Malignancies Patients with sinonasal malignancy must have a very highly detailed imaging evaluation of the site of origin of the lesion. Spread to the orbit, nasopharynx, infratemporal fossa, or intracranially *must* be documented or excluded to ensure proper treatment planning (Question 1).

Patient 4 showed spread to the cavernous sinus via the infraorbital nerve, inferior orbital fissure, and pterygopalatine fossa. Patient 5 showed spread via the greater and lesser palatine foramina and posterior superior alveolar neurovascular bundle to the pterygopalatine fossa (Question 3). Perineural spread can occur with any lesion but it is most common in adenocystic carcinoma. Recurrent carcinoma, sar-

CHECKLIST—PARANASAL SINUSES, NASAL CAVITY, FACIAL BONES (CASE 3.4) *(continued)*

	Seen	Nl	Abnl	Remarks
LOWER				
Soft tissue of face (fat, muscles)	√	√		
Nasal bones	√	√		
Nasolacrimal canal			√	Invaded by tumor
Nasal septum			√	Upper possibly involved by tumor
Middle meatus (lower)			√	Involved by tumor
Inferior meatus			√	Upper involved by tumor
Inferior concha/turbinate			√	Upper abnormal
Maxillary sinus (contents, walls)			√	Tumor and obstruction
Groove for posterior superior alveolar neurovascular bundle			√	Involved
Posterior choanae			√	Tumor on right
Nasopharynx (NP checklist as needed)			√	Early involvement on right
Clivus	√	√		
Sphenopalatine foramen			√	Filled with tumor
Pterygopalatine fossa			√	Filled with tumor
Pterygoid plates			√	Eroded
Infratemporal fossa (retroantral fat)			√	Invaded
Distal maxillary neurovascular bundle			√	Involved by tumor
Hard palate (greater and lesser palatine foramina)	√	√		
Maxillary alveolar ridge	√	√		
Maxillary (anterior nasal) spine				
Maxillary tuberosity				
Buccinator muscle				
Buccinator space				
Zygomatic arch	√	√		
Mandible				

Problem III

(Case histories and questions on p. 74)

Case 3.6 (Fig. 3.10)

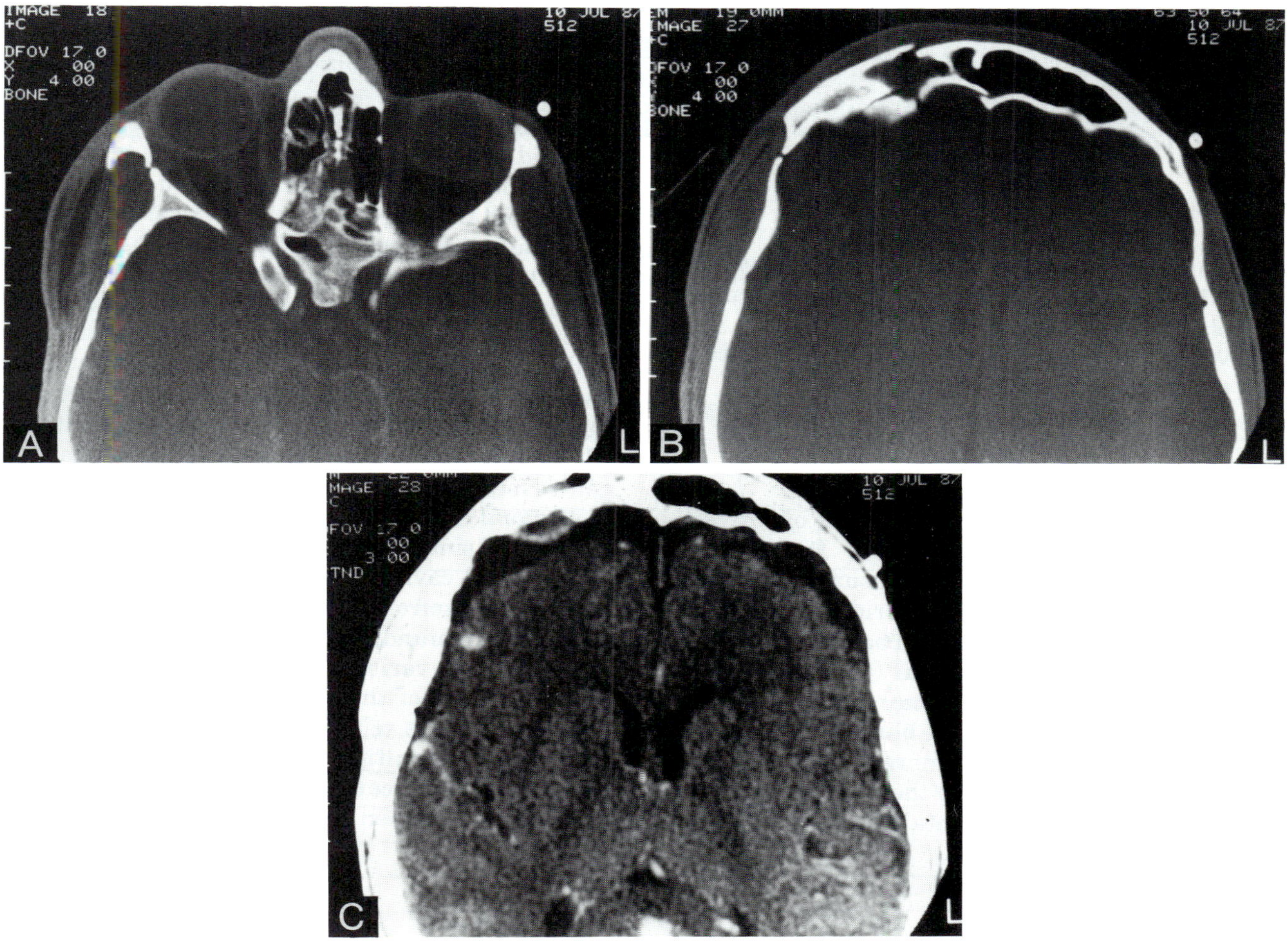

Figure 3.10*A–C*

Case 3.7 (Fig. 3.11)

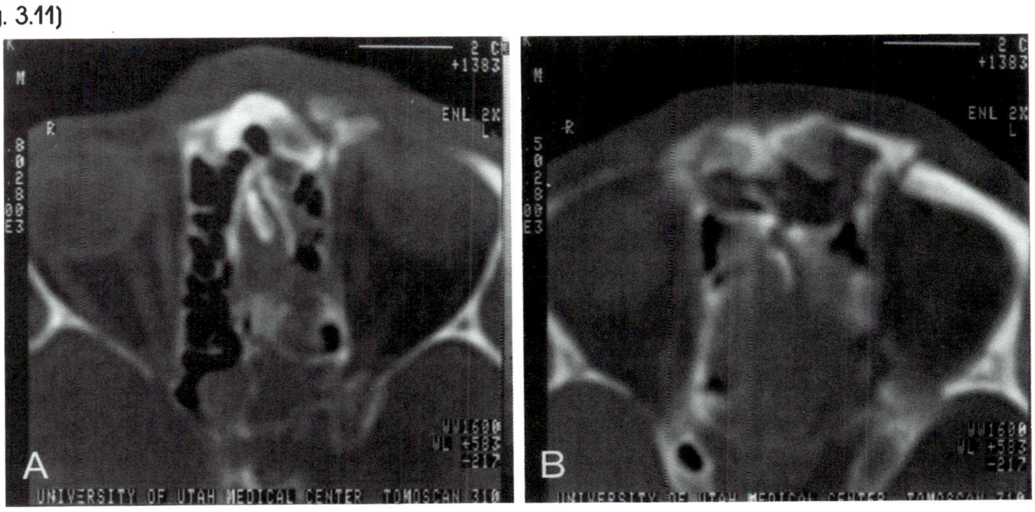

Figure 3.11*A* and *B*

Case Histories

Case 3.6 Patient sustained facial and head injuries in a motor vehicle accident. The initial CT done to evaluate the brain showed no brain injury but there was subtle evidence of facial fractures. This repeat exam was done.

Case 3.7 Another patient suffering facial injury

duct can lead to frontal mucocele as a delayed complication. Such injuries may also herald delayed CSF rhinorrhea, and if the cribriform plate is obviously injured patients may be started on antibiotics even in the absence of clinical evidence of CSF rhinorrhea.

Patient 6 has an orbital frontal fracture (Question 1). Pneumocephalus was present (on films not shown), indicating that the fracture involved a sinus (or the

SUGGESTED READINGS

Books, Chapters, Reviews

Mancuso AA, Hanafee WN: *Computed Tomography and Magnetic Resonance Imaging of the Head and Neck*. Baltimore, Williams & Wilkins, 1985.

Osborn AG: The nose. In Bergeron RT, Osborn AG, Som PM (eds): *Head and Neck Imaging—Excluding the Brain* St. Louis, CV Mosby, 1984, pp 143–172.

Osborn AG: The pterygopalatine (sphenomaxillary) fossa. In Bergeron RT, Osborn AG, Som PM (eds): *Head and Neck Imaging—Excluding the Brain*. St. Louis, CV Mosby, 1984, pp 172–185.

Som PM: The paranasal sinuses. In Bergeron RT, Osborn AG, Som PM (eds): *Head and Neck Imaging—Excluding the Brain*. St. Louis, CV Mosby, 1984, pp 1–142.

Articles

Paling MR, Black WC, Levine PA, Cantrell RW: Tumor invasion of the anterior skull base: a comparison of MR and CT studies. *J Comput Assist Tomogr* 164:811–816, 1987.

On allergic aspergillosis of the sinuses:

Kopp W, Fotter F, Steiner H: Aspergillosis of the paranasal sinuses. *Radiology* 156:715–716, 1985.

On endoscopic nasal surgery:

Kennedy DW, Zinreich ST, Rosenbaum AE: Functional endoscopic sinus surgery. *Arch Otolaryngol* 111:576–582, 1985.

Stammberger H: Endoscopic endonasal surgery—concepts in treatment of recurring rhinosinusitis. *Otolaryngol—Head Neck Surg* 94:143–155, 1986.

Teatini G, Simonetti G, Salvolini V, et al: Computed tomography of the ethmoid labyrinth and adjacent structures. *Ann Otol Rhinol Laryngol* 96:239–249, 1987.

Terrier F, Weber W, Ruefenacht D, et al: Anatomy of the ethmoid. *AJR* 144:493–500, 1985.

Zinreich SJ, Kennedy DW, Rosenbaum AE: Paranasal sinuses: CT imaging requirements for endoscopic surgery. *Radiology* 163:769–755, 1987.

On esthesioneuroblastoma:

Levine PA, McClean WC, Cantrell RW: Esthesioneuroblastoma: the University of Virginia experience 1960–1985. *Laryngoscope* 96:742–746, 1986.

On orbital frontal and frontoethmoid fractures.

Denneny JC, Davidson WD: Combined otolaryngological and neurosurgical approach in treating sinus factures. *Laryngoscope* 97:633–637, 1987.

Duvall AJ, Porto DP, Lynos D, et al: Frontal sinus fractures analysis of treatment results. *Arch Otolaryngol Head Neck Surg* 113:933–935, 1987.

Guyon JJ, Brant-Zawadzki, Seiff SR: CT demonstration of optic canal fractures. *AJR* 143:1031–1034, 1984.

Harris L, Marano GD, McCorkle D: Nasofrontal dust: CT in frontal sinus trauma. *Radiology* 165:195–198, 1987.

Levine SB, Rowe LD, Keane WM, et al: Evaluation and treatment of frontal sinus fractures. *Otolaryngol Head Neck Surg* 95:19–22, 1986.

Lipkin AF, Woodson GF, Miller HL: Visual loss due to orbital fracture. *Arch Otolaryngol Head Neck Surg* 113:81–83, 1987.

Weymuller EA: Blindness and LeFort III fractures. *Ann Otol Rhinol Laryngol* 93:2–5, 1984.

4

Parotid and Submandibular Glands

INDICATIONS

Diffuse inflammatory disease or autoimmune disease of the parotid gland and submandibular glands is best studied by conventional sialography. Acute, possibly suppurative sialadenitis is, however, an absolute contraindication to conventional sialography. If an abscess, stones, or major duct obstruction must be excluded in an acutely inflamed gland then contrast-enhanced CT should be done (Table 4.1). Oily contrast should not be used for conventional sialography. CT scanning combined with opacification of the gland via parotid duct injection (so-called CT sialography) is no longer done; this technique was largely abandoned in 1981–1982.

Parotid region masses may be evaluated by CT or MRI. Suggested triage to different imaging modalities is outlined in Table 4.1. In our hands CT is an all-around better study but MRI can be used in many patients without the small risks due to iodinated contrast use and with potentially better contrast resolution. Magnetic resonance imaging fails to detect stones or ductal ectasia and may not give as clear an indication of the inflammatory nature of a mass or aggressiveness at its margins. Magnetic resonance imaging and CT are nonspecific histologically (except for lipomas); parotid mass lesions always require very careful cytologic-histologic evaluation. This may be done via fine-needle aspiration (FNA) biopsy before imaging; however, at the University of Florida clinical data combined with imaging (CT/MRI) has been found to be more effective in evaluating parotid region masses than routine needle biopsy, since the imaging findings are more likely to alter therapy (Table 4.2). Needle biopsy is used only when its results are likely to change management. The decision to do FNA biopsy may be based on clinical and/or imaging findings (Table 4.2). Successful FNA biopsy requires an aggressive, experienced cytopathology department as much as effective imaging of the parotid region requires detailed knowledge of the referring physician's needs in managing such patients.

In parotid region masses the basic goals of the imager are to:

1. Determine whether the "mass" is intrinsic or extrinsic to the parotid gland.
2. Define the location of the facial nerve with respect to the mass. (The evaluation of patients with facial nerve dysfunction is discussed in Chapter 5 and evaluation of the parotid is certainly an important part of that study in many cases.)
3. Decide whether the mass is aggressive or nonaggressive.

The intrinsic versus extrinsic issue is usually a simple one, but it has the greatest potential to alter management in many cases of parotid region masses. Differential diagnosis of parotid region masses is presented in Table 4.3. With good technique and interpretive skills one can now define the relationship of intrinsic (and extrinsic) masses to the major divisions of the facial nerve as well as the main trunk even though the nerves themselves are not routinely visible. Aggressive versus nonaggressive differentiation depends on the margin of a mass, invasion of surrounding structures, and presence of CT/MRI-positive lymph nodes. Aggressive morphology is usually associated with inflammatory lesions and malignancies or a combination of the two; however, benign neoplasms may have aggressive margins and malignancies may appear smoothly marginated. Magnetic resonance imaging sometimes renders a less graphic picture of an aggressive margin than contrast-enhanced CT, but the better contrast resolution of MRI at lesion-muscle interfaces sometimes proves important. Neither MRI nor CT is tissue specific. Imaging should be used mainly to *avoid* "lumpectomy" in parotid lesions and to help protect the facial nerve. One must constantly be reminded that a biopsy of the parotid gland *is* a superficial parotidectomy or at minimum a resection of the mass with a wide cuff of normal parotid tissue. Dissemination of disease will frequently follow removal of benign or malignant parotid lesions if an adequate margin of normal parotid tissue has not been taken. This is a highly unfavorable result that can eventually lead to needless loss of facial nerve function or failure to cure a malignancy.

The submandibular region is usually studied for a mass lesion arising either within or extrinsic to the submandibular gland (Table 4.4). Once the location of the mass has been determined, its aggressive or nonaggressive nature can be evaluated by the same criteria as those outlined for parotid region masses. Of course the facial nerve is not at risk, but the relationship of the mass to the lingual nerve, mandible, and floor of the mouth can be defined. Such data may alter management decisions and help anticipate extent of functional loss to be expected in patients when surgery is indicated. Differential diagnosis of a mass in this region is fairly broad once a lymph node or submandibular gland origin have been

Table 4.1
Parotid Abnormalities—Imaging following Clinical Triage

- Rule out ductal pathology, confirm Sjögren's, Mikulicz' syndromes
  - Routine sialography with nonionic ionic, iso-osmolar contrast. *Do not* do this study during acute episode of sialadenitis. *Do not* use oil-base contrast for this exam.
- Diffuse, acute inflammatory process; rule out abcess, stones, gross ductal disease
  - CT with I.V. contrast[a]
- Mass ? etiology and extent with possible inflammatory component in history; i.e., if presence of stones, dilated ducts, or calcification would help in diff. diagnosis
  - CT with I.V. contrast[a]
- Mass ? etiology and extent, *no* inflammatory component in history
  - MRI or CT
    - All information necessary for disposition from one study (CT or MRI)
      - Any other appropriate workup
        - Disposition
    - Supplemental information necessary from alternative study (CT or MRI)
      - Do alternative study → Any other appropriate workup

[a]*Note:* CT-assisted sialography (i.e., contrast injected into the parotid duct) is no longer done for mass lesions and is contraindicated in an acutely inflamed salivary gland.

Table 4.2
Parotid Masses—Integrated Evaluation with FNA Biopsy and Imaging

Parotid region mass

- 1) Obviously superficial or in tail of gland region 2) Facial nerve not at risk 3) Deep margin obvious on PE 4) Nonpulsatile
  - Suspect node
    - or → FNA biopsy
    - Observe
  - Suspect intrinsic lesion
    - or → FNA biopsy
    - Remove with wide margin of normal parotid ("superficial" parotidectomy)
  - FNA biopsy
    - Disposition
      - → Observe
        - Final disposition based on clinical situation and resolution/nonresolution
      - → Remove with wide margin of normal parotid ("superficial" parotidectomy)
        - Final disposition based on histopathology
- 1) High in or around gland 2) Facial nerve at risk 3) Deep margin uncertain on PE 4) Pulsatile
  - CT or MRI[a]
    - Intrinsic nonaggressive, superficial to facial nerve
      - → Remove with wide margin of normal parotid ("superficial" parotidectomy)
    - Intrinsic aggressive and/or deep
      - FNA biopsy
        - Disposition
    - Extrinsic
      - Further imaging, angiography and biopsy as needed
        - Disposition

[a]See algorithm in Table 4.1

excluded. Computed tomography and MRI can aid tremendously in anticipating the etiology of the mass prior to the usual surgical resection.

TECHNIQUE

Specific CT protocols for both the parotid and submandibular regions are presented in Table 4.5. Since masses in these regions frequently turn out to be from extraglandular sources (e.g., parapharyngeal space, neck, floor of the mouth) other protocols should be consulted as soon as this becomes apparent so that all pertinent data are gathered without having to return the patient for additional examinations. Patients being evaluated for facial nerve dysfunction of uncertain etiology are best handled by algorithms suggested in Chapter 5.

Study of the parotid gland does not require routine evaluation of all cervical nodes, and the usual extent of the examination (zygoma to hyoid) will cover primary drainage sites. The gantry should be kept parallel to the IOML and changed only to avoid fillings. A study of the parotid need never be significantly degraded by fillings if done on units with 20° or more of gantry tilt. Maintaining at least the more cephalad sections parallel to the IOML will ensure that surgical landmarks for the facial nerve are not artificially distorted. Sections should always be a maximum of 3 to 4 mm thick. In patients with an inflammatory component in the history a set of 3 mm thick by 5 mm increment sections may be done without contrast before proceeding to a postcontrast contiguous 3-mm slice technique. This may also be done in mass lesions but is probably not worth the effort in an overwhelming majority of cases. Coronal sections may occasionally be useful for evaluating the undersurface of the temporal bone and descending facial canal, but axials almost always suffice. Raw data should be saved and reprocessed for bone detail whenever subtle bone destruction is questioned.

The submandibular region should be studied with the gantry angled along the inferior margin of the body of the mandible. This will help orient sections relative to the mylohyoid muscle. The mylohyoid is a major anatomic landmark in the region and separates the floor of the mouth from the neck. Coronal sections can be used to further define pathology relative to the mylohyoid when axial sections are inconclusive. Contiguous 3- to 4-mm sections and contrast are always used. Raw data are reprocessed in bone algorithms as necessary, usually for questions of sub-

Table 4.3
Differential Diagnosis of Parotid Region Masses

Parotid origin
- Congenital—first branchial cleft cyst, lymphangioma, hemangioma
- Inflammatory—cellulitis, abscess, acquired inflammatory cyst, autoimmune, viral, sarcoid, benign lymphoepithelial proliferation
- Benign tumor—benign mixed, Warthin, oncocytoma, lipoma, adenoma
- Malignant tumor—carinoma, including mucoepidermoid, adeno, adenoidcystic, acinous, squamous cell (primary and nodal metastases), ex pleomorphica, undifferentiated, lymphoma, oncocytic

Nonparotid origin
- Lymph nodes—reactive, metastatic (skin, cancer most common), melanoma, tuberculosis
- Masseter muscle—hypertrophy, neoplasm
- Mandible—benign and malignant tumors
- Masticator space—dental abscess, cellulitis, tumors
- Parapharyngeal space—neural origin tumors, paraganglioma, benign mixed tumor, lipoma, rhabdomyosarcoma, other mesenchymal origins, abscess, second branchial cleft cyst
- Pharynx—direct spread of carcinoma (rare presentation)
- Upper cervical spine—benign, malignant (metastases) neoplasms
- Upper neck—lymphangioma (cystic hygroma), hemangioma, lipoma (extraparotid)
- Facial nerve—neural origin, perineural spread of nonparotid malignancy

Table 4.4
Differential Diagnosis of Submandibular Region Masses

Submandibular gland origin
- Congenital—cysts
- Inflammatory—cellulitis, abscess, mucocele, giant stone
- Benign tumor—benign mixed, others rare
- Malignant tumor—carcinomas, including mucoepidermoid, adeno, adenoidcystic, undifferentiated, ex pleomorphica, invasion by extranodal spread of squamous cell carcinoma to submandibular node

Non–submandibular gland origin
- Neck and face (congenital)—second branchial cleft cyst, lymphangioma (cystic hygroma), hemangioma, dermoid, epidermoid, teratoma
- Lymph node—reactive, metastatic, lymphoma
- Mandible (masticator space)—abscesses, benign and malignant tumors
- Floor of mouth—congenital (see above), neural origin tumors, abscess, cellulitis, ranula (plunging or diving), minor salivary gland tumors (benign and malignant), carcinoma
- Parotid region—mass in parotid tail mimicking submandibular gland origin, extraparotid Warthin tumor

tle mandibular destruction. The lingual plate of the mandible is easy to evaluate, whereas subtle bone destruction along the undersurface of the mandibular body is difficult to detect on axial CT or MRI; coronals may prove useful in this situation.

Magnetic resonance imaging studies of the submandibular region are frequently degraded by jaw motion and swallowing. Physical attempts at immobilization frequently worsen the situation and may aggravate marginal claustrophobia. Still MRI studies can prove highly informative even when slightly to mildly degraded by motion. In the parotid region motion artifact poses little or no problem in the upper two-thirds of the gland. Sections through the tail occasionally suffer losses as a result of motion problems discussed above.

Both regions are studied with standard head coils or more localized volume-type receiver coils; the latter should allow for complete visualization of surrounding structures of interest. Surface coils (i.e., flat receiver coils) placed directly on the face offer little benefit over volume designs and may cause poor visualization of deeper anatomy and/or pathology. These may be used to produce highly spatially resolved images in very selected circumstances. Certainly localized flat receiver coils should *not* be used routinely.

The patient's head should be positioned so that the IOML is perpendicular to the table top. A preliminary localizing view can be done to choose the optimal plane of study if desired. Standard 2DFT, Rf refocused, spin echo pulse sequences are used. Three-dimensional Fourier transform may be useful for 2- to 3-mm sections in subtle cases involving the facial nerve and skull base region. Gadolinum-DTPA will probably not offer much over plain MRI in evaluation of the major salivary glands but its potential will be investigated. It can be anticipated that paramagnetic contrast will diminish lesion conspicuity because of diminished lesion-fat contrast. Fat suppression pulse techniques may actually prove more useful than Gd-DTPA for increasing lesion conspicuity. Flow-sensitive pulse sequences might prove useful in selected cases that may have a vascular etiology. Other basic technical factors are as follows:

FOV: 18 TO 24 cm
SLT: 5 mm (3 mm in selected region of interest)
Acquisition matrix: 160 to 192 × 256 or 256 × 256
General approach
- Acquisition 1: Axial single echo 500 to 700/20 to 30
- Acquisition 2: Axial dual echo 2000/30 to 100*
- Acquisition 3: Optional coronal, single echo, pulse sequence chosen based on #1 and #2.
- Acquisition 4: Concentrated 3-mm sections, another plane, fat suppression, gradient echo, neck survey†

*TE range allows for selection of spin density–T_2-weighted pair or "mixed" and T_2-weighted pair as desired.
†Selection highly dependent on clinical situation and findings on initial acquisitions.

Table 4.5
CT Protocols—Parotid and Submandibular Regions

Area Under Study	Extent of Study	Gantry Angle	Slice Thickness	FOV (CM)	Coronals	Bone Algorithm Used	Contrast/ Comment
PAROTID REGION							
a) Mass—? etiology	a) Zygoma to hyoid	a) Parallel to IOML; if fillings present angle just enough to avoid them	a) 3 mm	a) 15–18	a) Rarely	a) Only if mandibular origin or involvement is noted on soft tissue algorithm	a) If mass is nodal full node survey may be indicated; if parapharyngeal or skull base in origin, see those protocols. Contrast always used.
b) Mass—known/ suspected benign parotid tumor (FN biopsy, clinical exam)	b) Zygoma to hyoid	b) As in (a)	b) 3 mm	b) 15–18	b) No	b) No	b) Do not survey nodes. Contrast always used.
c) Mass—known or suspected parotid malignancy	c) Zygoma to hyoid and survey nodes to low neck	c) As in (a) for parotid then angle parallel to mandibular body for node survey	c) 3 mm (parotid), 3 mm by 5-mm increments for neck survey	c) 15–18	c) Occasionally for skull base descending facial canal	c) If skull base or mandibular spread seen on soft tissue algorithm	c) Low incidence of nodal metastases but survey is worthwhile even in "low-grade" mucoepidermoid. Contrast always used.
d) Mass—possible inflammatory etiology (for ductal disease do routine sialography)	d) Zygoma to hyoid	d) As in (a)	d) 5 mm precontrast, 3 mm postcontrast	d) 15–18	d) No	d) No	d) Precontrast optional, but may be helpful; depends on individual case (see (e)); postcontrast always used.
e) Abscess vs. cellulitis	e) Zygoma to hyoid and lower as needed	e) As in (a) then parallel to mandibular body for lower sections	e) 3 mm (parotid), 5 mm or 3 mm by 5-mm increments for lower sections	e) 15–18	e) No	e) Occasionally for mandible	e) *Avoid* sialography in an acutely inflamed salivary. I.V. contrast always used.
SUBMANDIBULAR GLAND (SMG) REGION							
Extrinsic mass vs. intrinsic SMG pathology	Mandibular alveolar ridge to hyoid; survey neck and nodes as needed	Parallel to mandibular body	3 mm	15–18	Occasionally	Rarely	If nodal mass present, survey neck and consider surveying upper pharynx; if inflammatory consider precontrast survey of SMG region by 5 mm

(Use checklists in Appendix A as a study aid)

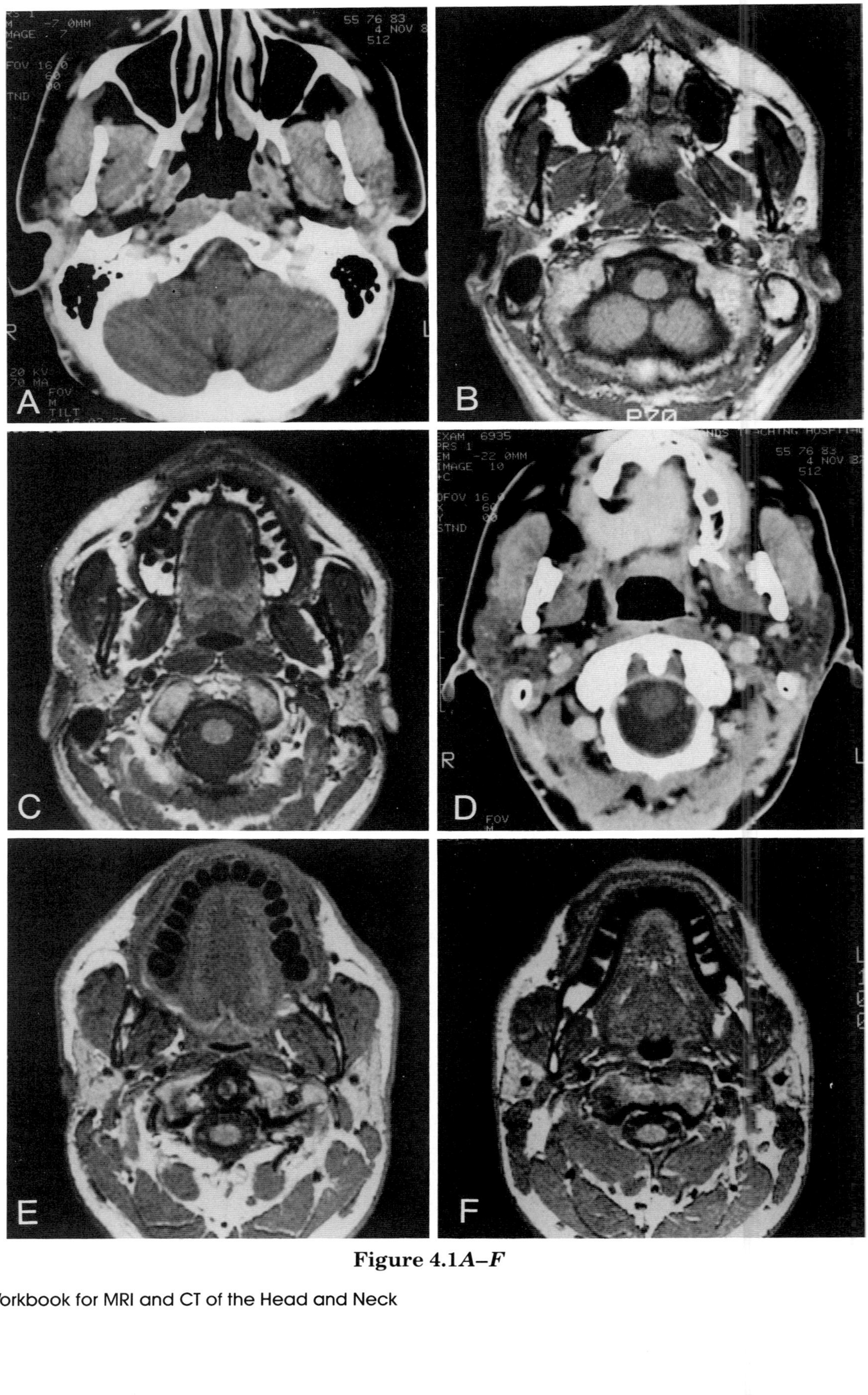

Figure 4.1*A–F*

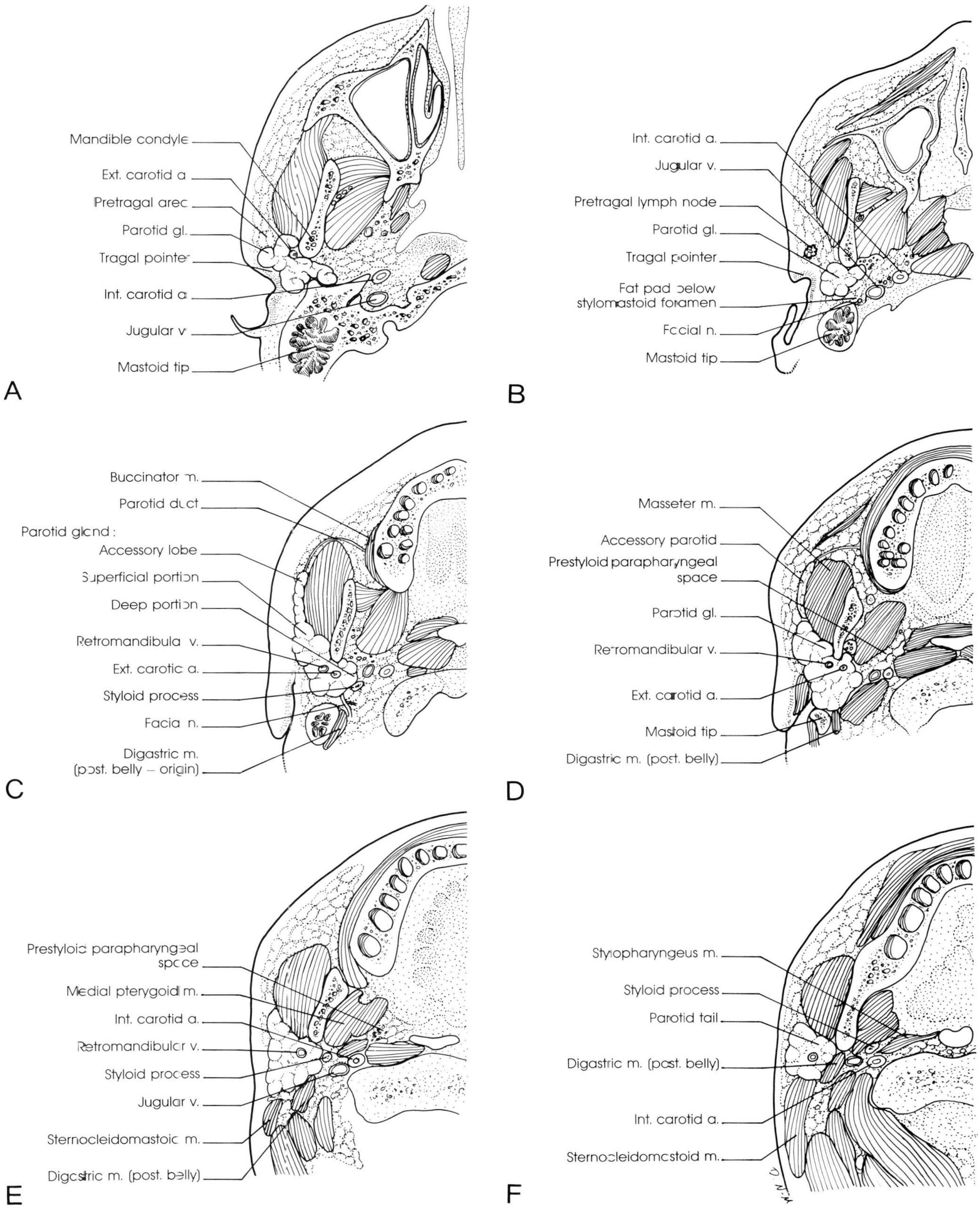
Mandible condyle
Ext. carotid a
Pretragal area
Parotid gl.
Tragal pointer
Int. carotid a
Jugular v
Mastoid tip
A
Int. carotid a.
Jugular v.
Pretragal lymph node
Parotid gl.
Tragal pointer
Fat pad below stylomastoid foramen
Facial n.
Mastoid tip
B
Buccinator m.
Parotid duct
Parotid gland:
Accessory lobe
Superficial portion
Deep portion
Retromandibula v.
Ext. carotid a.
Styloid process
Facia n.
Digastric m. (post. belly – origin)
C
Masseter m.
Accessory parotid
Prestyloid parapharyngeal space
Parotid gl.
Retromandibular v.
Ext. carotid a.
Mastoid tip
Digastric m. (post. belly)
D
Prestyloid parapharyngeal space
Medial pterygoid m.
Int. carotid a.
Retromandibular v.
Styloid process
Jugular v.
Sternocleidomastoid m.
Digastric m. (post. belly)
E
Stylopharyngeus m.
Styloid process
Parotid tail
Digastric m. (post. belly)
Int. carotid a.
Sternocleidomastoid m.
F

Figure 4.2*A–F*

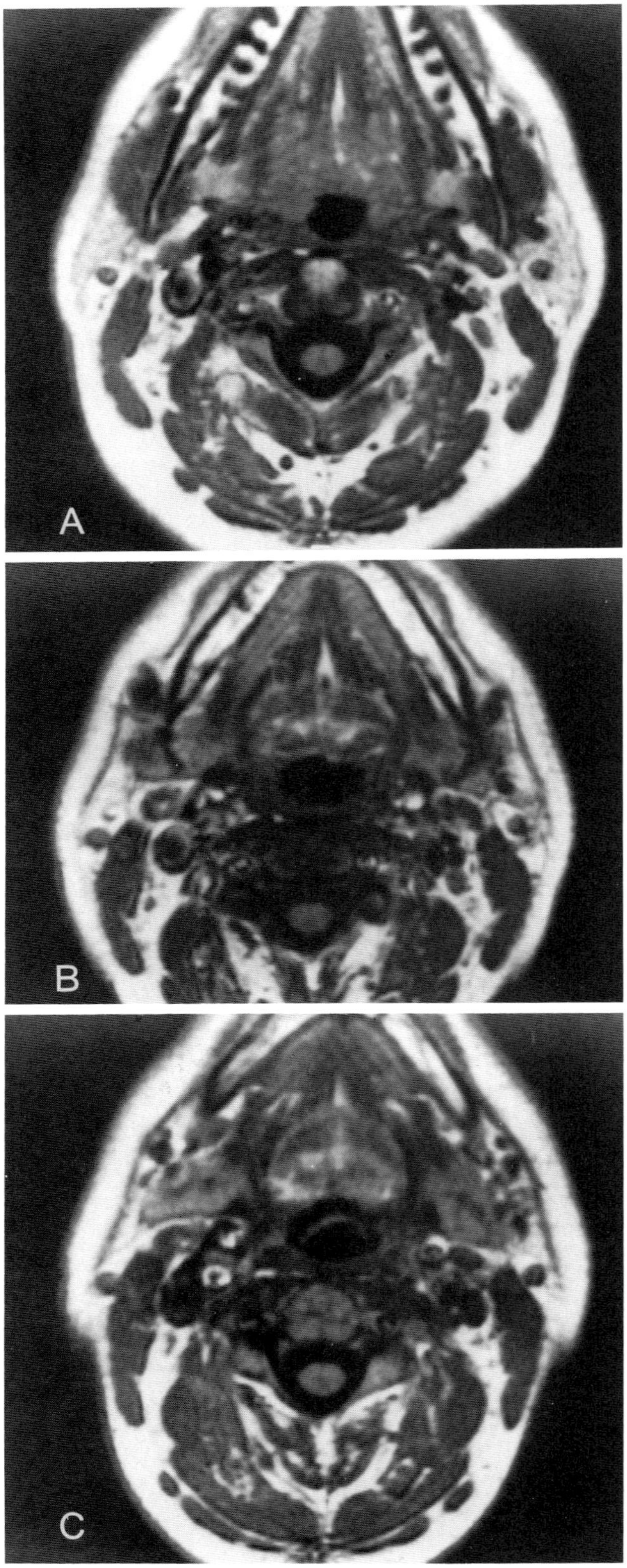

Figure 4.3*A–C*

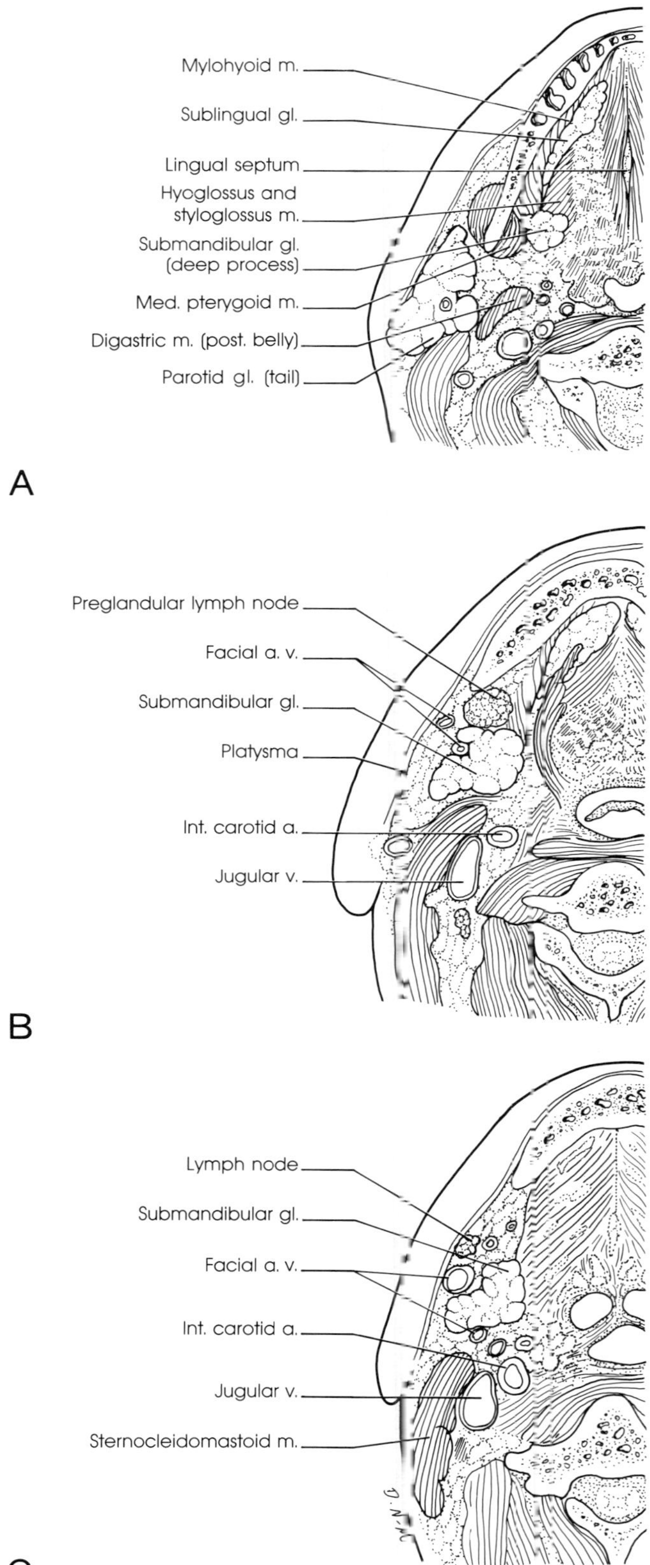

Figure 4.4*A–C*

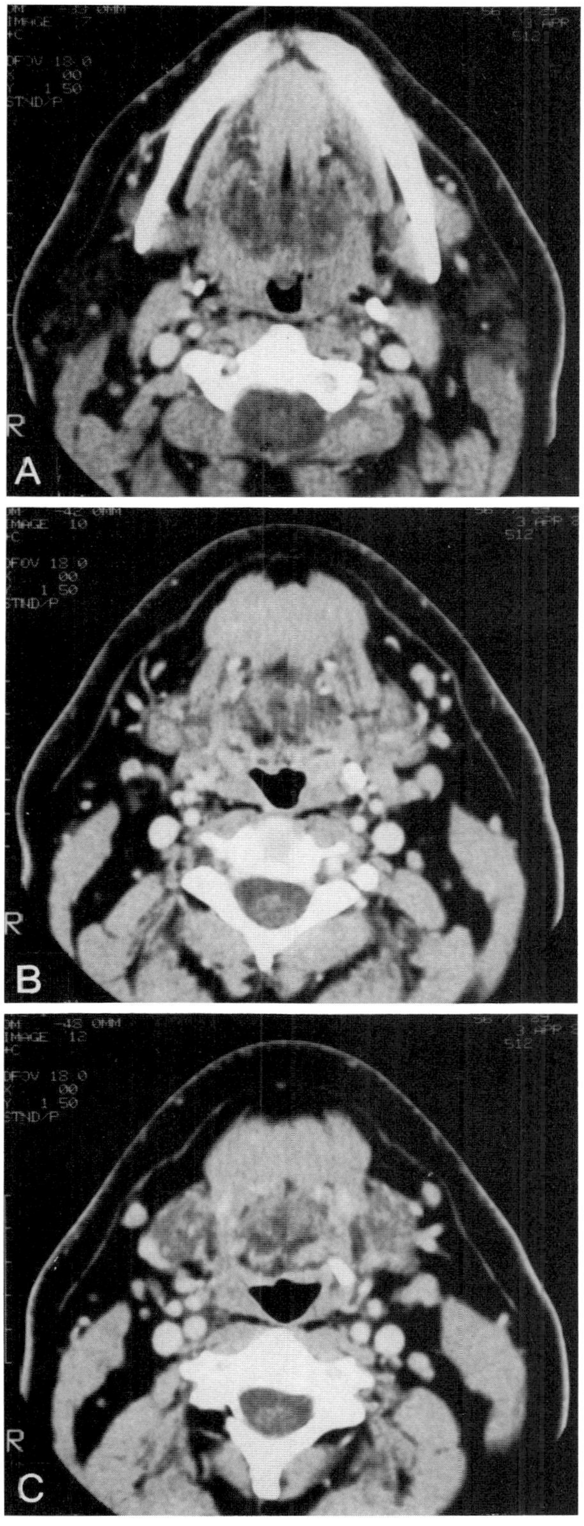

Figure 4.5*A–C*

CASES

Use checklists in Appendix A to analyze the following cases.

Problem I

Case 4.1 (Fig. 4.6*A–D*)

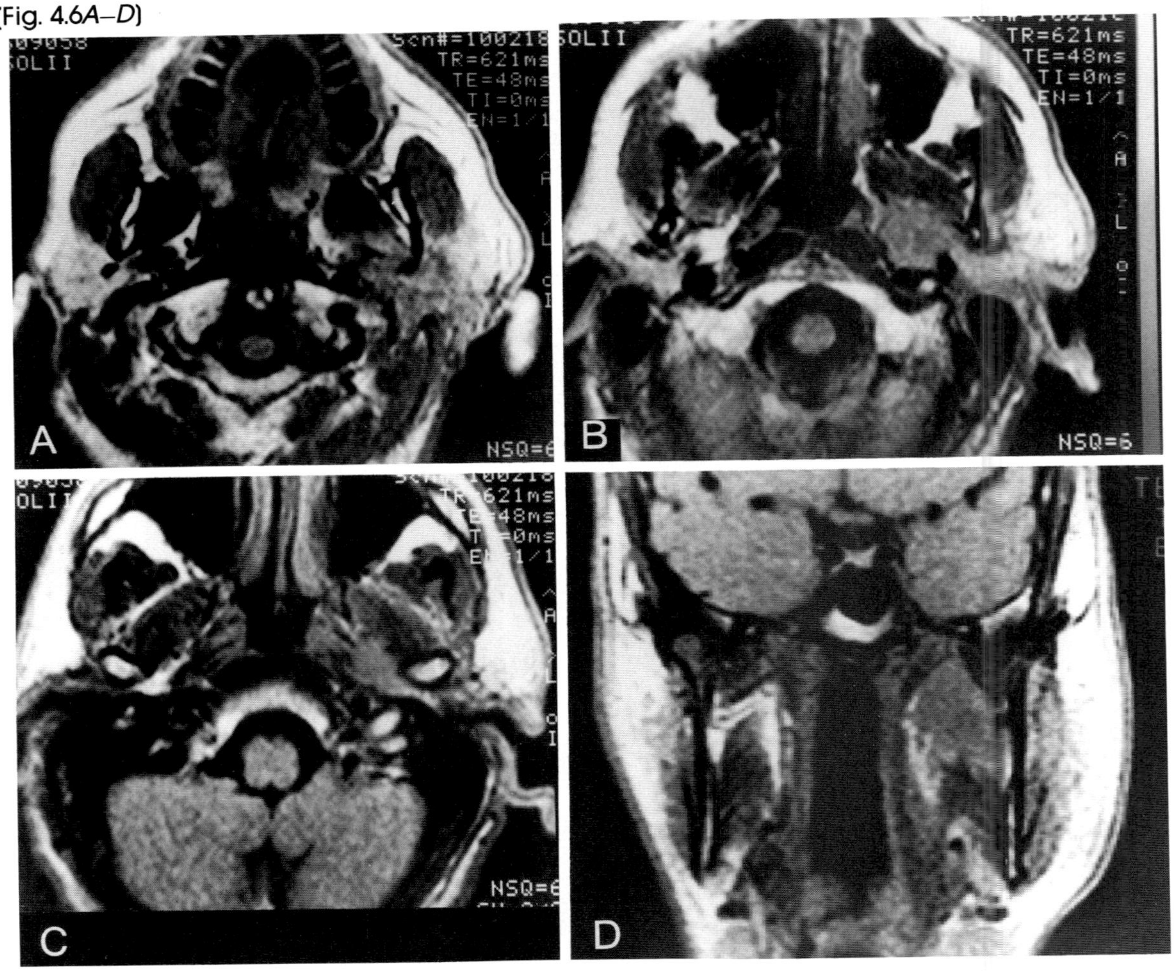

Figure 4.6*A–D*

Case 4.2 (Fig. 4.7*A* and *B*)

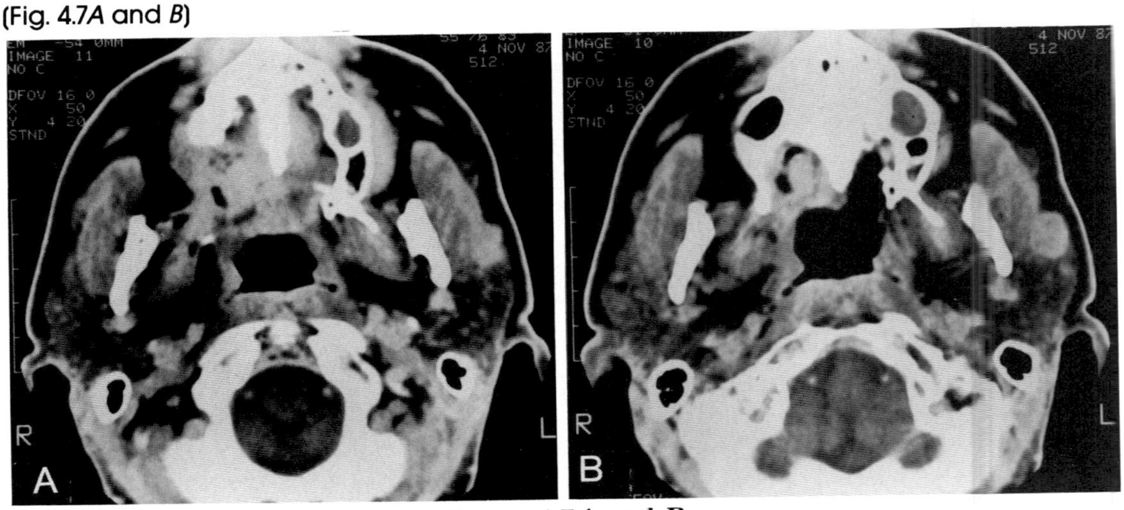

Figure 4.7*A* and *B*

Case 4.3 (Fig. 4.8*A* and *B*)

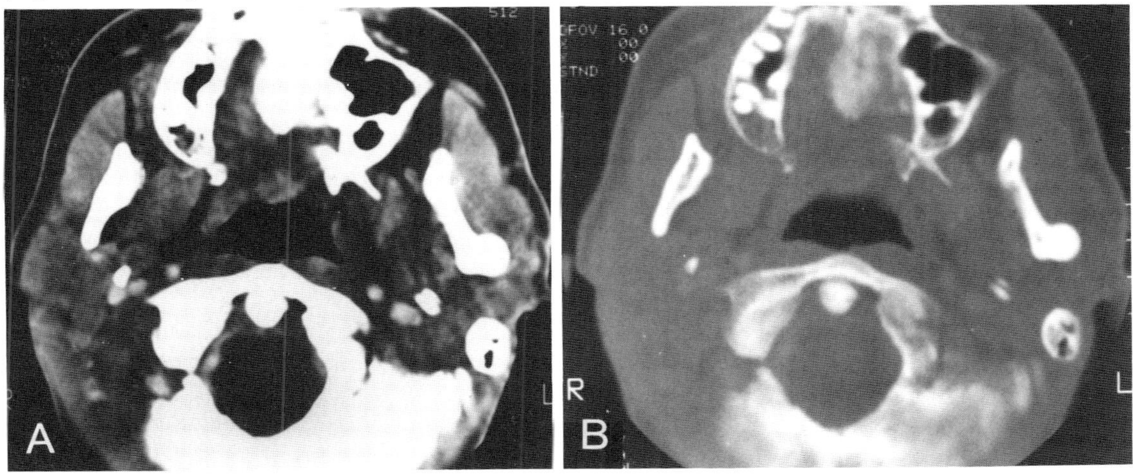

Figure 4.8*A* and *B*

Case Histories

Case 4.1 A 30-year-old male with a parotid region mass. Facial nerve function is normal.

Case 4.2 A 40-year-old male with a parotid region mass. Facial nerve function is normal.

Case 4.3 A 50-year-old female with a parotid region mass. No prior imaging. Before being referred to our institution patient had needle biopsy and excision of a "parotid mass." Both returned normal parotid tissue.

Questions

1. For each case establish whether the mass is intrinsic or extrinsic to the parotid gland.
2. If the mass is intrinsic describe its relation to the main trunk and distal branches of the facial nerve as well as you can.
3. On the basis of morphology or other factors decide whether needle biopsy would alter the therapy in each patient.
4. Anatomic issue: What imaging landmarks identify the course of the main trunk of the facial nerve?

Discussion

Problem I—Parotid Region Masses In Cases 4.1 and 4.2 the lesions are intrinsic to the parotid gland, and in Case 4.3 the mass is extrinsic and due to an osteochondroma of the mandible (Question 1). In patient 1 the mass lies predominantly below the main trunk of the facial nerve but definitely involves the deep portion of the gland and in fact extends far into the parapharyngeal space so that even though function is normal the nerve will likely be sacrificed at surgery if the tumor proves to be malignant. In Case 4.2 the main trunk of the nerve is free of tumor since the tumor lies distal to the splitting of the main trunk (see anatomic issue discussion below); however, one can predict that sacrifice of the zygomatic and buccal branches may be required if an adequate margin of resection is to be assured (Question 2). Thus lesion *must* be removed with an adequate cuff of normal tissue. Since there is no parotid tissue medial to the lesion a margin of muscle must be taken. Masses in this location usually displace the more peripheral divisions of the facial nerve laterally. The branch(es) will be stretched and sometimes adherent to the mass, making paresis or sacrifice necessary in some cases. It is best if the patient knows about this possibility preoperatively. If the branch were displaced medially it would almost assure sacrifice in order to avoid subtotal resection. When parotid lesions such as this benign mixed tumor are located more centrally in the gland a complete excision with a wide cuff of normal tissue is almost always possible without damage to the facial nerve or its branches.

Needle biopsy obviously added nothing in Case 4.3 because the lesion was extrinsic. In Case 4.1 the lesion appears highly aggressive and infiltrates the parapharyngeal space to near the skull base. Needle biopsy should be done to establish whether the lesion is malignant because one might consider doing radiotherapy before surgery. Radiotherapy when used in parotid lesions, however, usually *follows* gross total resection. In Case 4.2 needle biopsy would add nothing to the patient's management. The same operative procedure will be done regardless of histology. The lesion will be removed with a wide cuff of normal parotid tissue with an attempt made to preserve the facial nerve. This lesion turned out to be a benign mixed tumor and, as suggested by CT, the main trunk and lower division of the facial nerve were saved as well as the zygomatic branch; however, the buccal branch had to be sacrificed to ensure adequate margins. At the University of Florida it has been our experience that imaging (CT or MRI) will change management or provide other useful clinical data far more often than will fine-needle biopsy in parotid region masses.

Anatomic Issue: The Facial Nerve The facial nerve exits the stylomastoid foramen and passes through a small fat pad that is always visible on high-resolution MRI and CT images. The main trunk then courses obliquely forward. The surgeon finds the nerve by identifying the tragal "pointer" (it points to the facial nerve) and digastric muscle. The surgeon knows (and so should you) that the main trunk of the nerve will lie 10 to 15 mm caudal to the tragal pointer and lateral to the posterior belly of the digastric muscle. The nerve usually courses lateral to the retromandibular vein. All of these surgical landmarks can be seen on MRI and CT and used to judge the relationship of masses to the nerve. In our experience it is unusual to confidently identify the nerve itself within the parotid gland, but it should be clear from the prior discussion that this is not necessary. Within the gland the nerve splits into major divisions at the pes anserinus. With a little study and practice it becomes possible to accurately predict the relationship of masses to the major branches of the facial nerve. One must learn these anatomic landmarks in order to become an effective consultant to parotid surgeons. One can then also properly advise inexperienced surgeons about the dangers inherent in approaching a parotid region mass and when necessary go so far as to suggest appropriate referral of the patient to a more experienced surgical colleague.

CHECKLIST—PAROTID REGION (CASE 4.1)

	Seen	Nl	Abnl	Remarks
UPPER Pinna		√		
Pretragal soft tissues and nodes		√		
Zygomatic arch	No			
Masseter muscle		√		
Mandible—head		√		
Mandible—condyle		√		
Condylar fossa—temporomandibular joint	No			
External auditory canal—cartilaginous portion		√		
External auditory canal—bony portion		√		
Mastoid portion of temporal bone		√		
Facial canal—descending portion		√		
Stylomastoid foramen	No			
Styloid process		√		
Fat pad below stylomastoid foramen			√	Obliterated
Digastric groove		√		
Insertion of posterior belly of digastric muscle			√	Tumor subjacent
Tragal pointer		√		
Prestyloid parapharyngeal space			√	Infiltrated to within 5 mm of skull base
Carotid artery		√		
Jugular vein		√		Flow artifact
MID Subcutaneous fat			√	Indurated
Masseter muscle			√	Post. portion edematous or invaded
Mandible—ramus		√		Adjacent tumor
Buccinator space		√		
Parotid duct	No			
Parotid tissue—accessory lobe	No			
Parotid gland—superficial portion			√	Involved with tumor
Parotid gland—deep portion			√	Involved with tumor
Retromandibular vein			√	Compressed, displaced
External carotid artery			√	Displaced
Expected course of facial nerve			√	Involved with tumor
Intraparotid nodes		√		None visible
Mastoid tip		√		Tumor adjacent
Styloid process		√		
Posterior belly digastric muscle			√	Probably involved
Prestyloid parapharyngeal space			√	Invaded
Carotid artery			√	Displaced
Jugular vein			√	Displaced, compressed
Medial pterygoid muscle			√	Invaded
Course of mandibular nerve			√	Upper part probably involved by tumor

Normal Anatomy–Temporal Bone
(Use checklists in Appendix A as a study aid)

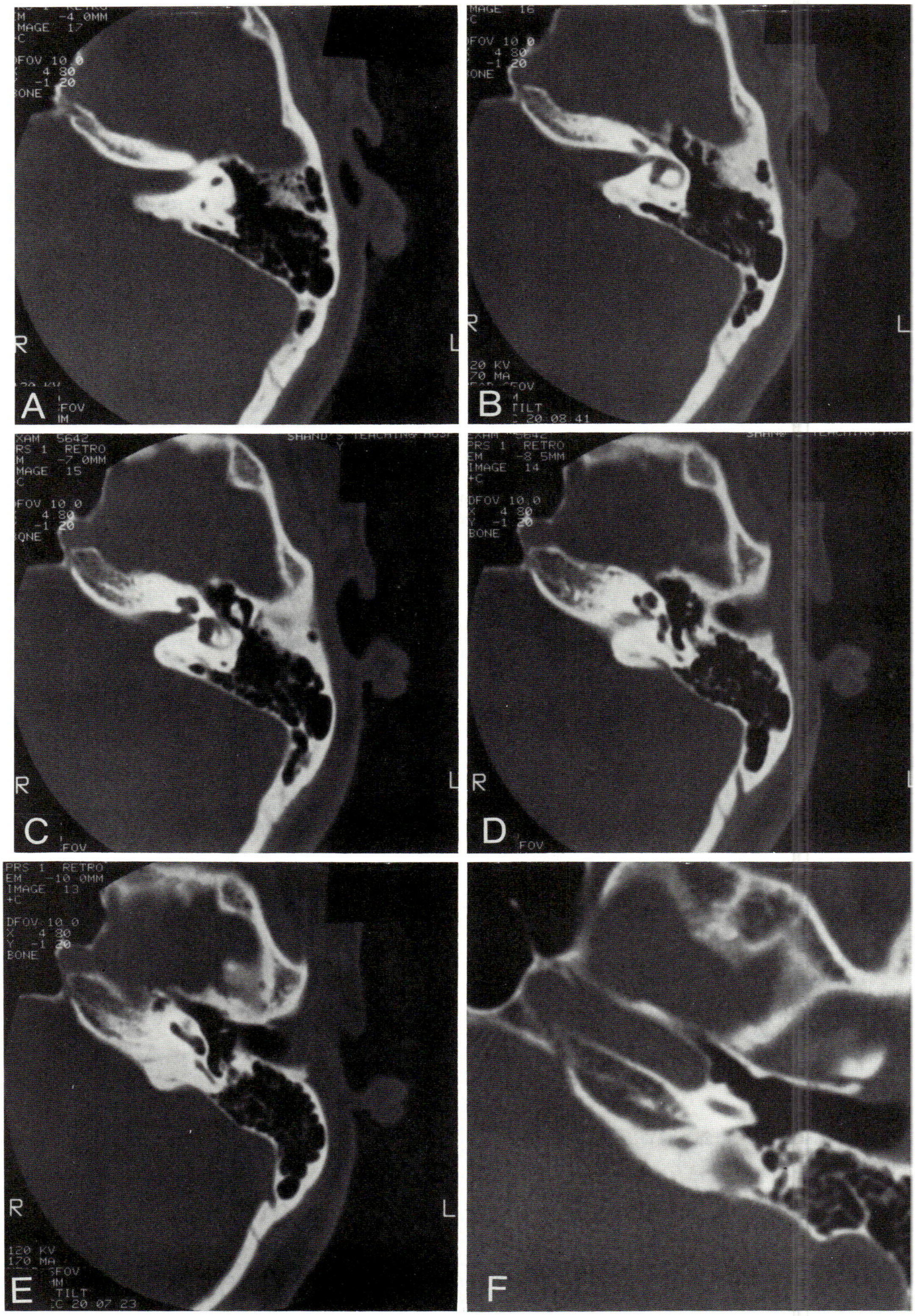

Figure 5.1*A–F*

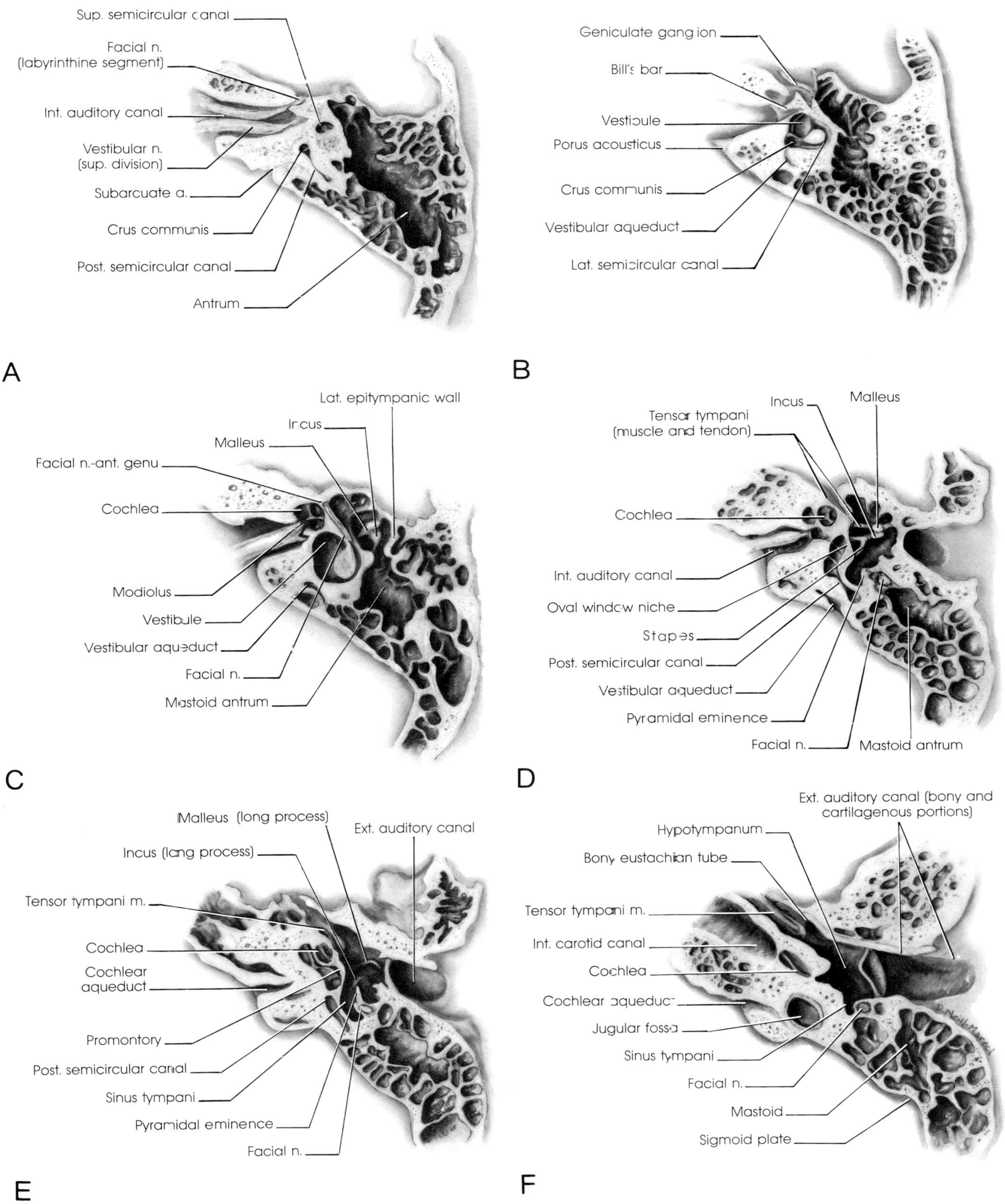
Sup. semicircular canal
Facial n. (labyrinthine segment)
Int. auditory canal
Vestibular n. (sup. division)
Subarcuate a.
Crus communis
Post. semicircular canal
Antrum
A
Geniculate ganglion
Bill's bar
Vestibule
Porus acousticus
Crus communis
Vestibular aqueduct
Lat. semicircular canal
B
Lat. epitympanic wall
Incus
Malleus
Facial n.-ant. genu
Cochlea
Modiolus
Vestibule
Vestibular aqueduct
Facial n.
Mastoid antrum
C
Incus
Malleus
Tensor tympani (muscle and tendon)
Cochlea
Int. auditory canal
Oval window niche
Stapes
Post. semicircular canal
Vestibular aqueduct
Pyramidal eminence
Facial n.
Mastoid antrum
D
Malleus (long process)
Ext. auditory canal
Incus (long process)
Tensor tympani m.
Cochlea
Cochlear aqueduct
Promontory
Post. semicircular canal
Sinus tympani
Pyramidal eminence
Facial n.
E
Ext. auditory canal (bony and cartilagenous portions)
Hypotympanum
Bony eustachian tube
Tensor tympani m.
Int. carotid canal
Cochlea
Cochlear aqueduct
Jugular fossa
Sinus tympani
Facial n.
Mastoid
Sigmoid plate
F

Figure 5.2A–F

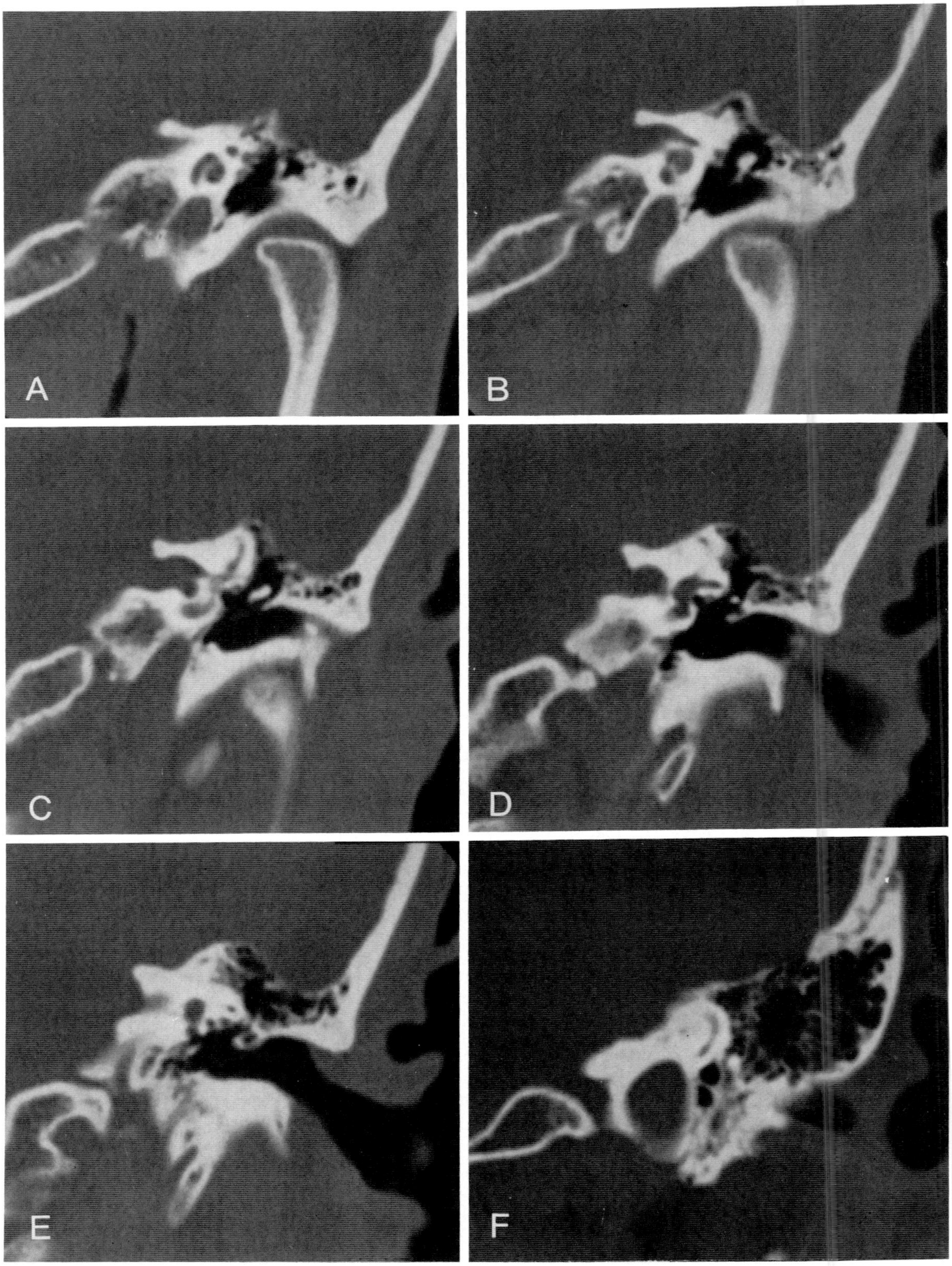

Figure 5.3*A–F*

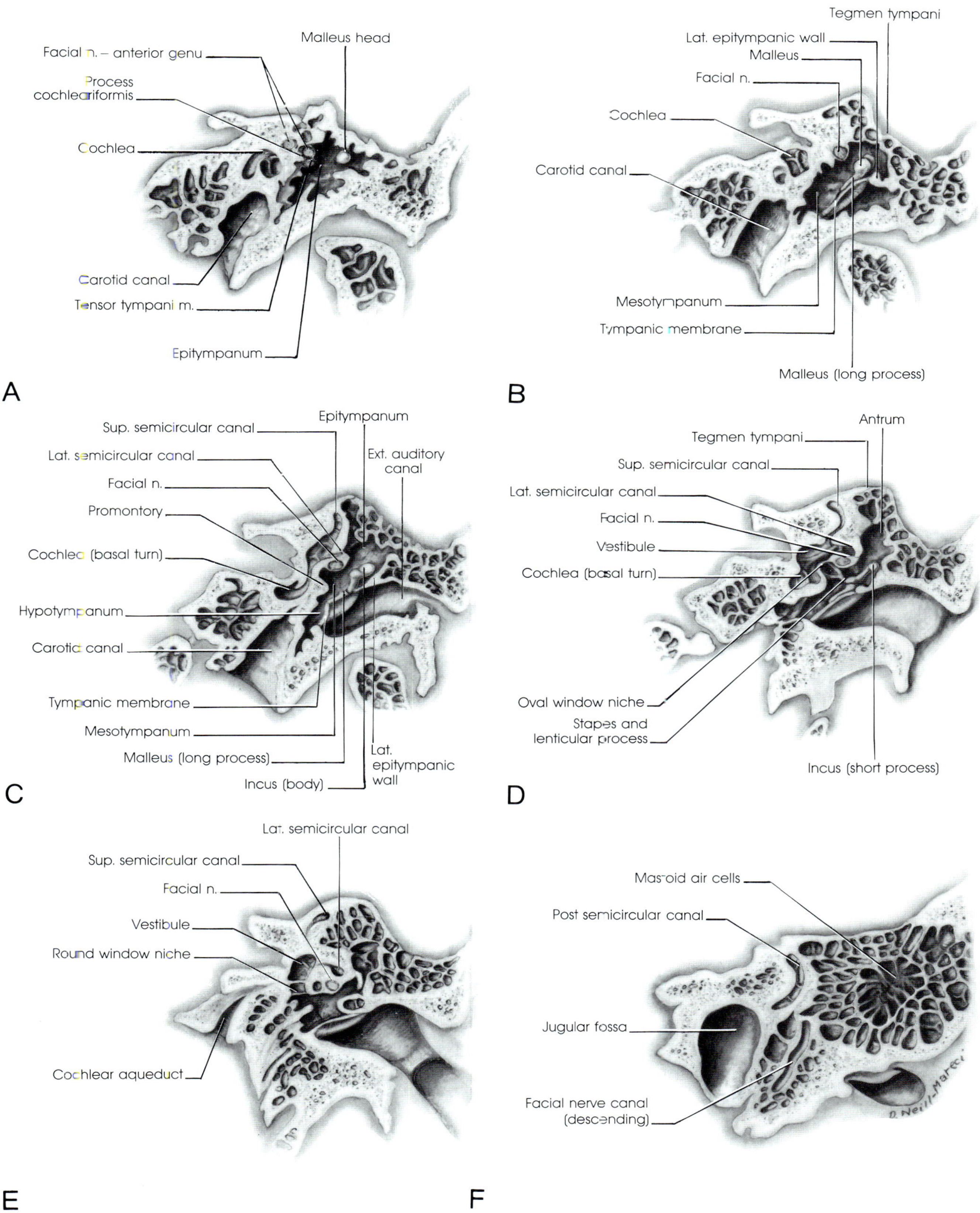
Malleus head
Facial n. – anterior genu
Process cochleariformis
Cochlea
Carotid canal
Tensor tympani m.
Epitympanum
A
Tegmen tympani
Lat. epitympanic wall
Malleus
Facial n.
Cochlea
Carotid canal
Mesotympanum
Tympanic membrane
Malleus (long process)
B
Epitympanum
Sup. semicircular canal
Lat. semicircular canal
Facial n.
Promontory
Cochlea (basal turn)
Hypotympanum
Carotid canal
Tympanic membrane
Mesotympanum
Malleus (long process)
Incus (body)
Ext. auditory canal
Lat. epitympanic wall
C
Antrum
Tegmen tympani
Sup. semicircular canal
Lat. semicircular canal
Facial n.
Vestibule
Cochlea (basal turn)
Oval window niche
Stapes and lenticular process
Incus (short process)
D
Lat. semicircular canal
Sup. semicircular canal
Facial n.
Vestibule
Round window niche
Cochlear aqueduct
E
Mastoid air cells
Post semicircular canal
Jugular fossa
Facial nerve canal (descending)
D. Neill-Marecic
F

Figure 5.4*A–F*

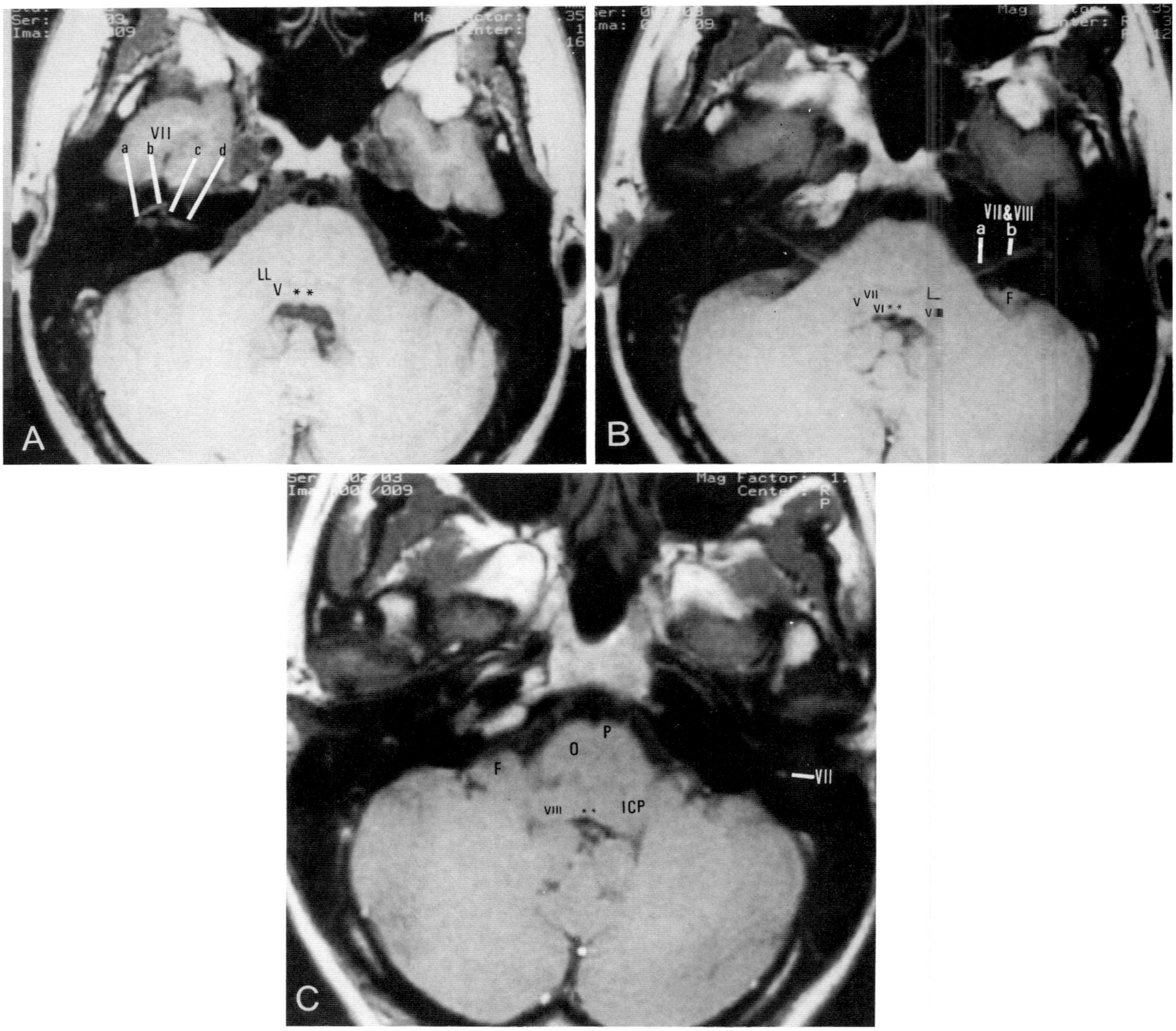

Figure 5.5*A–C*

Figure 5.5. *A,* at the mid to upper pons. Several segments of the facial nerve (VII) are visible, including: *d,* canalicular; *c,* labrynthine; *b,* anterior or first genu; *a,* tympanic or horizontal. *LL,* lateral lemniscus; *V,* trigeminal nerve nucleus; **, median longitudinal fasciculus. *B,* at the lower pons–pontomedullary junction. Cisternal (*a*) and canalicular (*b*) segments of VIIth and VIIIth nerves are shown. Positions of cranial nerve nuclei are indicated by appropriate Roman numerals. *LL,* lateral lemniscus; *F,* flocculus; **, median longitudinal fasciculus. *C,* just below pontomedullary junction–upper medulla. Descending segment of facial nerve (VII). *VIII,* vestibular nucleus; **, median longitudinal fasciculus; *F,* flocculus; *ICP,* inferior cerebellar peduncle; *O,* olivary nucleus; *P,* pyramid.

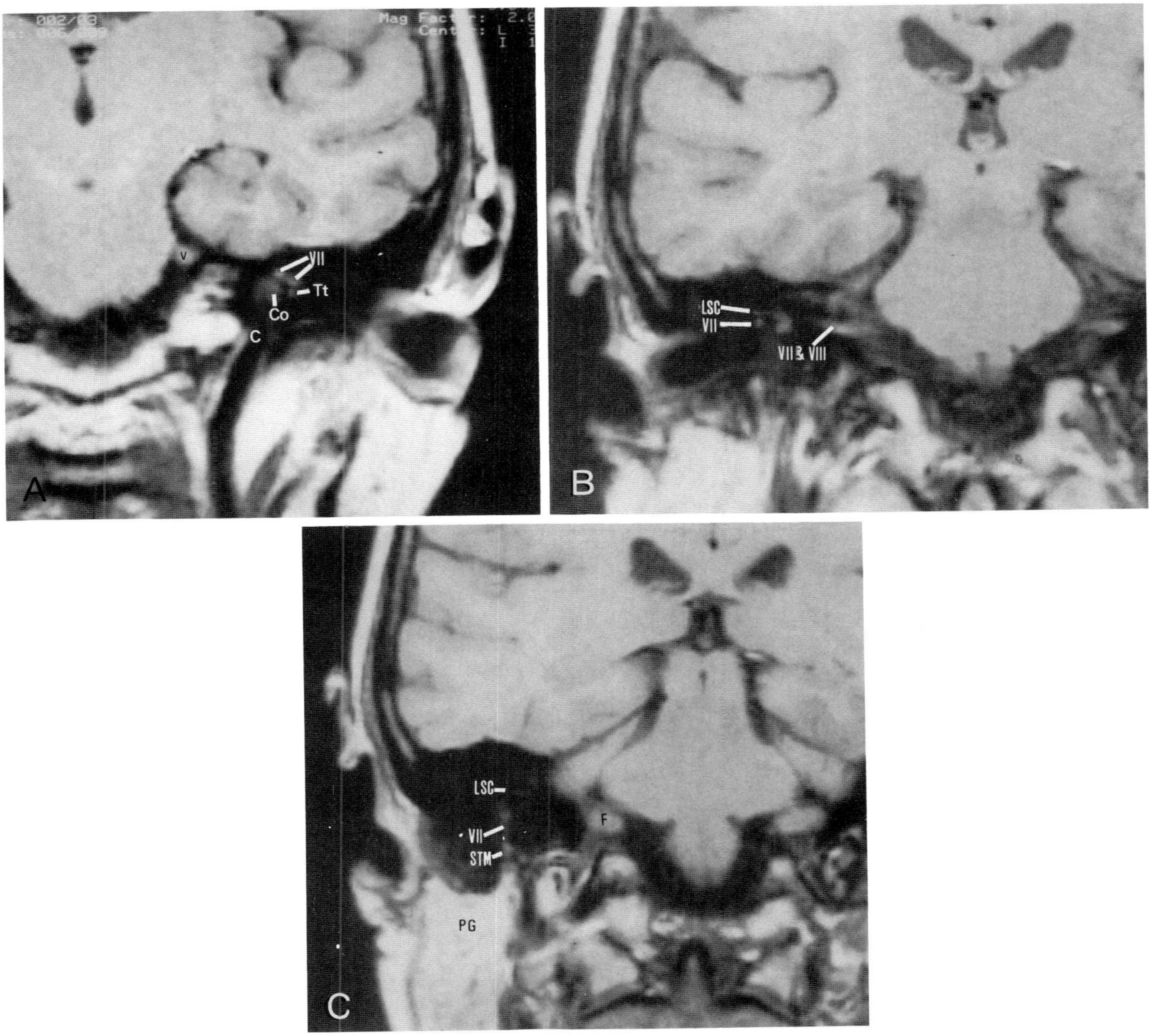

Figure 5.6*A–C*

Figure 5.6 *A*, coronal section through anteriormost portion of cerebellopontine angle cistern. *V*, trigeminal nerve; *VII*, anterior genu of the facial nerve; *Tt*, tensor tympani muscle; *Co*, cochlea; *C*, carotid artery. *B*, coronal section through the mid-cerebellopontine angle cistern. VIIth and VIIIth cranial nerves enter the internal auditory canal. *LSC*, lateral semicircular canal; *VII*, tympanic or horizontal segment of facial nerve. *C*, coronal section through the posterior cerebellopontine angle cistern. *F*, flocculus; *LSC*, lateral semicircular canal; *VII*, descending segment of facial nerve; *STM*, stylomastoid foramen; *PG*, parotid gland.

CASES

Use checklists in Appendix A to analyze the following cases.

PROBLEM I

Case 5.1 (Fig. 5.7*A–C*)

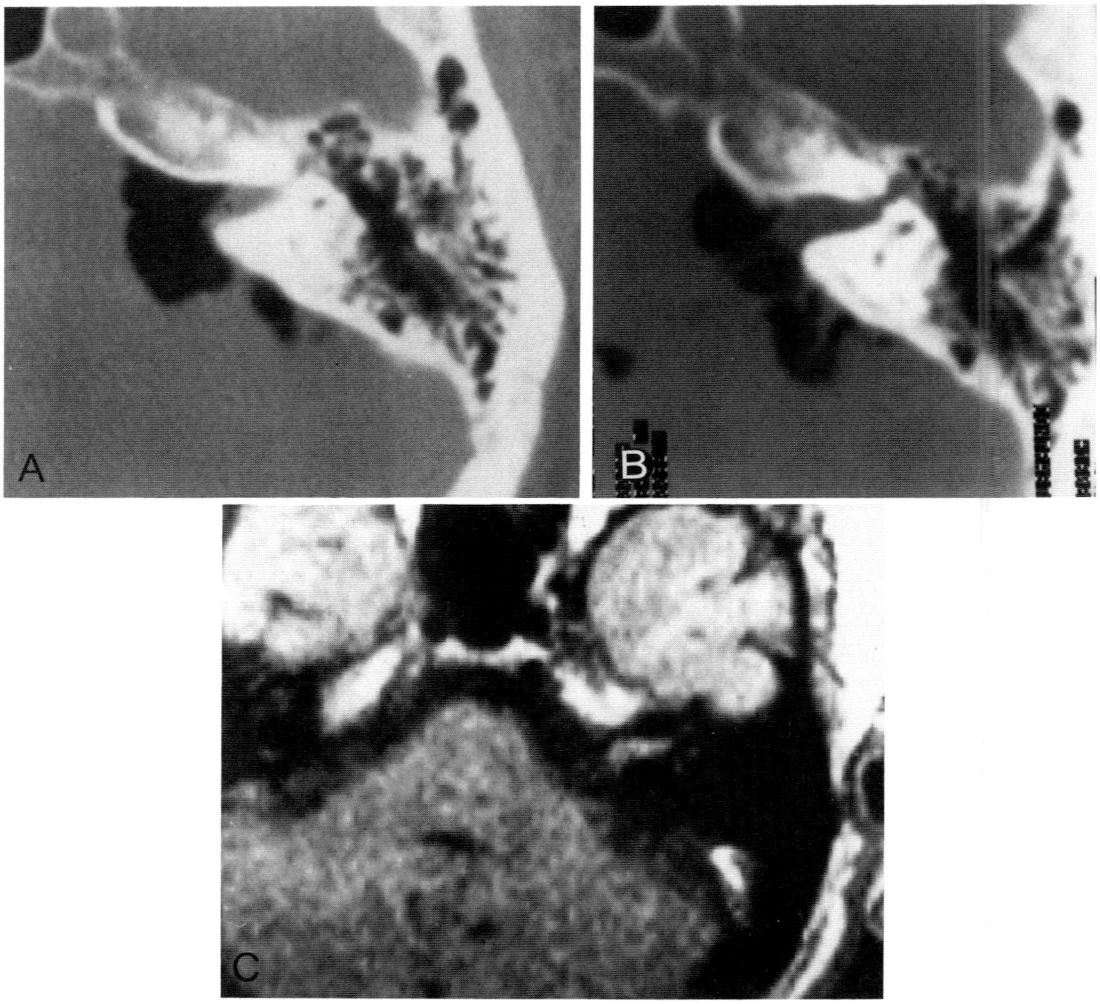

Figure 5.7*A–C*

CASE HISTORY

Case 5.1 A 65-year-old male with sensorineural hearing loss and vertigo. Prior CT was negative so CPA air cisternography (*A*) was done at another institution. About 6 weeks later MRI was done at our institution (*C*), and followed by another cisternogram (*B*) at the neurosurgeon's request.

Questions

1. Looking at the first cisternogram alone, could it be a false positive? Defend your answer.
2. Is it likely that this is an acoustic neuroma? What would explain the rapid increase in size between the two exams?
3. What is the imaging exam of choice for evaluating patients with retrocochlear sensorineural hearing loss?
4. What is the best pulse sequence in this setting for showing causative extra-axial pathology? Intra-axial? Would Gd-DTPA help?
5. Anatomic issue: Briefly describe the central relationships of the auditory-vestibular pathways.

Discussion

Problem I—Imaging Evaluation of the Auditory-Vestibular Pathways Air or positive-contrast cisternography have little role left in neuroimaging except in highly selected cases or when MRI cannot be done. This case arose in the time period (1985–1986) when the validity of the detection of intracanalicular lesions by MRI was still in question, mainly by our clinical colleagues. The air study in this patient (Case 5.1) was from another institution and showed lack of filling of the left IAC, but a meniscus rather than a bulging configuration is seen at the air-lesion interface. Our interpretation was that this could represent a lesion or incomplete displacement of the CSF in the IAC (Question 1). About 4 to 6 weeks later the MRI exam showed the mass to be filling the IAC and extending slightly beyond the porus acousticus. A confirmatory air study was then done the day after the MRI and showed additional extension along the labyrinthine segment of the facial nerve. This lesion was enlarging too rapidly to be an acoustic neuroma unless there had been hemorrhage. The patient did not have an abrupt onset of symptoms to suggest bleeding, and there was no clear MRI evidence of hemorrhage. We suggested that a lesion other than acoustic neuroma (e.g., metastasis or inflammation) be considered (Question 2); the neurosurgeons, forewarned, biopsied the "fleshy"-appearing lesion, which turned out to be metastatic, poorly differentiated carcinoma.

Magnetic resonance imaging is unequivocally the primary imaging exam for the posterior fossa in general and for patients with sensorineural hearing loss in particular (Question 3). A very high-resolution, thin section, 2DFT or 3DFT, T_1-weighted pulse sequence is the one of choice for detection of extra-axial CPA and intracanalicular lesions (Question 4). Gadolinium-DTPA can make the exam nearly infallible for detection of such lesions. A T_2-weighted pulse sequence should be done to look for intra-axial pathology if the initial sequences (with or without paramagnetic contrast) show no reason for the patient's symptoms (Question 4).

Anatomic Issue: The Auditory-Vestibular and the Cochleovestibular Pathways The end organ for the cochlear and vestibular nerves is the membranous labyrinth of the inner ear. The conglomerate VIIIth nerve travels in the IAC and then the CPA cistern inferior to the middle cerebellar peduncle (Figs. 5.5 and 5.6). It enters the dorsal and lateral aspect of the brainstem at the pontomedullary junction just anterior to the inferior cerebellar peduncle. The vestibular nuclei lie near the floor of the fourth ventricle and the cochlear nucleus lies more laterally (near the entry zone of the nerve) at the same level. The cochlear nucleus projects to the cortex via mainly dorsal lateral (lateral lemniscus) pathways that terminate in the medial geniculate body and inferior colliculi. The vestibular pathways are extremely complex, projecting to other nuclei throughout the brainstem and cerebellum. Within the brainstem one of the most important of these tracts is the median longitudinal fasciculus (MLF). The MLF has a central role in assuring coordinated eye movements and must be scrutinized in all patients with nystagmus, "dizziness," and other indications of possible vestibular pathway dysfunction.

Case 5.2 (Fig. 5.8*A–D*)

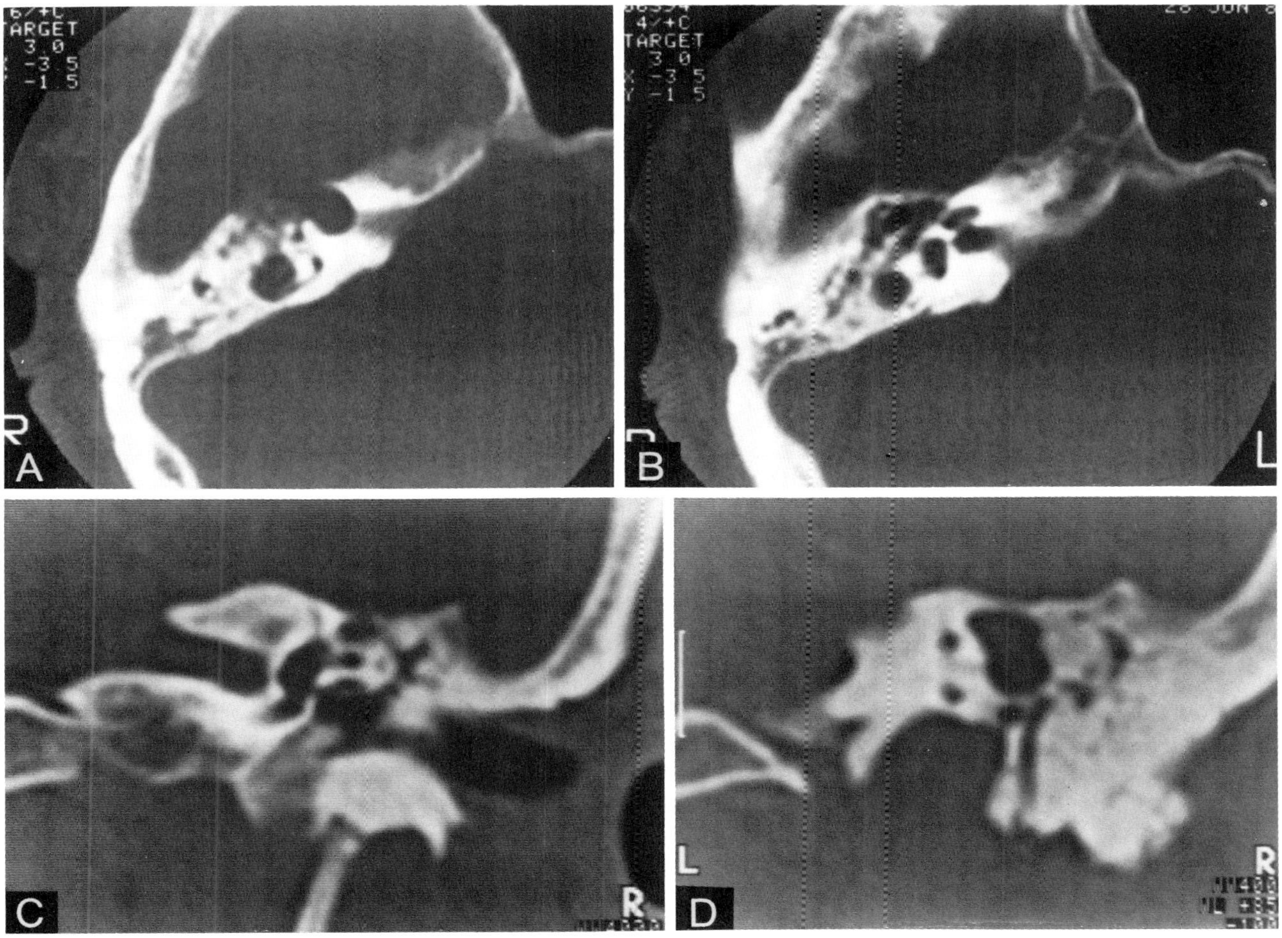

Figure 5.8*A–D*

CASE HISTORY

Case 5.2 Patient with a facial nerve paresis and outside *axial* CT (*A* and *B*) said to show a facial neuroma. Coronal CT sections were done the evening before planned intracranial approach to this lesion at our institution (*C* and *D*). Magnetic resonance imaging was suggested but not done.

Questions

1. Look at the axial sections and decide whether you agree with the stated interpretation.
2. Look at the coronal sections done subsequently and state the most likely diagnosis.
3. Can MRI help in this situation? If so, given two pulse sequences and one plane which would you choose?
4. Why is a neuro-otologist or neurosurgeon well served by knowing a lesion may represent an epidermoid or dermoid?
5. Anatomic issue: Describe the entire course of the facial nerve in detail.

Discussion

Problem II—Lesions of the Course of the Facial Nerve through the Temporal Bone The axial sections in Case 5.2 show a lesion tunneling around and through the bone of the otic capsule but not really following the facial canal (Question 1). This was an exam from an outside institution and no coronals were done. Coronals done at our institution clearly show that the lesion is not of facial nerve origin and the pattern seen is most suggestive of a primary cholesteatoma (no prior history of middle ear disease and the tympanic membrane was normal) (Question 2). Secondary cholesteatoma or erosive granulation tissue (chronic erosive otitis media) can cause similar findings. Magnetic resonance imaging can help in showing the full extent of disease and in differential diagnosis. Coronal sections are most informative and should be done with T_1 and T_2-weighting. This may help to distinguish cholesterolosis from acquired or congenital cholesteatoma and may indicate that drainage via tympanomastoid rather than intracranial surgery is indicated (Question 3). Also, forewarned, the neurosurgeon or neuro-otologist can be even more careful to avoid spillage of cholesteatomatous debris into the subarachnoid space if an intracranial approach to the lesion becomes a necessary part of the treatment plan (Question 4).

Anatomic Issue: The Facial Nerve The facial nerve nucleus lies near the pontomedullary junction. The nerve exits the lower pons traveling obliquely cephalad (cisternal segment) to enter the IAC. The nerve travels in the anterior superior quadrant of the IAC. It exits the canal by going anterolaterally through a small canal adjacent to Bill's bar (labyrinthine segment) and makes a hairpin turn posteriorly (anterior or first genu) at the geniculate ganglion (Figs. 5.5 and 5.6). The greater superficial petrosal nerve runs anteromedially from here along the floor of the middle cranial fossa. The facial nerve then travels beneath the lateral semicircular canal in a small, variably mineralized bony canal (tympanic or horizontal segment). The chorda tympani from the lingual nerve joins the tympanic segment in the middle ear. The facial nerve then turns inferiorly (posterior or second genu) to enter a usually very well mineralized descending facial canal. A branch at or near the posterior genu innervates the stapedius muscle. The nerve exits the stylomastoid foramen and travels, in a fat pad, to its course through the parotid gland and beyond (Chapter 4). One must understand all of this anatomy to properly evaluate patients with facial nerve dysfunction.

In our experience perineural spread of skin or parotid cancer is the most common neoplasm affecting the facial nerve. Secondary involvement by cholesteatoma is unusual, but not rare. Neurinoma and hemangioma are the most common benign lesions involving the nerve, but both are uncommon.

Case 5.3 (Fig. 5.9*A–F*)

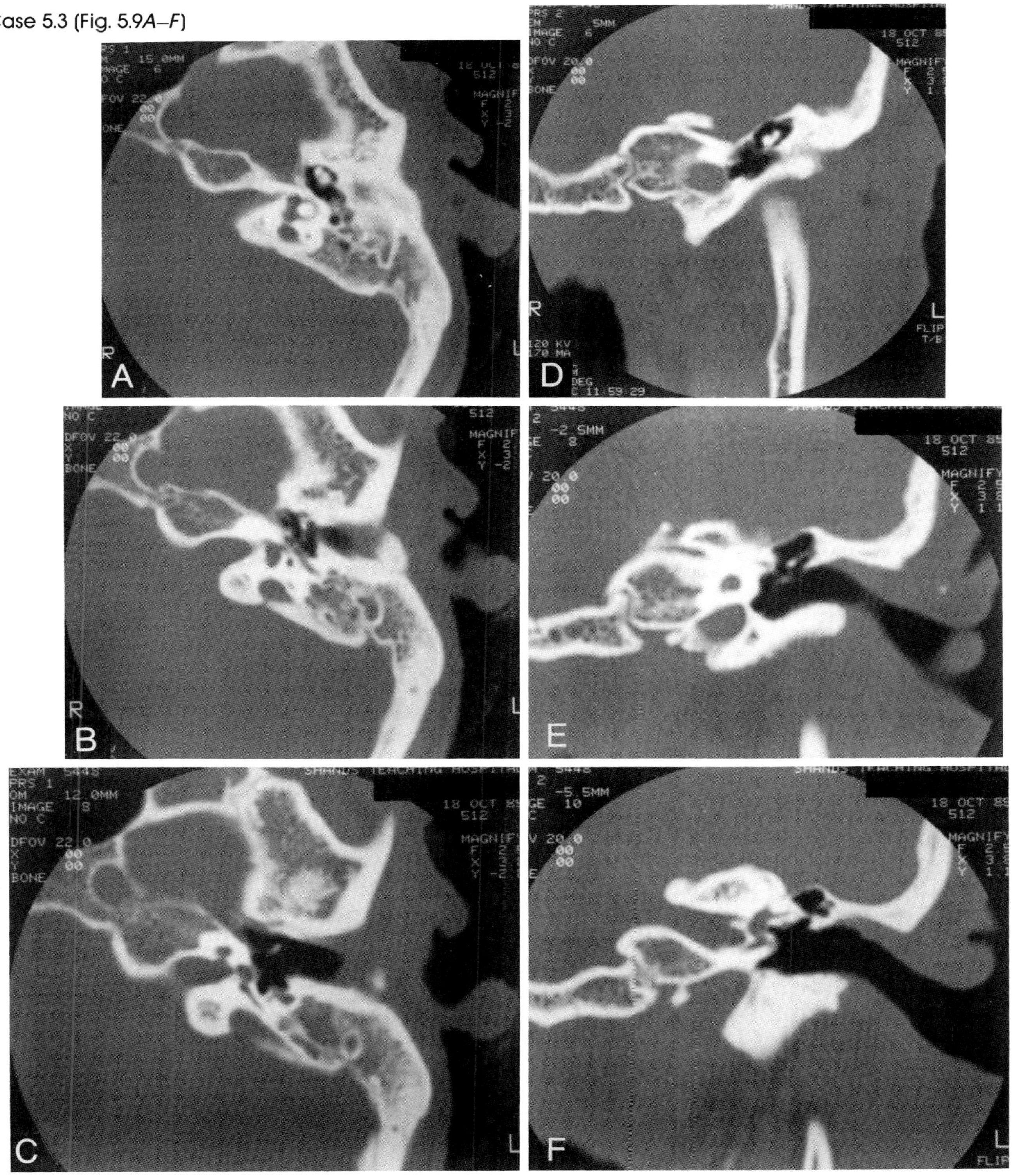

Figure 5.9*A–F*

Case 5.4 (Fig. 5.10)

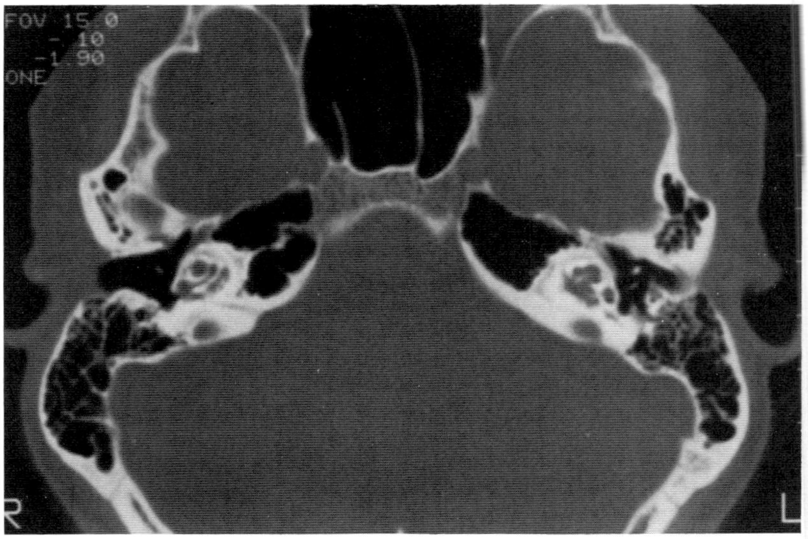

Figure 5.10

CASE HISTORIES

Case 5.3 Child with possible congenital anomalies of the ear.

Case 5.4 Candidate for a cochlear implant.

Questions

1. Enumerate all the things that you should specifically comment on in your report to the referring clinician.
2. State what abnormalities are present in each patient.
3. Are coronal sections necessary in all cases?
4. Anatomic issue: What is the vestibular aqueduct? What is its course and normal size range?

DISCUSSION

Problem III—Congenital Hearing Loss Patients with congenital hearing loss often present for imaging to help determine its cause and whether surgical intervention has any role in therapy. It is essential to evaluate the auditory pathways from one end to the other and report *specifically* on *each* of the following points:

1. External auditory canal—stenosis versus atresia, soft tissue or bony.
2. Size of middle ear cleft.
3. Status of ossicles and oval window.
4. Course of facial nerve.
5. Are there inner ear anomalies (cochlear, vestibular, respective aqueducts) or abnormalities (e.g., otosclerosis, obliterative labyrinthitis)?
6. Is there evidence of congenital cholesteatoma?
7. Adjunctive data: extent of mastoid aeration; positions of sigmoid plate, jugular fossa, carotid canal.

Case 5.3 is somewhat unusual in that there are mixed inner and middle ear anomalies. The middle ear develops mainly from first branchial apparatus structures, whereas the inner ear develops from the primitive otocyst. Their basic formation is slightly separated in embryologic life so that anomalies are usually isolated. The specific findings are described in the accompanying filled-out checklist (Question 2).

The patient in Case 5.4 also had congenital hearing loss and was being evaluated for possible cochlear implantation. In this situation the report should include comment on the following (Question 1):

1. Is there congenital anomaly of any kind (see above)?
2. Is the cochlea normally formed?
3. Is there evidence of obliterative labyrinthitis or otosclerosis?
4. Is there evidence of a mass lesion (e.g., congenital cholesteatoma)?
5. Status of the round window.
6. Adjunctive data, including: any evidence of middle ear disease that could be active; aeration and development of mastoid; positions of the jugular fossa, carotid canal, sigmoid plate.

This patient had bilateral otosclerosis that was mainly in its osteolytic phase (Question 2). Indications and contraindications for cochlear implantation are changing matters. The diagnostic imager must provide the highest quality studies that will in turn contain the required information. These imaging data will be combined with *many* clinical criteria to determine whether cochlear implantation is possible.

Coronal sections are necessary in the majority of cases being evaluated for these indications. Axials alone may be used in *screening* for congenital anomalies. Coronals are always done in cochlear implant patients for definitive study of the round window (Question 3).

Anatomic Issue: The Vestibular Aqueduct The vestibular aqueduct is the bony canal for the endolymphatic sac or duct. It runs from the posterior surface of the temporal bone just superior and lateral to the jugular fossa to the crus communis (junction of the ampullary ends of the posterior limb of the superior semicircular canal and superior limb of the posterior semicircular canal). It should measure less than 2.5 mm in size; if larger there is a high likelihood of associated anomalies of the membranous and/or bony labyrinth. The predictive value of an abnormally small canal for assessing risk in Meniere's disease patients is highly controversial.

CHECKLIST—TEMPORAL BONE (CASE 5.3)

	Seen	Nl	Abnl	Remarks
UPPER				
Mastoid—periantral air cells			√	Underdeveloped
Epitympanic recess—upper antrum			√	Antrum not developed
Koerner's septum			√	Not seen
Otic capsule bone (arcuate emminence)	No			
Arcuate tunnel	No			
Superior semicircular canal	No			Ampullary end dilated
Inferior semicircular canal (superior limb)			√	Ampullary end dilated
Common crus			√	Bulbous
Lateral semicircular canal			√	Foreshortened
Vestibular aqueduct			√	Markedly dilated
Internal auditory canal		√		Slightly deformed
Facial canal—labyrinthine segment			√	Slightly deformed but not well seen
Bill's bar			√	Area deformed
Facial canal—anterior genu			√	Slightly deformed
Petrous apex		√		
UPPER-MID				
Mastoid—periantral air cells			√	Underdeveloped
Sigmoid plate		√		
Epitympanic recess		√		
Lateral wall epitympanic recess (scutum)		√		
Aditus ad antrum			√	Small
Mastoid antrum			√	Underdeveloped
Koerner's septum			√	Not visible
Malleus—head		√		
Incus—body and short process			√	Anomalous, ? anklyosed to lateral wall
Facial canal—tympanic (horizontal) segment		√		
Facial canal—posterior genu		√		
Pyramidal eminence		√		
Tensor tympani semicanal	No			
Otic capsule bone		√		
Vestibule			√	? Slight deformity
Oval window niche		√		
Posterior semicircular canal		√		
Vestibular aqueduct			√	Markedly enlarged
Cochlea including modiolus			√	Grossly deformed
Internal auditory canal		√		Slightly deformed
Petrous apex		√		

continued

CHECKLIST—TEMPORAL BONE (CASE 5.3) *(continued)*

	Seen	Nl	Abnl	Remarks
MID-LOWER Mastoid air cells			√	Underdeveloped
Sigmoid plate		√		
External auditory canal—bony portion		√		
External auditory canal—cartilaginous portion		√		
Tympanic membrane	No			
Mesotympanum		√		
Malleus—long process			√	? Ankylosed to ant. wall, deformed
Incus—long process			√	Deformed
Stapes—crura			?	Thickened; not well seen
Tensor tympani semicanal		√		
Tensor tympani muscle and tendon		√		
Facial canal—descending portion		√		
Sinus tympani		√		
Otic capsule bone		√		
Vestibule			?	? Slight deformity
Posterior semicircular canal		√		
Cochlea			√	Grossly deformed
Petrous apex		√		
Cochlear aqueduct	No			

Case 5.5 (Fig. 5.11*A*–*D*)

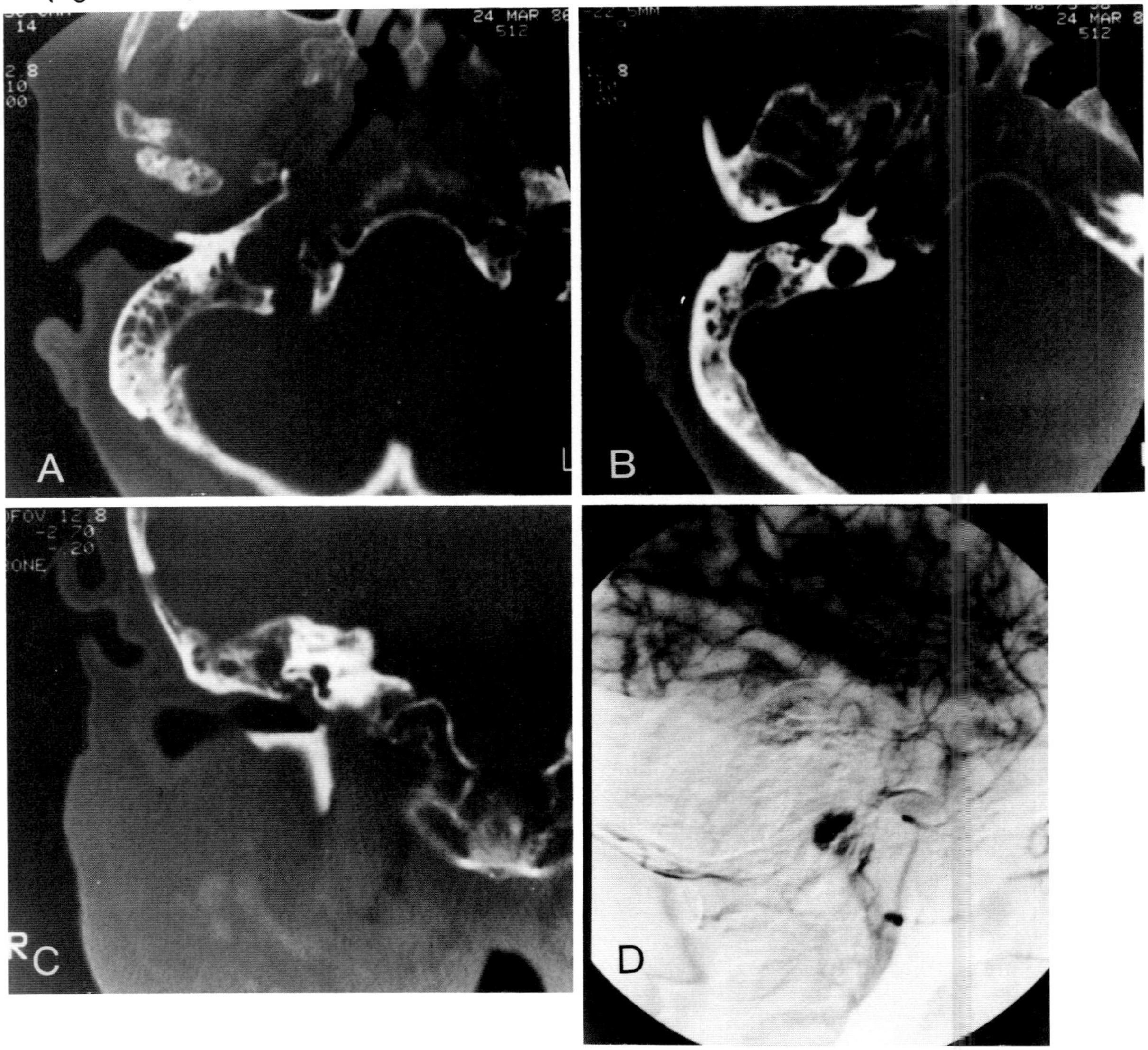

Figure 5.11*A*–*D*

Case History

Case 5.5 A 70-year-old female with pulsatile tinnitus and bluish-red mass behind the tympanic membrane. Cranial nerve exam is normal.

Questions

1. How does one distinguish between a high jugular bulb and a paraganglioma (glomus jugulare type)?
2. What is the frequency of high jugular bulbs (i.e., those seen at and above the level of the external auditory canal or round window)? What is the significance of the finding? What is a jugular diverticulum?
3. What is your final diagnosis in this case?
4. Anatomic issue: What structures go through the jugular fossa?

Discussion

Problem IV—Assessment of Patients with Objective Pulsatile Tinnitus and Middle Ear Mass Patients with a "noise in the ear" frequently come to imaging. They must be triaged into basic groups, including: (*a*) subjective versus objective tinnitus, (*b*) pulsatile versus nonpulsatile tinnitus, and (*c*) association of the sound with a middle ear mass. Imaging may then be directed in a manner similar to that shown in Table 5.4. A high jugular bulb (fossa) lies at the level of the inferior margin of the tympanic ring or round window or above; it may be present as a normal variant in up to 24% of the population (Question 2). In a high jugular bulb the jugular spur should be intact and the bony margins of the jugular fossa remain smooth and well corticated, except at perhaps their margin with the hypotympanum, where dehiscence is not infrequent. A glomus jugulare–type paraganglioma will almost always erode the margins of the jugular fossa as well as the jugular spur by the time of presentation (Question 1). A jugular diverticulum is a further outpouching of the jugular vein that further distorts the configuration of the jugular bulb and surrounding structures (e.g., inner ear, internal auditory canal) but does not fray the edges of surrounding bone (Question 2).

The patient in Case 5.5 has a paraganglioma—glomus tympanicum type *coincident* with the *normal variation* of a high jugular bulb and dehiscence of the bony wall between the jugular fossa and hypotympanum. An angiogram was necessary to be absolutely sure that this was not a glomus jugulare growing into the hypotympanum. Surgery confirmed this diagnosis (Question 3).

Anatomic Issue: Structures of the Jugular Fossa The jugular fossa is divided into compartments by a bony or fibrous septum. The larger pars venosum contains the jugular vein and cranial nerves X and XI; the much smaller pars nervosa contains the IXth cranial nerve. The jugular fossae may show great variation from side to side in the same patient, and one should avoid suggesting that this is a pathologic change unless there is bone erosion or compelling clinical evidence that this may be a source of symptomatology.

CHECKLIST—TEMPORAL BONE (CASE 5.5)

	Seen	Nl	Abnl	Remarks
LOWER Mastoid air cells			√	Opacified
Sigmoid plate		√		
External auditory canal—bony portion		√		
External auditory canal—cartilaginous portion		√		
Tympanic membrane		√		
Hypotympanum			√	Round 4 × 4 mm mass and opacified
Malleus—long process	No			
Incus—long process	No			
Eustachian tube—bony portion			√	Mass at proximal end
Facial canal—descending portion		√		
Stylomastoid foramen	No			
Fat pad below stylomastoid foramen	No			
Sinus tympani			√	Opacified
Otic capsule bone		√		
Cochlea		√		Only distal basal turn seen
Round window	No			
Cochlear aqueduct	No			
Petrous apex		√		But osteoporotic
Carotid canal		√		But osteoporotic
Jugular fossa (pars nervosa, venosum) spur		?		High but normally corticated; ? dehiscent
Jugular tubercle			√	Osteoporotic

SUGGESTED READINGS

Books, Chapters, Reviews

Bergeron RT: The temporal bone. In Bergeron RT, Osborn AG, Som PM (eds): *Head and Neck Imaging—excluding the Brain*. St. Louis, CV Mosby, pp 728–846.

Mafee MF: Acoustic neuroma and other acoustic nerve disorders: role of CT and MRI: an analysis of 238 cases. In Harnsberger HR (ed): *Seminars in Ultrasound, CT and MR*. New York, Grune & Stratton, 1987, vol 8, no 3, pp 256–283.

Mancuso AA, Hanafee WN: *Computed Tomography and Magnetic Resonance Imaging of the Head and Neck*. Baltimore, Williams & Wilkins, 1985, Chap 5, pp 88–138.

Swartz J: *Imaging of the Temporal Bone*. Stuttgart, Thieme Medical Publishers, 1986.

Teresi L, Lufkin R, Nitta K: MRI of the facial nerve: normal anatomy and pathology. In Harnsberger HR (ed): *Seminars in Ultrasound, CT and MRI*. New York, Grune & Stratton, 1987, vol 8, no 3, pp 240–255.

Vignaud J, Jardin C, Rosen L: *The Ear—Diagnostic Imaging*. Paris, Masson Publishing, 1986.

Articles

On the facial nerve:

Curtin HD, Wolfe P, Snyderman N: The facial nerve between the stylomastoid foramen and the parotid: computed tomographic imaging. *Radiology* 149:165–169, 1983.

Daniels DL, Czervionke LF, Rojunas KW: Facial nerve enhancement in MR imaging. *AJNR* 8:605–607, 1987.

Disbro MA, Harnsberger HR, Osborne AG: Peripheral facial nerve dysfunction: CT evaluation. *Radiology* 155:659–663, 1985.

Gentry LR, Jacoby CG, Turski PA, et al: Cerebellopontine angle–petromastoid mass lesions: comparative study of diagnosis with MR imaging and CT. *Radiology* 162:513–520, 1987.

Kalovidouris A, Mancuso AA, Dillon W: A CT-clinical approach to patients with symptoms related to the V, VII, IX–XII cranial nerves and cervical sympathetics. *Radiology* 151:671–676, 1984.

On pulsatile tinnitus:

Levine SB, Show JB: Pulsatile tinnitus. *Laryngoscope* 97:401–406, 1987.

On acoustic neuromas:

House JW, Waluch V, Jackler RK: Magnetic resonance imaging in acoustic neuroma diagnosis. *Ann Otol Rhinol Laryngol* 95:16–20, 1986.

Valvassori GE, Morales FG, Palacios E, et al: MR of the normal and abnormal internal auditory canal. *AJNR* 9:115–119, 1988.

On evaluation of congenital anomalies:

Jahrsdoerfer RA, Yeakley JW, Hall JW, et al: High-resolution CT scanning and auditory brain stem response in congenital aural atresia: patient selection and surgical correlation. *Otolaryngol Head Neck Surg* 93:292–298, 1985.

Swartz JD, Faerber EN: Congenital malformations of the external and middle ear: high-resolution CT findings of surgical import. *AJR* 144:501–506, 1985.

On precochlear implant evaluation:

Harnsberger HR, Dart DJ, Parkin JL, et al: Cochlear implant candidates: assessment with CT and MR imaging. *Radiology* 164:53–57, 1987.

Jackler RK, Luxford WM, Schindler RA, et al: Cochlear patency problems in cochlear implantation. *Laryngoscope* 97:801–805, 1987.

Mafee MF, Valvassori GE, Deitch RL: Use of CT in the evaluation of cochlear otosclerosis. *Radiology* 156:703–708, 1985.

Rosenberg RA, Cohen NL, Reede DL: Radiographic imaging for the cochlear implant. *Ann Otol Rhinol Laryngol* 96:300–304, 1987.

Swartz JD, Mandell DM, Faerber EN: Labyrinthine ossification: etiologies and CT findings. *Radiology* 157:395–398, 1985.

Miscellaneous:

Rosenberg RA, Hammerschlag PE, Cohen NL, et at: Cholesteatoma vs. cholesterol granuloma of the petrous apex. *Otolaryngol Head Neck Surg* 94:322–327, 1986.

6

Nasopharynx, Parapharyngeal Space, Skull Base, Cranial Nerves V and IX–XII, and Sympathetics

INDICATIONS

The skull base and nasopharynx form a crossroads between classical neuroradiology and the newer subspecialty of head and neck radiology, which deals more with the extracranial head and neck. It is at this juncture that the regional anatomy becomes extraordinarily complex, clinical situations overlap, and millimeters often make a substantial difference in diagnosis and management. The complexity of the clinical-diagnostic situation can lead to a high rate of significant error for the inexperienced or unwary observer. General indications for studies in this area are listed in Table 6.1.

Magnetic resonance imaging has become a primary tool for many indications this region because the pathology here may arise in or affect the brainstem, cerebellum, cisterns of the posterior fossa, skull base, and structures below the skull base (see Tables 6.2 through 6.9). Magnetic resonance imaging is well suited to the task of imaging this region because of its capacity to resolve subtle intra-axial pathology, show tumor-muscle interfaces, and demonstrate cisterns of the posterior fossa—all in multiple planes. It does not typically suffer the motion degradation in these areas that occurs so frequently in the oropharynx, hypopharynx, and larynx. Computed tomography does provide better bone detail, but MRI is sensitive to skull base involvement and CT need only be used as a supplement to MRI for detection of subtle bone destruction or further characterization of a lesion of uncertain etiology. Computed tomography is better than MRI for staging cervical metastatic disease, but this is less critical in nasopharyngeal cancer metastases than in those from other primary sites since the neck is always presumed to be involved and usually managed with radiation therapy alone in patients with primary nasopharyngeal carcinoma. Magnetic resonance imaging provides a reasonable screening-type staging of the neck, and supplemental CT can be used whenever necessary to clarify details that might aid therapeutic decisions (e.g., subtle evidence of capsular penetration and extranodal spread that might require combined radiation therapy and surgical management).

Juvenile angiofibromas and paragangliomas are two relatively common lesions that involve the nasopharynx, skull base, and parapharyngeal space. Both of these tumors are highly vascular. Magnetic resonance imaging can identify the flow void in larger feeding vessels of these and other "vascular" lesions; however, its sensitivity in this regard is unknown and it certainly does *not* eliminate the need for confirmatory angiography in many cases. Flow-sensitive techniques such as gradient echo combined with 3DFT acquisition may improve the ability of MRI to establish the high-flow nature of a lesion. Contrast-enhanced CT with dynamic techniques can strongly suggest a high-flow lesion but also only replaces angiography in selected cases. Even with this limi-

Table 6.1
Indications for CT-MRI of the Nasopharynx, Parapharyngeal Space, Skull Base, Cranial Nerves V and IX–XII, and Sympathetics[a]

By disease category:
Congenital
choanal atresia (CT)
skull base anomalies—bone detail (CT)
skull base anomalies with meningoencephalocele, etc. (MRI)[b]
Inflammatory (CT)
abscess versus cellulitis—parapharyngeal, retropharyngeal, masticator spaces
malignant otitis externa, rhinocerebral mucormycosis or aspergillosis
Tumor—benign and malignant
histology known, ? extent (MRI)
? histology and/or site of origin (MRI)
? subtle skull base destruction, MRI negative (CT)
post-therapy, ? recurrence (MRI)
By clinical presentation:
Mass—? site of origin, etiology and extent (MRI; CT if bone detail is necesary)
Any specific cranial nerve deficit (MRI)
Trigeminal neuralgia—atypical facial pain (MRI)
Otalgia (CT)
Trismus (CT or MRI)
Glossopharyngeal neuralgia (MRI)
Vocal cord paresis (MRI)
Swallowing difficulties without pain (MRI)
Horner's syndrome (MRI)
Unilateral serous otitis media unresponsive to medical management (MRI)
Metastatic cervical adenopathy, mid and upper neck, ? primary site (CT)
Sleep apnea (MRI)

[a]Study in parentheses suggested as the one to begin with for specific indication.
[b]CT with positive contrast cisternography might be necessary.

tation MRI remains a reasonable first choice for evaluating parapharyngeal masses; the coronal images are extremely useful for preoperative planning. Computed tomography and/or angiography should be used for *initial* diagnosis and management decisions whenever the need arises. Magnetic resonance imaging alone can then frequently be used for follow-up.

Cranial nerves V and IX–XII and the cervical sympathetics wind their way from the brainstem, through the skull base, and finally on to the entire head and neck region (of course in the reverse direction for the sympathetics) (Tables 6.3 through 6.9). Magnetic resonance imaging is ideally suited to the evaluation of patients presenting with symptomatology referable to the origins and entire course of the cranial nerves and upper sympathetic trunk. It is very important to triage these patients so that unnecessary studies are avoided and necessary ones are properly focused. Diagnostic algorithms and suggestions for triage are presented in Tables 6.3 through 6.9. These are meant to be guidelines and certainly can be modified to fit shifting technological capabilities and different practice settings. It is, however, extraordinarily important to have this or a similar approach so that all anatomic regions of interest in patients with cranial nerve deficits, especially those beyond the skull base, are examined completely.

It should be apparent that CT and MRI are exceptional imaging tools for the problems just discussed. They do not, however, make histologic diagnoses (except for lipomas). They often narrow the potentially broad differential diagnosis (Table 6.2) to two choices and frequently suggest but one plausible diagnosis when viewed in the entire clinical context. Computed tomography- or MRI-guided aspiration biopsy may be used for histologic confirmation in cases in which surgical confirmation might prove difficult or unnecessarily morbid (see Chapter 1). In confirmation of paragangliomas, juvenile angiofibromas, and other highly vascular lesions angiography may be considered the "biopsy" in some cases. The keys to evaluating problems in this region are a sound algorithmic approach, good clinical information, and a clear working knowledge of the anatomy and pathology.

Table 6.2
Differential Diagnosis of Parapharyngeal and Deep Face Masses by Site of Origin

Parapharyngeal space (prestyloid)
- Congenital—atypical second branchial cleft cyst
- Inflammatory—abscess, cellulitis, malignant otitis externa, mucormycosis, parasitic cysts
- Benign tumor—mixed tumor from minor salivary glands or deep lobe of parotid, neural origin, lipoma, hemanigioma, fibrous origin, leiomyoma
- Malignant tumor—carcinoma of minor salivary gland or deep lobe parotid origin, squamous cell carcinoma, sarcoma (rhabdomyosarcoma), lymphoma, neuroblastoma, metastases to retropharyngeal node

Parapharyngeal space (poststyloid, carotid sheath)
- Inflammatory—abscess, cellulitis, malignant otitis externa, mucormycosis (and other fungi)
- Benign tumors—paraganglioma, neural origin, lipoma, meningioma
- Malignant tumors—metastases to retropharyngeal node, squamous cell carcinoma, lymphoma, neuroblastoma, sarcoma (neural origin)
- Vascular—tortuous carotid, carotid aneurysm, arteriovenous malformation

Infratemporal fossa and masticator space
- Inflammatory—odontogenic cellulitis, abscess, parasitic cysts, mucormycosis
- Benign tumor—neural origin, lipoma, leiomyoma, hemangioma
- Malignant tumor—spread from oropharyngeal/oral cavity squamous cell carcinoma, sarcoma (MFH, rhabdomyosarcoma, neural origin), lymphoma, minor salivary gland carcinoma

Retropharyngeal space
- Inflammatory—cellulitis/abscess, reactive noninfected fluid collections, reactive adenopathy (retropharyngeal nodes)
- Benign tumor—lipoma
- Malignant tumor—retropharyngeal nodal metastases (squamous cell carcinoma, lymphoma, others are rare)
- Vascular—hematoma, tortuous carotid, carotid aneurysm, arteriovenous malformation

Prevertebral space
- Inflammatory—cellulitis/abscess pyogenic or tubercular from vertebral osteomyelitis-diskitis
- Benign tumor—osseous origin (osteoblastoma, aneurysmal bone cyst), chordoma
- Malignant tumor—vertebral metastasis, primary bone tumor (Ewing's sarcoma, myeloma)
- Vascular—vertebral artery aneurysm, arteriovenous malformation
- Traumatic/degenerative—large osteophytes

Table 6.3
Trigeminal Nerve—Clinical Triage

High Yield	Low Yield
Atypical facial pain Progressive history Multiple cranial nerves involved Additional symptoms (e.g., trismus, otalgia) "Hard" supportive neurologic findings Prior history of cancer (e.g., skin of face, remote sites)	Typical trigeminal neuralgia[a] Stable complaints Strictly subjective complaints with vague localization Otherwise negative past medical history Likely myofacial, temporomandibular joint, or tension headache patient[b]

[a]Even though low yield, patients with typical "tic douloureux" should be studied especially if rhizotomy is planned.
[b]It is often difficult to decide if this group of patients warrants imaging—a stable versus progressive history is usually the best determinant.

Table 6.4
Trigeminal Neuralgia—Imaging after Clinical Triage[a]

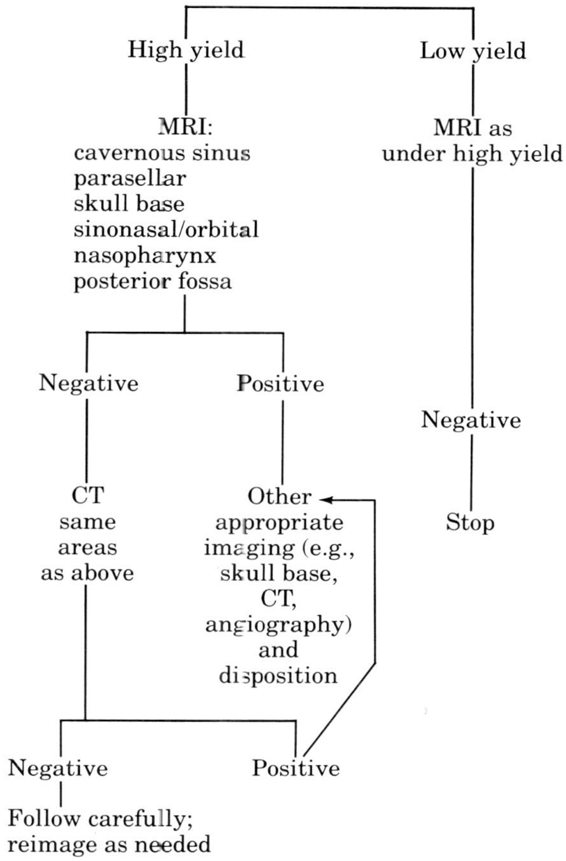

[a]High and low yield criteria are outlined in Table 6.3.

Table 6.5
Cranial Nerves IX–XII—Clinical Triage

High Yield	Low Yield
More than one nerve affected	Otalgia that is stable or indistinguishable from myofacial pain, temporomandibular joint syndromes
"Hard" neurologic findings	Isolated vocal cord paresis
Progressive history	Lack of associated findings
Past history of treated malignancy	Complaints stable—i.e., not progressive
Progressive otalgia with other symptoms (e.g., dysphagia) or smoking, alcohol abuse	Negative past medical history
Vocal cord paresis with associated findings (e.g., brachial plexopathy, other cranial nerves out)	

Table 6.6
Cranial Nerves IX–XII—Imaging after Clinical Triage

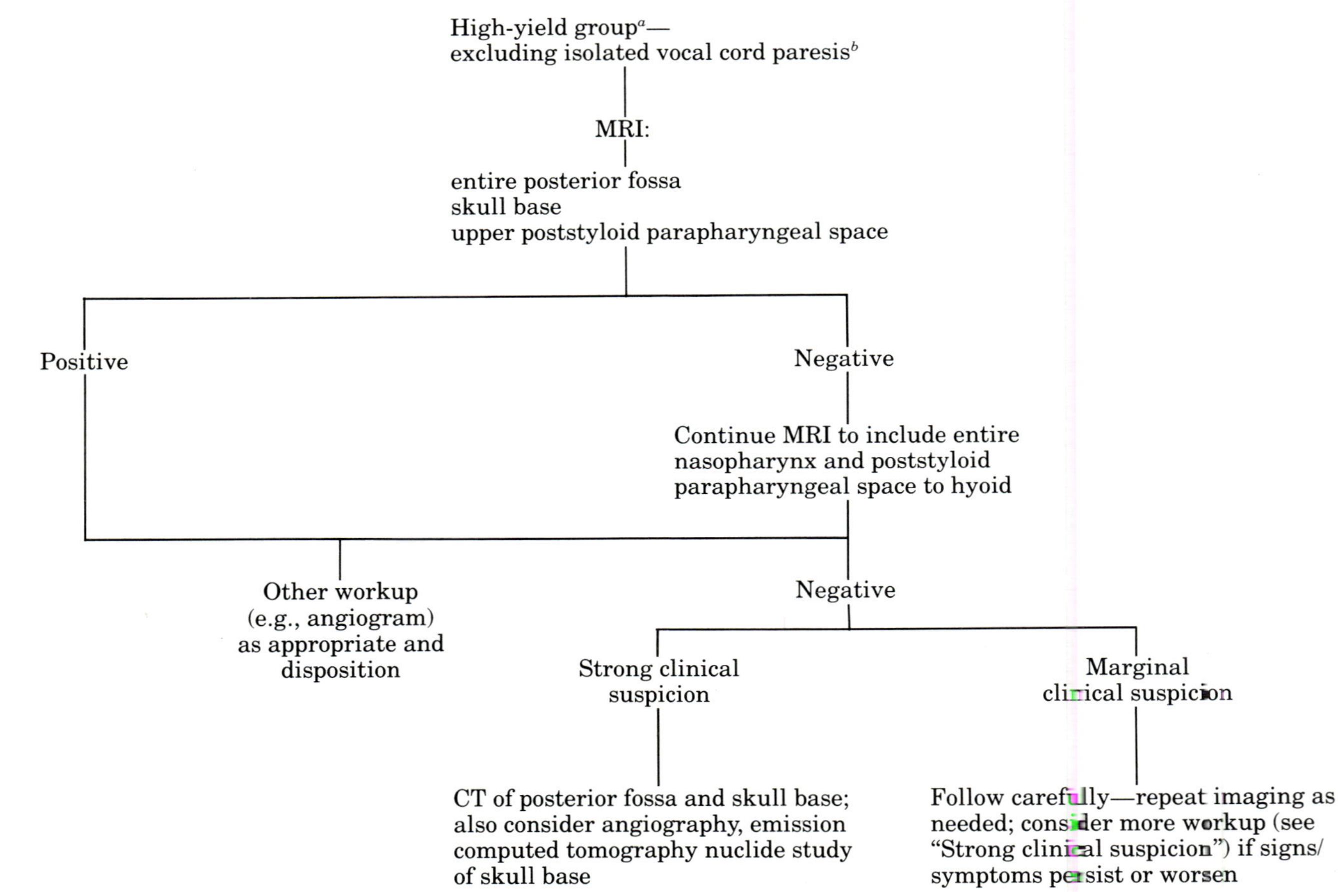

[a]See Table 6.5 for triage to high- and low-yield groups.
[b]See separate algorithm (Table 6.7) for vocal cord paresis.

Table 6.7
Imaging Patients with Vocal Cord Paresis of Uncertain Etiology

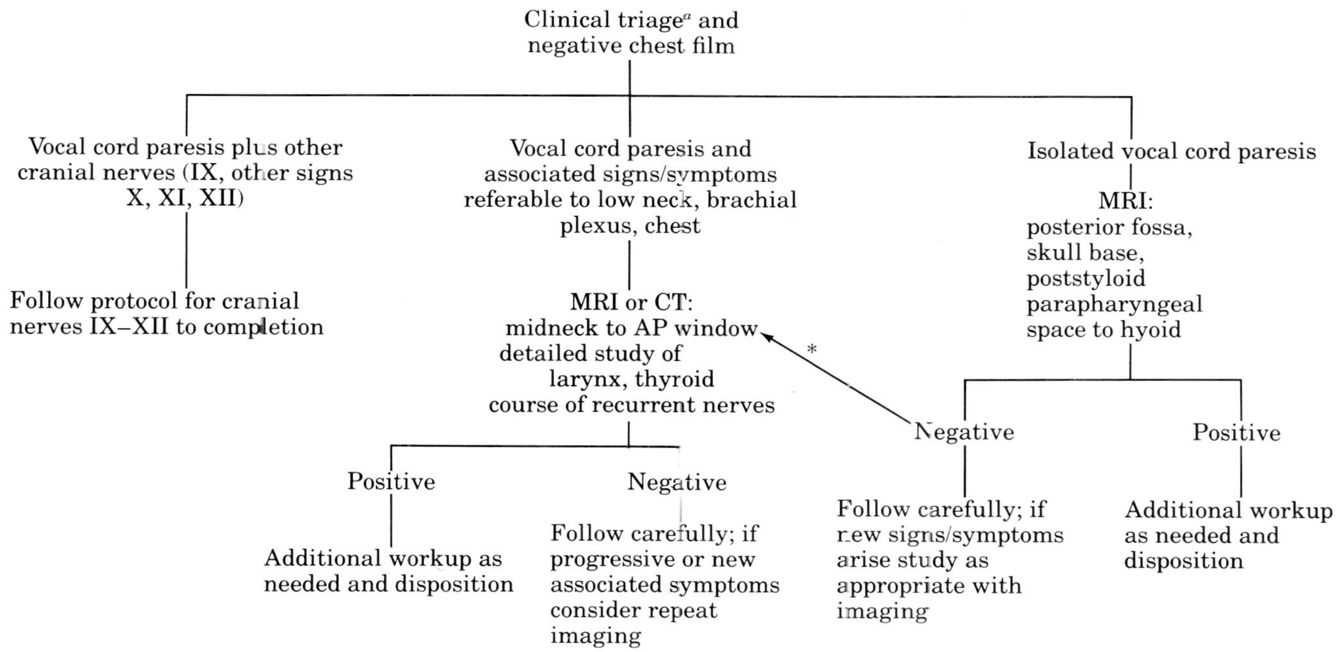

[a]See Table 6.6; this also assumes complete cranial nerve exam and indirect laryngoscopy have been performed by competent observers.
*Imaging in isolated, "idiopathic" vocal cord paresis is a low-yield situation; this part of pathway is optional and must be evaluated on a cost-benefit basis in individual patients.

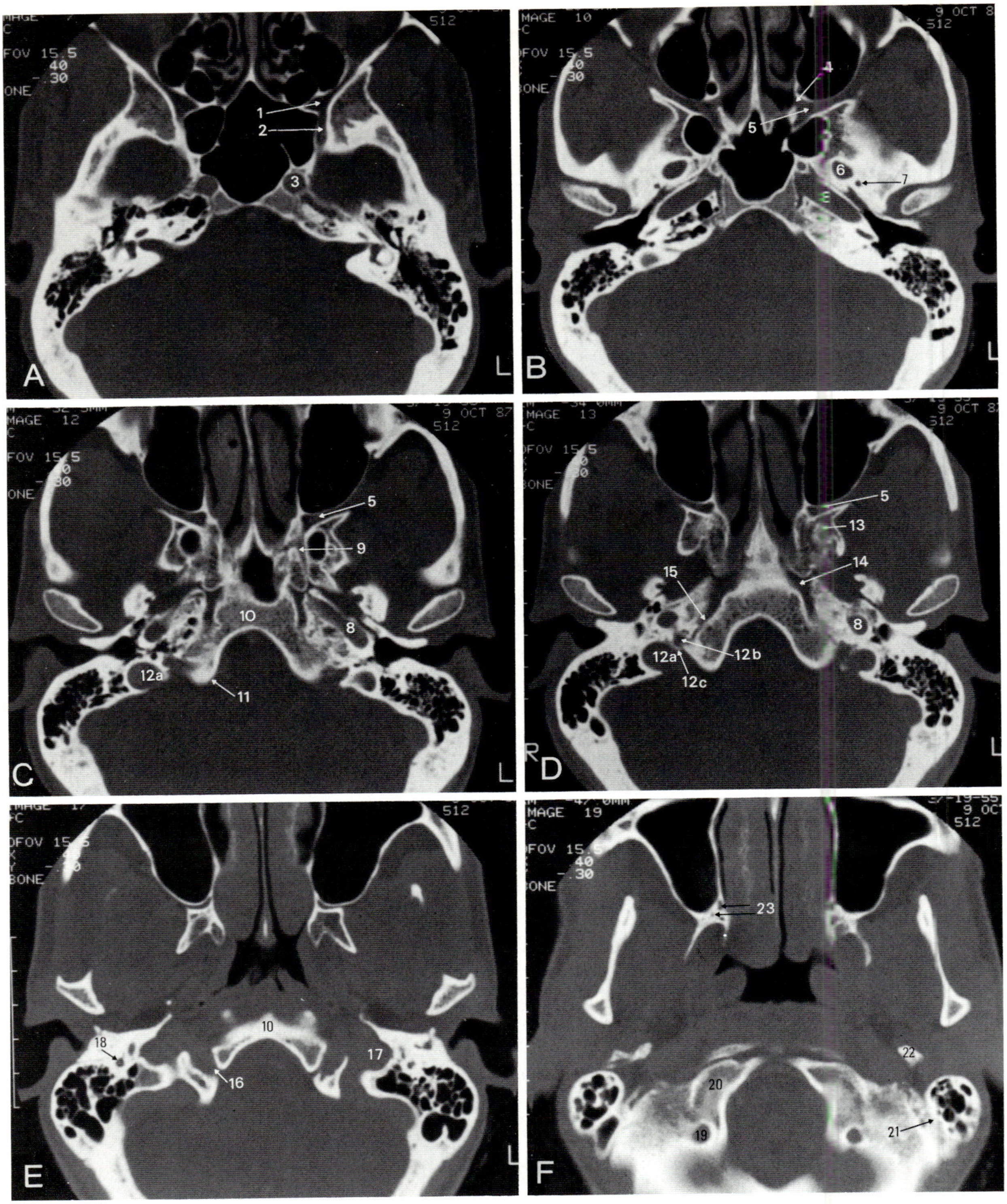

Figure 6.3*A–F*

Figure 6.3*A–F*. Key: *1,* inferior orbital fissure; *2,* foramen rotundum; *3,* carotid; *4,* sphenopalatine foramen; *5,* pterygomaxillary fossa; *6,* foramen ovale; *7,* foramen spinosum; *8,* carotid canal; *9,* Vidian canal; *10,* clivus; *11,* jugular tubercle; *12a,* jugular fossa–pars vascularis; *12b,* jugular fossa–pars nervosa; *12c,* jugular "spur"; *13,* pterygoid process; *14,* foramen lacerum region; *15,* petro-occipital fissure; *16,* hypoglossal canal; *17,* jugular foramen; *18,* stylomastoid foramen; *19,* condylar canal; *20,* occipital condyle; *21,* mastoid notch (digastric groove); *22,* styloid process; *23,* course of nerves from greater and lesser palatine foramina.

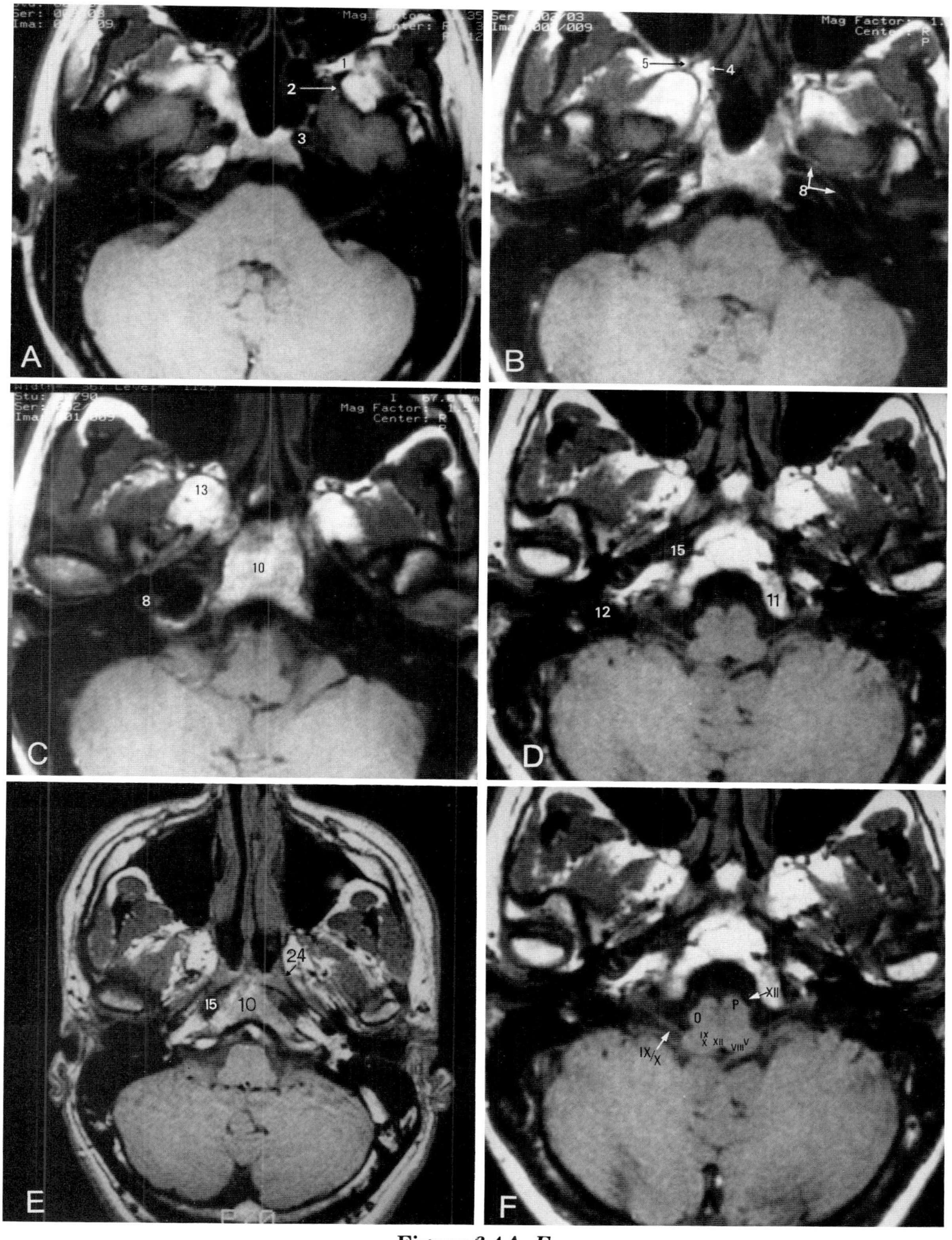

Figure 6.4*A–F*

Figure 6.4*A–F*. Key: *1,* inferior orbital fissure; *2,* foramen rotundum; *3,* carotid; *4,* sphenopalatine foramen; *5,* pterygopalatine fossa; *8,* carotid canal; *10,* clivus; *11,* jugular tubercle; *12,* jugular fossa; *13,* pterygoid process; *15,* petro-occipital fissure; *24,* pharyngobasilar fascia; *o,* olive; *P,* pyramid; *V,* medullary portion of sensory nucleus of trigeminal nerve; *VIII,* lower aspect of vestibular nucleus; *IX,* glossopharyngeal nucleus and cisternal course of nerve; *X,* vagal nuclei and cisternal course of nerve; *XII,* hypoglossal nucleus and cisternal course of nerve.

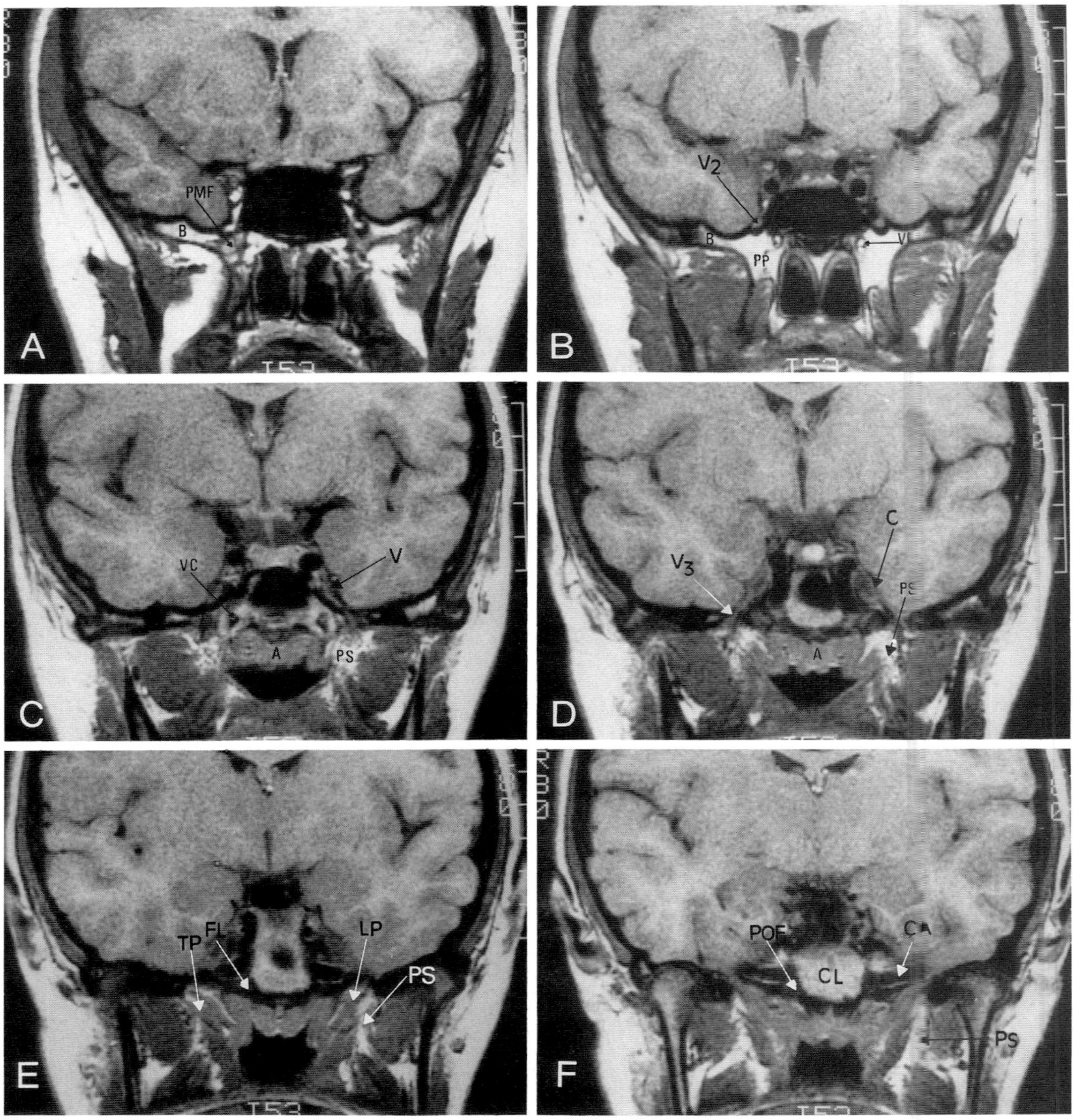

Figure 6.5*A–F*

Figure 6.5*A–F*. Key: *PMF,* pterygomandibular fossa; *B,* basisphenoid (floor middle cranial fossa); *PP,* pterygoid process; *VC,* Vidian canal; V_2, second division of trigeminal nerve in foramen rotundum; *V,* trigeminal ganglion in cavernous sinus; *PS,* parapharyngeal space; *A,* adenoidal pad; V_3, third division of trigeminal nerve in foramen ovale; *C,* cistern of trigeminal nerve and ganglion; *FL,* foramen lacerum; *TP,* tensor veli palatini muscle; *LP,* levator veli palatini muscle; *CA,* carotid artery (in carotid canal); *CL,* clivus; *POF,* petro-occipital fissure.

CASES

Use checklists in Appendix A to analyze the following cases.

Problem I

(Case histories and questions on p. 139)

Case 6.1 (Fig. 6.6*A–D*)

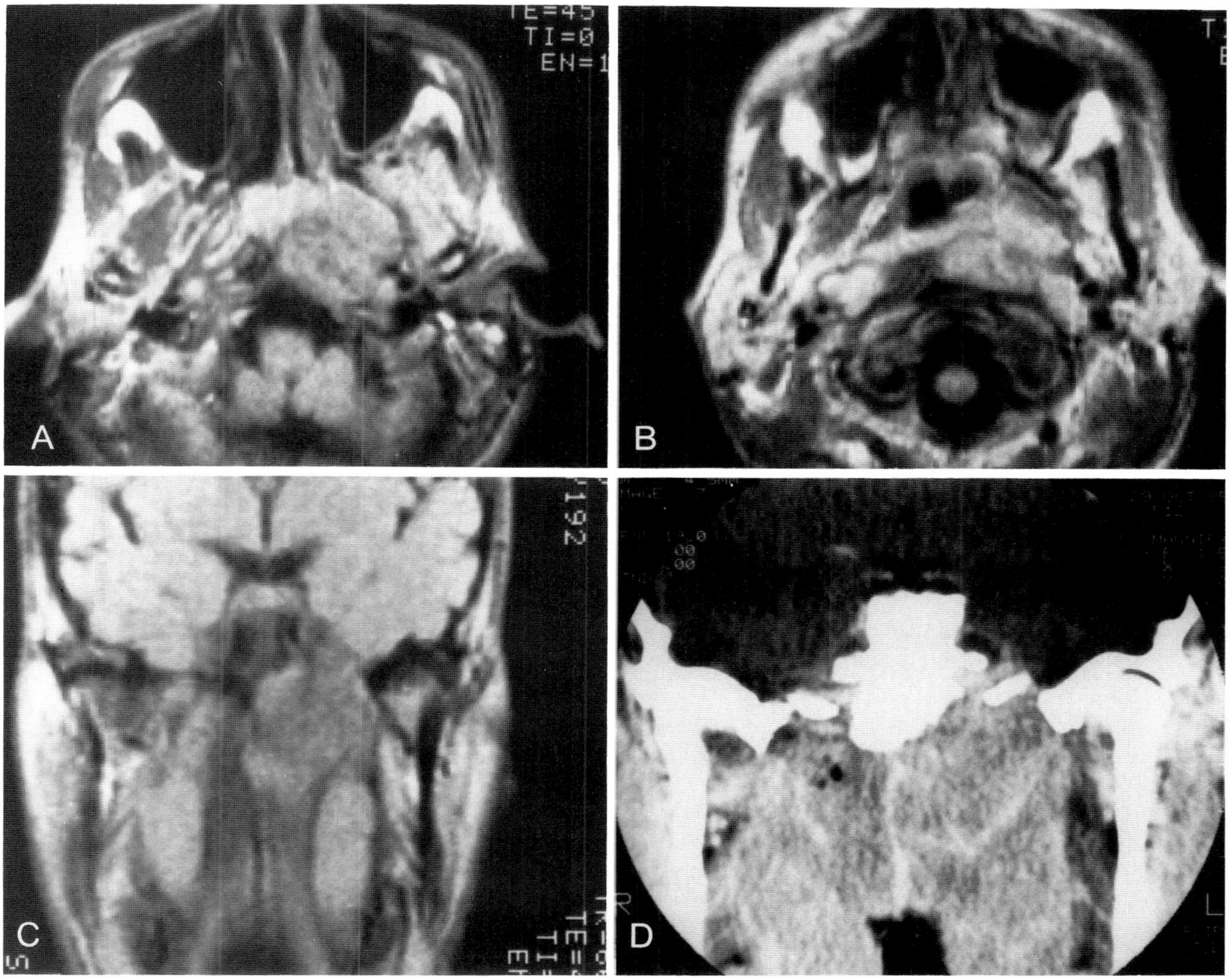

Figure 6.6*A–D*

Case 6.2 (Fig. 6.7*A–D*)

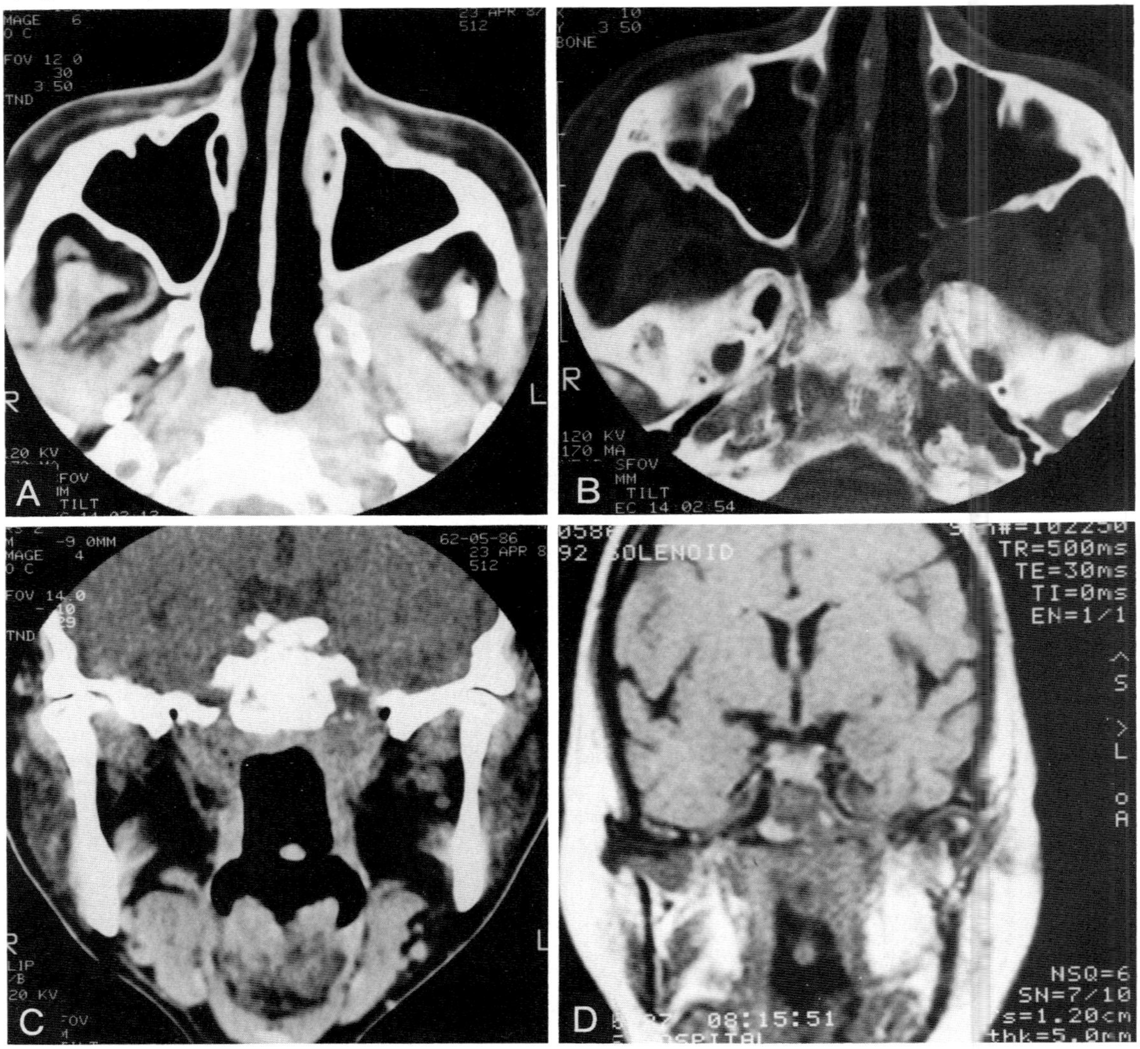

Figure 6.7*A–D*

Case 6.3 (Fig. 6.8*A–D*)

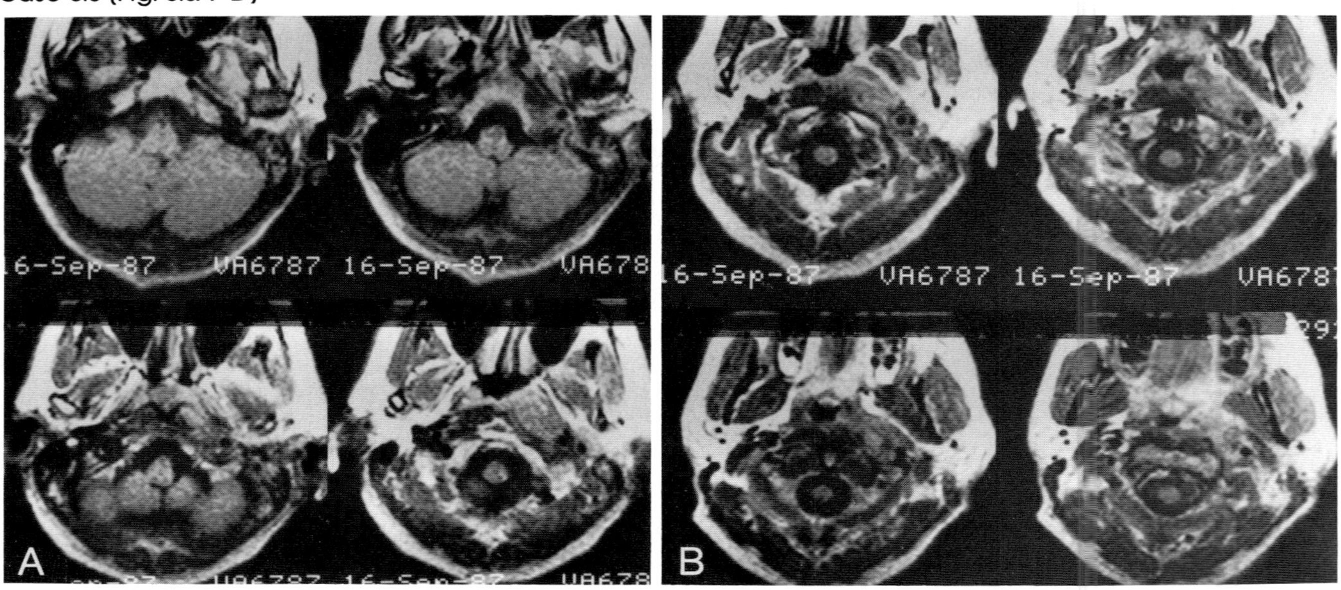

Figure 6.8*A* and *B*

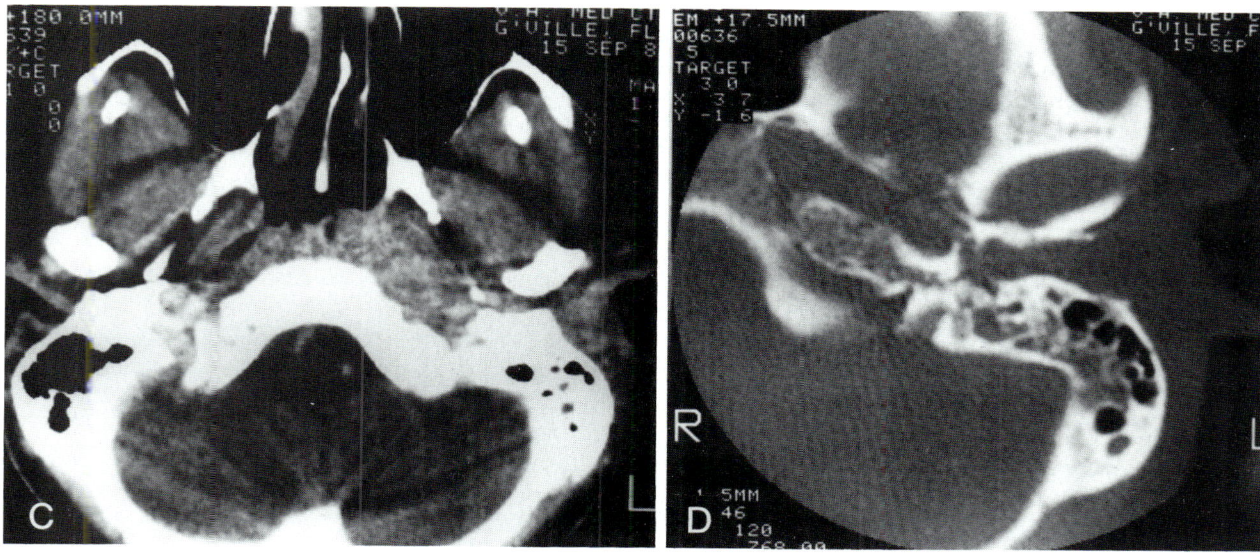

Figure 6.8*C* and *D*

Case Histories

Case 6.1 A 35-year-old male with left serous otitis media, facial pain, and failure to elevate left side of palate.

Case 6.2 A 65-year-old woman with left-sided facial pain and numbness

Case 6.3 A 78-year-old male with a mass around the external auditory canal.

Questions

1. Explain why patients in Cases 6.1 and 6.2 have facial pain and in what dermatome(s) it is likely distributed.
2. Give three reasons why the patient in Case 6.1 might not be able to elevate his palate. Why is there serous otitis media?
3. The patient in Case 6.3 was noted to have multiple cranial nerve deficits after the CT and MRI were done. Predict which were out and give the reason why.
4. If you had just one acquisition to use in a known nasopharyngeal lesion, what would you do?
5. Give your best diagnosis in each case. One of the patients is diabetic. Which one?
6. Anatomic issue: What goes *through* the foramen lacerum?

Discussion

Problem I—Clinical Presentations of Nasopharyngeal Pathology Both patients 1 and 2 have infiltrating masses that involve the skull base, which can produce headaches and deep facial pain. Both processes also involve the course of the second, and in patient 1 the third, division of the trigeminal nerve (Question 1). Dermatomes involved would likely correspond to those nerves. In Case 6.1 the mass also involves the pharyngeal wall musculature and is quite bulky. There are associated retropharyngeal nodes that might compress any of cranial nerves IX through XII and the sympathetics. Each of these circumstances could lead to failure of palatal elevation (Question 2). The serous otitis media may be due to eustachian tube dysfunction and/or obstruction.

Careful review of the findings in Case 6.3 (outlined in the checklist below) shows that the mass in the external auditory canal was only the "tip of an iceberg." Infiltrating mass had spread to just below the stylomastoid foramen (VIIth nerve) as well as the skull base, jugular fossa, and poststyloid parapharyngeal space (nerves IX through XII and sympathetics). Mild VIIth, Xth, and XIIth nerve deficits were confirmed (Question 3).

A coronal, relatively T^1-weighted image would be the best single pulse sequence for evaluating nasopharynx. This would allow for evaluation of the skull base and cavernous sinus as well as cephalocaudal and medial-lateral extent of tumor. It would also allow for a gross assessment of whether the lesion might be vascular (see Chapter 1) (Question 4).

Case 6.1 is a straightforward carcinoma of the nasopharynx with skull base invasion and bilateral retropharyngeal adenopathy. Case 6.3 is a highly unusual spread pattern of nasopharyngeal cancer. This may have been a primary in the eustachian tube. This case could have been mistaken for a diabetic with malignant otitis externa. The patient in Case 6.2 is actually the diabetic with invasive mucormycosis in the sphenoid sinus, pterygopalatine fossa, and nasopharynx. Considered inoperable, she was given amphotericin and hyperbaric treatment. A recent gallium single-photon emission computed tomography exam showed no evidence of active inflammation and CT findings have been stable for 12 months.

Anatomic Issue: The Foramen Lacerum This "foramen" is in fact plugged with cartilage in life. The carotid artery courses above it rather than through it (the latter is a common misconception). The area around the foramen lacerum, however, is a favored point of attack of nasopharyngeal carcinoma. The mucosa at the top of the fossa of Rosenmueller lies just subjacent to this part of the skull base, as does the fat of the upper prestyloid parapharyngeal space. The tensor and levator veli palatini muscles take origin from this region. Cancer follows each of these paths to invade the skull base in and about the petroclival junction and foramen lacerum region. Lymphomas, on the other hand, seem to spread along the carotid, within the carotid canal, while eroding bone in this region. Eventually such tumors reach the cavernous sinus via these routes. Only small, distal branches of the ascending pharyngeal artery and some sympathetic nerves normally go *through* the foramen lacerum.

CHECKLIST—NASOPHARYNX (CASE 6.3)

	Seen	Nl	Abnl	Remarks
HIGH Skull Base and Middle Cranial Fossa Parasellar—cavernous sinus	√	√		
Sphenoid sinus	√	√		
Foramen lacerum	No			
Foramen ovale	No			
Inferior petrous apex—carotid foramen and canal			√	Infiltrating mass around carotid
Petroclival junction			√	Infiltrated—eroded posteriorly
Clivus			√	Early erosion left side
Jugular foramen		√		
Superior and inferior orbital fissures		√		Inferior normal; superior not seen
Sphenopalatine foramen		√		
Pterygopalatine fossa		√		
Pterygoid processes (base)		√		
Temporomandibular joints		√		
Middle ear			√	Opacified, ? invaded
Mastoid			√	Probable mucosal thickening
Facial nerve canal—descending portion		√		
Deep Origins of tensor and levator veli palatini muscles			√	Probably infiltrated
Parapharyngeal space			√	Infiltrated on left
Pharyngobasilar fascia			√	Infiltrated on left
Infratemporal fossa and masticator space (temporalis and lateral pterygoid muscles)		√		
Other Nasal cavity		√		
MID Superficial Soft Tissues Eustachian tube orifice			√	Involved with mass from deep aspect
Torus tubarius			?	? Involved with mass from deep aspect
Lateral pharyngeal recesses			√	Infiltrated from deep aspect
Adenoidal tissue			√	Probable tumor on left
Deep Structures and Spaces Tensor and levator veli palatini muscles			√	Infiltrated
Parapharyngeal space			√	Infiltrated
Infratemporal fossa and masticator space (medial pterygoids)		√		
Prevertebral muscles				Infiltrated on left
Retropharyngeal nodes			√	Enlarged on left
Carotid sheath (poststyloid parapharyngeal space)			√	Infiltrated on left
Pterygoid plates		√		
Pterygopalatine fossa		√		

continued

CHECKLIST—NASOPHARYNX (CASE 6.3) *continued)*

	Seen	Nl	Abnl	Remarks
Other Nasal cavity		√		
Maxillary sinuses		√		
Mandible		√		
Deep portion of parotid			√	Minimally infiltrated
Clivus			√	Early erosion left
Stylomastoid foramen		√		but tumor very close
Mastoid tip			?	
Foramen magnum		√		
LOWER Superficial Soft Tissues Soft palate		√		
Adenoidal tissue			√	Invaded on deep aspect
Deep Structures and Spaces Levator veli palatini and pharyngeal wall musculature			√	Infiltrated on left
Parapharyngeal space			√	Infiltrated on left
Infratemporal fossa and masticator space (medial pterygoid muscle)		√		
Pterygoid plates		√		
Buccinator space		√		
Carotid sheath			√	Infiltrated on left
Prevertebral muscles			√	Infiltrated on left
Retropharyngeal nodes			√	Enlarged on left
Other Parotid (deep and superficial portions)		√		
Maxillary sinuses		√		
C_1 and spinal canal		√		
Mandible		√		

Problem II
(Case histories and questions on p. 144)

Case 6.4 (Fig. 6.9*A–E*)

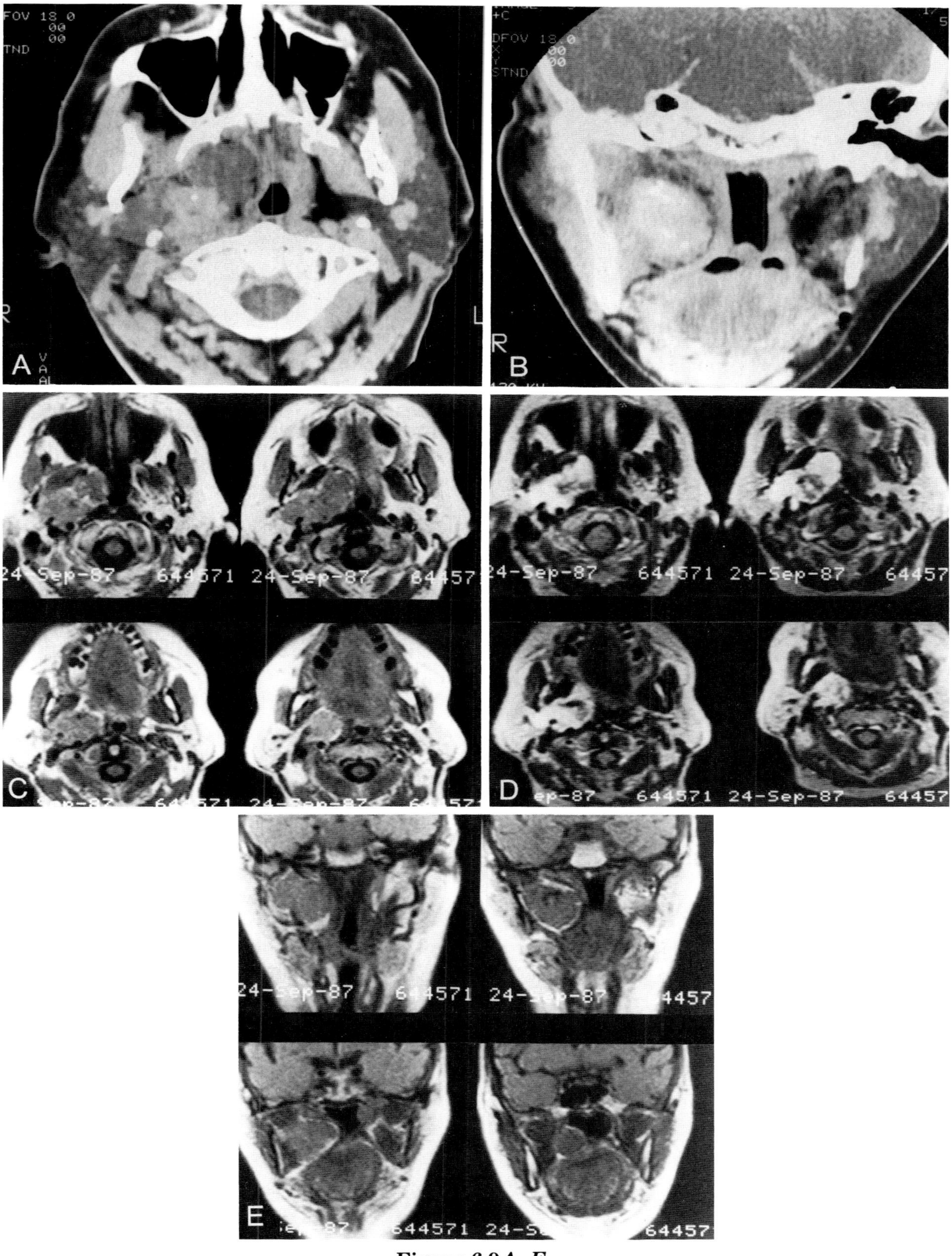

Figure 6.9*A–E*

Cases

Use checklists in Appendix A to analyze the following cases.

Problem I

Case 7.1 (Fig. 7.5 *A* and *B*)

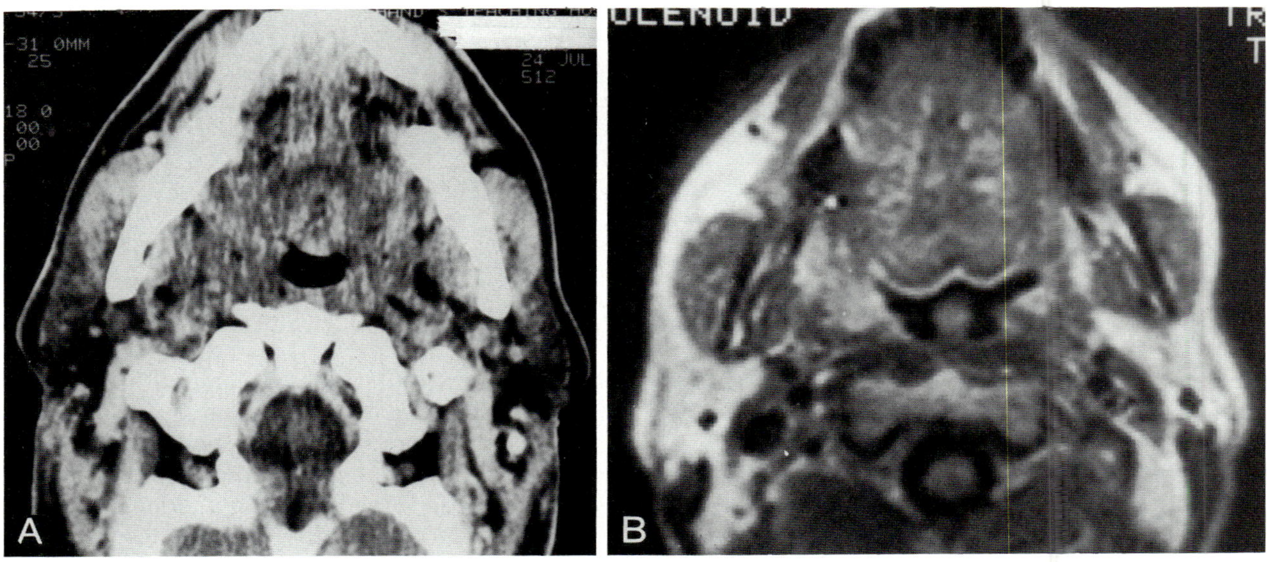

Figure 7.5 *A* and *B*

Case History

Case 7.1 A 54-year-old male with a 3-month history of an enlarged right upper neck node and, upon detailed questioning, mild, intermittent otalgia. Needle biopsy of the node showed squamous cell carcinoma. Complete exam by expert head and neck surgeons showed no evidence of primary tumor.

Questions

1. Name four common modes of clinical presentation of patients with clinically inapparent (on careful physical exam) malignancies of the upper aerodigestive tract.
2. Name the four most common sites of origin of these so-called occult primary tumors.
3. State your diagnoses for Case 7.1.
4. Anatomic issue: How do you deal with the marked amount of superficial assymmetry visible on scans through the oropharynx?

Discussion

Problem I—"Clinically Occult" Primary Tumor Presenting as a Neck Node and Otalgia The patient in Case 7.1 has a deeply infiltrating mass in the right glossotonsillar sulcus manifest by extension into the parapharyngeal space through the superior constrictor muscle (Question 3). The finding is a little more obvious on MRI and it is our practice to confirm subtle CT findings with supplemental MRI in such cases. This patient went on to have panendoscopy and speculative biopsies of the nasopharynx, tonsil, tongue base, and pyriform sinus that were negative (read on); these are the most frequent sites of "occult" primary tumors of the upper aerodigestive tract (Question 2). Because of the CT and MRI findings deeper excisional biopsies of the lower pole of the tonsil–glossotonsillar sulcus were done. These revealed squamous cell carcinoma, allowing the patient's subsequent therapy to be properly focused. Occult primary tumors account for a very small percentage of upper aerodigestive tract neoplasia; however, diagnosis is often delayed in spite of compelling clinical findings, because the lesions lie beneath intact mucosal surfaces. These patients may present with cervical metastatic disease, otalgia, atypical facial pain, or specific cranial nerve deficits (Question 1). Precise and focused imaging directed by clear and complete clinical data can help avoid needless delays in diagnosis of such cancers.

Anatomic Issue: Variability of Superficial Soft Tissues of the Oropharynx Most of the normal variation seen here is due to aggregates of lymphoid tissue (tonsils) in the faucial tonsils, glossotonsillar sucli, and tongue base–vallecula region. These aggregates may show focal calcification and fluid areas as well as variations in contour. One must look to the deep tissue planes for evidence of significant pathology. Tonsillar masses that break through the superior constrictor to involve the parapharyngeal space are usually cancers. The same is true of those showing focal penetration of the tongue base intrinsic muscles or extension along the mylohyoid muscle or within the sublingual space. By discounting superficial asymmetry and emphasizing careful scrutiny of *deep* tissue planes you will improve your diagnostic accuracy in this region and sometimes add immeasurably to patient care. Poor interpretations here, however, can lead to disenchantment of referring clinicians and potentially increased morbidity. Much practice, meticulous scan techniques, and thorough familiarity with the normal anatomy and normal variations are essential for the best results.

Problem II

(Case history and questions on p. 162)

Case 7.2 (Fig. 7.6 *A–E*)

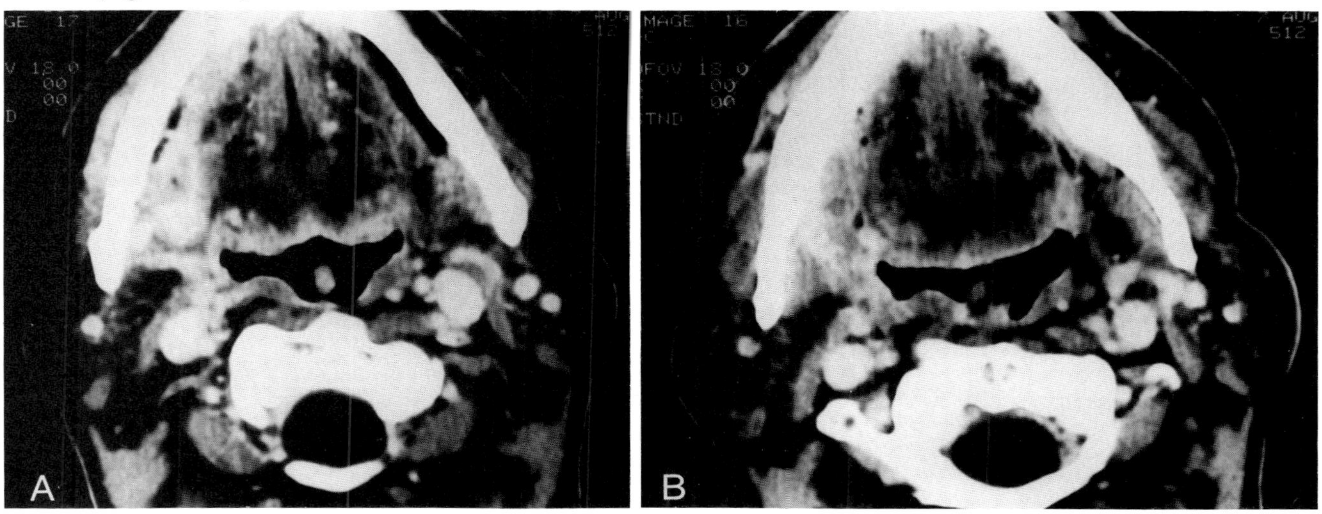

Figure 7.6 *A–B*

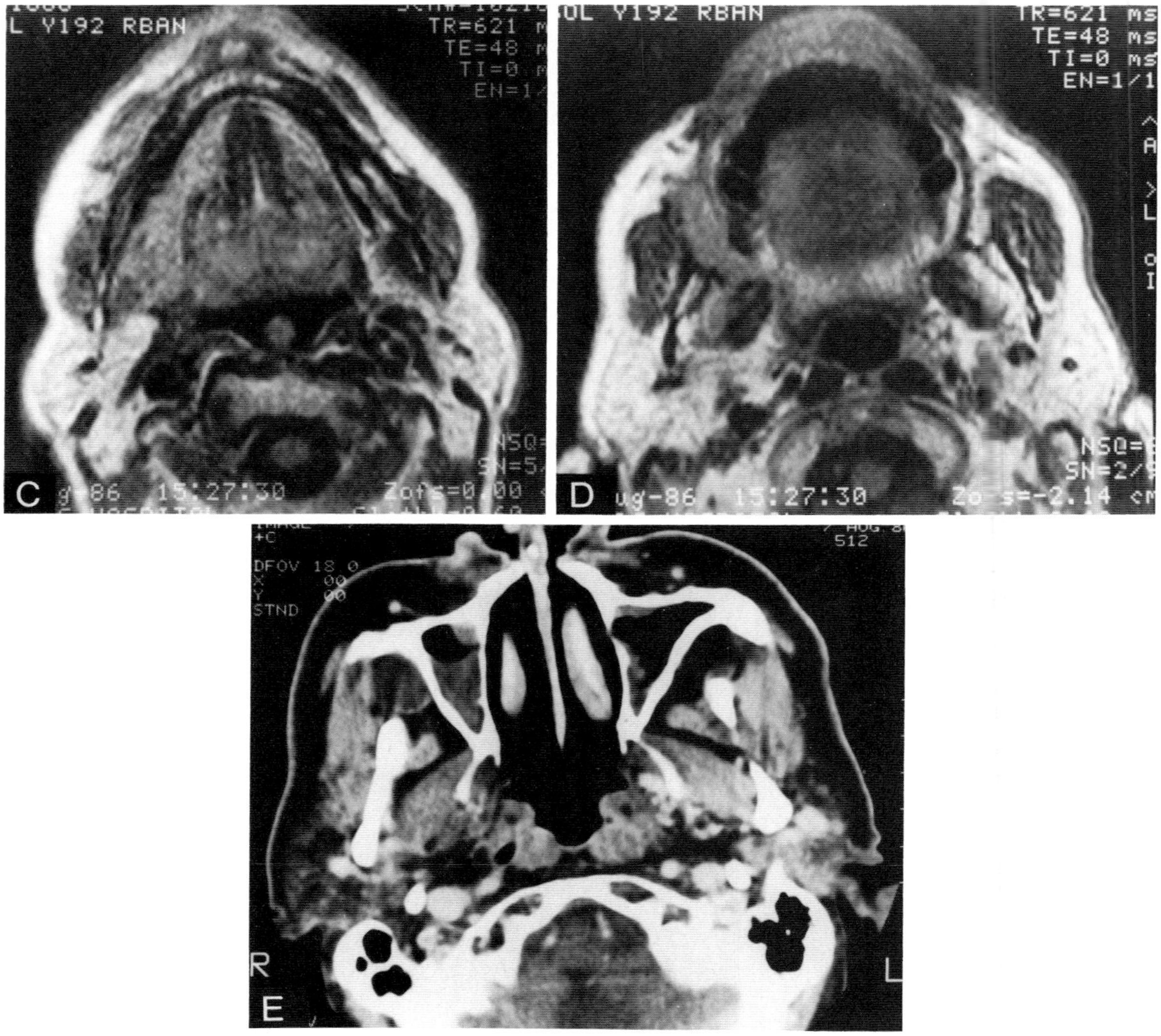

Figure 7.6 *C–E*

Case History

Case 7.2 A 60-year-old male with retromolar trigone carcinoma. Clinically lesion was staged as a "large T2 or small T3." The patient was somewhat anxious and prone to gagging, causing some limitation in the physical exam. Spread along the floor of the mouth was considered to be limited to the area just subjacent to the retromolar trigone.

Questions

1. The patient in Case 7.2 has two findings that significantly altered his surgical management. What are the findings and how might they alter management?
2. Anatomic issue: Describe the origins and extent of the pterygomandibular raphe.

Discussion

Problem II—Retromolar Trigone Cancer Spread Patterns The patient in Case 7.2 has a more advanced retromolar trigone cancer than was apparent clinically. Spread along the mylohyoid went well beyond the point where a segmental mandibular resection at the mental foramen would have provided an adequate margin; a hemimandibulectomy was done. Also the very extensive involvement of the pterygomandibular space predicted that the lingual nerve would need to be sacrificed (see Fig. 7.3). Both these situations were anticipated and this saved operative time as well as possible violation of the tumor during the portion of the procedure when the mandible was resected. The tumor also spread cephalad via the pterygomandibular raphe to involve the buccinator space. It ended just below the maxillary tuberosity, which is the usual upper margin of resection. Sometimes the primary tumor will spread higher than the buccinator space in the retroantral fat, requiring that a formal posterior maxillectomy be added to avoid a positive deep superior margin. In this patient there was a 2-cm buccinator lymph node, which necessitated the posterior maxillectomy for en bloc resection. Involvement of these intercalated lymph nodules is uncommon even in advanced gingivobuccal sulcus, alveolar ridge, and retromolar trigone cancers, but they must be looked for to ensure proper preoperative planning.

Anatomic Issue: The Pterygomandibular Raphe The pterygomandibular raphe forms a line of attachment for the buccinator and superior constrictor muscles; it is the junction of the oral cavity and oropharynx lying between the anterior tonsillar pillar and retromolar trigone (see Fig. 7.3). The raphe extends from the hamulus of the medial pterygoid plate to its attachment on the posteromedial aspects of the mandible just above the posterior edge of the mylohyoid muscle (see Fig. 7.3). More advanced (large T2 to T4) squamous cell carcinoma or other malignancies in this area may grow deep to or along the raphe. This can direct clinically occult cephalad spread to the upper buccinator space–lower infratemporal fossa. Submucosal caudal spread along the raphe to the mylohyoid muscle can result in contiguous occult spread anteriorly along the floor of the mouth or inferiorly to the soft tissues of the neck.

CHECKLIST—ORAL CAVITY, OROPHARYNX, FOM, TONGUE BASE, MANDIBLE (if lesion extends cephalad use nasopharynx checklists as well) (CASE 7.2)

	Seen	Nl	Abnl	Remarks
UPPER				
Superficial Soft Tissues				
Uvula		√		
Soft palate		√		
Tonsillar fossa (faucial tonsils)		√		
Upper gingivobuccal sulcus		√		
Deep Soft Tissues				
Parapharyngeal space		√		
Infratemporal fossa/masticator space			√	Node; tumor between pterygoid muscles/mandible
Oral tongue		√		
Buccinator muscle			√	Infiltrated
Buccinator space			√	Infiltrated
Carotid sheath		√		
Prevertebral muscles		√		
Retropharyngeal nodes		√		
Bones				
Hard palate	No			
Palatine foramina	No			
Pterygoid processes		√		Where seen
Maxillary alveolar ridge		√		
Maxillary tuberosity			?	? Erosion
Mandible (condyle, ramus, coronoid)			√	Tumor in masticator space
Upper cervical spine		√		
Other				
Parotid gland		√		
MID				
Superficial Soft Tissues				
Uvula (tip)		√		
Level of circumvallate papillae		√		
Anterior ⅔ (oral) tongue		√		
Mid-lower tonsillar fossa		√		
Upper glossotonsillar sulcus		√		
Lower gingivobuccal sulcus		√		
Deep Soft Tissues				
Parapharyngeal space			√	Infiltrated
Pterygomandibular space (lingual nerve)			√	Infiltrated
Infratemporal fossa/masticator space			√	Medial pterygoid m. infiltrated
Carotid sheath		√		
Prevertebral muscles		√		
Retropharyngeal nodes		√		
Bones				
Mandibular alveolar ridge	No			
Mandibular ramus, body, foramen			√	Eroded medially
Upper cervical spine		√		
Other				
Parotid (superficial and deep)		√		

continued

CHECKLIST—ORAL CAVITY, OROPHARYNX, FOM, TONGUE BASE, MANDIBLE (CASE 7.2) *(continued)*

	Seen	Nl	Abnl	Remarks
LOWER Superficial Soft Tissues Lower glossotonsillar sulcus		√		
Lingual tonsils		√		
Valleculae		√		
Pharyngoepiglottic folds		√		
Deep Soft Tissues Mylohyoid muscle			√	Almost entirely infiltrated
Genioglossus-geniohyoid muscles		√		Tumor adjacent
Lingual septum		√		
Sublingual space (lingual vessels)			√	Partially infiltrated
Hyoglossus-styloglossus muscles			√	Tumor invades posteriorly mainly styloglossus
Intrinsic tongue muscles (base)		√		
Anterior belly digastric		√		
Posterior belly digastric		√		
Carotid sheath (nodes)		√		
Prevertebral muscles				
Preepiglottic space		√		
Bones Mandible (body/angle)		√		Tumor adjacent
Mental foramen		√		
Hyoid		√		
Other Submandibular gland and space			√	Tumor may involve deep process
Submandibular-submental nodes	No			
Parotid—tail		√		

Case 7.3 (Fig. 7.7 *A–C*)

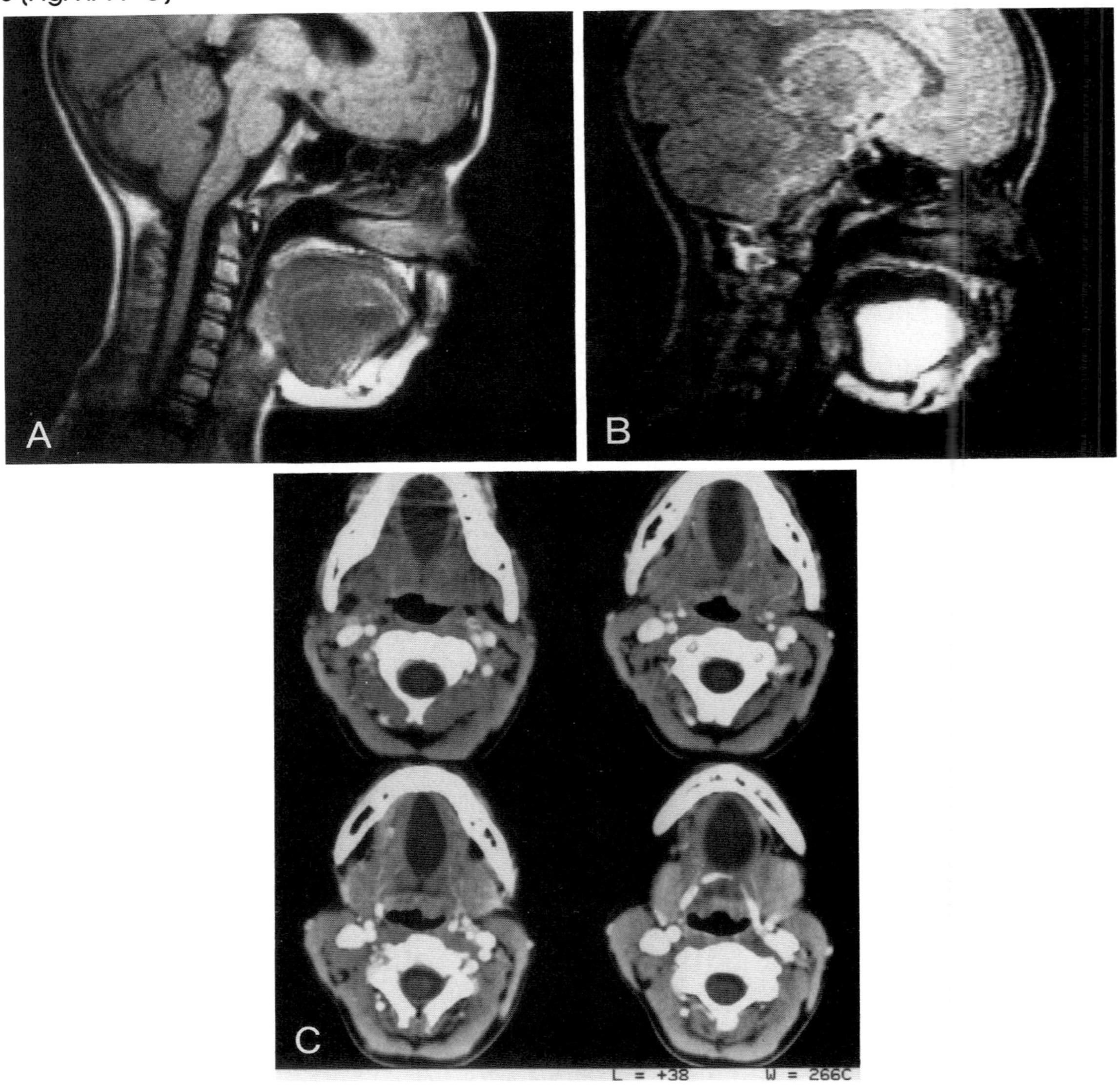

Figure 7.7 *A–C*

Case History

Case 7.3 An 11-year-old female who had a midline mass in the upper neck thought to be a thyroglossal duct cyst by the referring physician.

Questions

1. Do you agree with the suggested diagnosis?
2. Would you prefer CT or MRI for evaluating this particular patient?
3. Anatomic issue: What is the floor of the mouth?

Discussion

Problem III—Benign Masses in the Floor of the Mouth The patient in Case 7.3 does *not* have a thyroglossal duct cyst because this cystic mass lies well anterior to the pathway of the thyroglossal duct. The thyroglossal duct runs from the foramen cecum (midline in the tongue base) through the body of the hyoid bone and on to the thyroid gland. This mass splits the midline extrinsic tongue muscles and basically occupies the floor of the mouth (i.e., lies above the mylohyoid muscle). Its appearance and location suggests epidermoid cyst as the only plausible diagnosis (Question 1).

Magnetic resonance imaging or CT could be used to evaluate such masses, especially in pediatric patients. The usual relative advantages and disadvantages of each study in this situation have been discussed elsewhere (e.g., Chapter 1 and "Indications").

Anatomic Issue: The Floor of the Mouth The floor of the mouth is the mylohyoid muscle. This muscle slopes downward from the mylohyoid line of the mandible, its fibers on either side joining at a midline raphe and its posterior fibers attaching to the hyoid bone. The mouth lies above the mylohyoid muscle, the neck below. The arrangement just described is quite similar to that in the pelvic floor except that the hyoid is mobile to allow for the large movements of the tongue during swallowing. Above the mylohyoid muscle the floor of the mouth is subdivided by the extrinsic tongue muscles. The most obvious subdivisions are the sublingual spaces lying between the geniohyoid-genioglossus complex and the mylohyoid. The sublingual gland, lingual nerve, artery and vein, hypoglossal nerve, and submandibular duct course around and through these spaces and subdivide musculature.

changes suggestive of such spread. The multiplanar capabilities of MRI are potentially useful but not essential for evaluating most laryngeal and hypopharyngeal cancer. With 3-mm sections, proper gantry angle, and other technical "pointers" described subsequently one can almost always definitively evaluate the anterior commissure, subglottic region, and laryngeal ventricle with axial CT sections. Finally, CT is overall a better tool for evaluating cervical and retropharyngeal nodes. For all of these reasons CT remains the primary examination for laryngeal and hypopharyngeal pathology. Even in patients who cannot have iodinated contrast we begin with CT and use MRI only if necessary information seems to be lacking after the noncontrast CT exam.

Computed tomography and MRI provide useful clinical information in patients with cancer. A working knowledge of the spread patterns of laryngeal and hypopharyngeal cancer is most helpful for both supervising and interpreting studies in these patients. Patients with benign masses or traumatic or inflammatory lesions may also benefit for CT or MRI imaging. Specific indications and differential diagnoses are outlined in Tables 8.1 and 8.2.

Table 8.2
Differential Diagnosis of Laryngeal, Perilaryngeal, and Hypopharyngeal Masses

Congenital
Thyroglossal duct cyst, laryngocele
Inflammatory—autoimmune
Abscess, cellulitis, laryngopyocele, laryngocele, tuberculosis, syphilis, rheumatoid nodules, nonspecific granulomas, relapsing perichondritis, amyloidosis
Benign tumors
Hemangioma, enchondroma, paraganglioma (endolaryngeal), minor salivary gland origin, teratoma, lipoma, other mesenchymal origin
Malignant tumors
Squamous cell carcinoma, other carcinomas (minor or salivary gland origin), rhabdomyosarcoma, chondrosarcoma, metastases
Vascular
Tortuous carotid (posterior pharyngeal wall)
Traumatic
Old, displaced fractures that have healed with deformity
Retropharyngeal, prevertebral space origin
Neck origin

TECHNIQUE

Detailed CT protocols are presented by indication in Table 8.3. The larynx and hypopharynx should be studied with the neck comfortably extended. It is *absolutely essential* that the sections be made parallel to the true and false cords and laryngeal ventricle. This level should be identified on a lateral digital radiograph and the proper plane of section chosen. If the true cord, ventricle, or false cord level cannot be identified then the plane parallel to the C_{4-5} or C_{5-6} disk space should be used as an estimate. Scans should be done during breath-holding, so the preliminary digital radiograph should also be obtained at end inspiration. Scanning during breath-holding eliminates motion artifacts but it also causes the true and false cords to be pressed together because many patients will unconsciously perform a mild Valsalva maneuver at end inspiration. If this occurs and is interfering with interpretation then repeat scans in quiet respiration should be made from the false cords to midsubglottis; this will only be necessary in about 10 to 20% of the studies. Contiguous 3- to 4-mm sections are a must from 1 cm above the false cords to the bottom of the cricoid cartilage. Otherwise 3-mm thick by 5-mm increment sections may be used. *No* special maneuvers such as phonation or modified Valsalva are used.

Reformations are rarely more informative than a well-done axial study and if coronal or sagittal planes seem essential reformations or MRI can be done. Intravenous contrast is used in all cancer cases to evaluate both the primary and cervical nodes. It is also used in inflammatory lesions and benign masses but is not necessary for the evaluation of most patients with trauma or subglottic stenosis.

Magnetic resonance imaging should be done with a volume receiver coil especially designed to examine the neck. A half-saddle is a fairly standard approach. Flatter surface coils that have been designed for adequate penetration, such as angled loop gap resonators, may also be sufficient. A solenoid may be used if the main magnetic field is perpendicular to the patient. Whatever the receiver, it should be as well adapted as possible for study of the neck. The neck should be comfortably extended to bring the axial sections as parallel to the plane of the true cords as possible. If oblique angulation is available in software it should be used to ensure this optimal plane of the axial sections; of course, this requires a sagittal midplane preliminary acquisition for planning.

Standard 2DFT, Rf-refocused spin echo pulse sequences are used. Three-dimensional Fourier transform will probably routinely suffer too much motion to be of value in the larynx. Gradient echo techniques potentially provide some latitude for reducing motion artifacts but they are of no proven benefit in this region at this time. Flow-sensitive data from gradient echo techniques are unlikely to be of value in most laryngeal lesions. Gadolinium-DTPA may prove to be of value in patients with laryngeal and hypopharyngeal pathology for evaluating both the primary tumor and nodes. This remains speculative at present and is under study. More specific techniques are as follows:

FOV: 18 to 24 cm
SLT: 5 mm (3 mm in selected region of interest)
Acquisition matrix: 160 to 192 × 256 or 256 × 256
General exam—larynx and hypopharynx*

Acquisition 1: axial, single echo 650 to 700/45† or 500 to 700/20 to 30, center at true vocal-ventricle level

Acquisition 2:
- a) repeat #1 higher or lower if necessary *or*
- b) react to observations on first acquisitions, options including:
  1) another plane
  2) more T_2 weighting (2000/70 to 90)
  3) survey neck for nodes

---

*Examination of this area must be highly physician interactive so that no "routine" beyond this can be offered in good conscience. An average study requires three or four acquisitions.

†Optional 45-msec echo delay time improves tumor-muscle contrast while retaining tumor-fat contrast (see Chapter 1); this may be useful for showing early exolaryngeal spread.

Table 8.3
CT Protocols—Larynx and Hypopharynx

Area under Study	Extent of Study	Gantry Angle	Slice Thickness	FOV (cm)	Coronals	Algorithim	Contrast/ Comment
a) Benign mass or mass of uncertain etiology; inflammatory disease	a) 1 cm above hyoid to bottom of cricoid	a) Parallel to true vocal cord (TVC) or C_{4-5}/ C_{5-6} disk (obtain scout during suspended inspiration	a) 3 mm thick by 5-mm increments to FVC; contiguous 3 mm from FVC to bottom or cricoid; may want to repeat FVC-TVC in quiet respiration (see cancer protocol)	a) 14–16	a) Rarely	a) Acquire soft tissue; retro bone occasionally for cartilage detail	a) I.V. contrast always used
b) Trauma/blunt or penetrating	b) As in (a)	b) As in (a)	b) As in (a)	b) 14–16	b) No	b) As in (a)	b) I.V. contrast not used unless suspect abscess
c) Subglottic—tracheal stenosis	c) False vocal cord (FVC) to cricoid; always include trachea to thoracic inlet; often include trachea to carina	c) As in (a)	c) Contiguous 3 mm from FVC to thoracic inlet; 5-mm increments from thoracic inlet to carina as needed	c) 14–16	c) Coronal and sagittal reformation frequently used	c) As in (a)	c) I.V. contrast not used unless mass or abscess is suspected
d) Cancer	d1) 1 cm above hyoid to 1 cm above FVC	d1) Parallel to TVC or C_{4-5}/C_{5-6} disk (obtain scout during suspended inspiration	d1) 3 mm by 5-mm increments or 3 mm contiguous	d1) 14–16	Reformations for transglottic tumor may be done (evaluate ventricle) Sagittal reformation may be done for preepiglottic spread (PES) of anterior commissure spread	d1) Acquire soft tissue; retro bone occasionally for cartilage detail	d1) In supraglottic lesions look for tongue base/PES. In glottic lesions evaluate ventricle, subglottic extent carefully. In hypopharynx note extent in postcricoid-apex region and exolaryngeal spread. Contrast always used.
	d2) FVC to bottom of cricoid	d2) As in (a)	d2) 3 mm contiguous	d2) 14–16		d2) As in (a)	d2) In all lesions carefully evaluate cartilages. Contrast always used.
	d3) Optional: Repeat FVC to bottom of cricoid during quiet breathing	d3) As in (a). May want to retake scout in quiet breathing to reangle gantry and localize FVC-TVC level	d3) 3 mm contiguous	d3) 14–16	d3) No	d3) As in (a)	d3) Quiet breathing and suspended inspiration help in evaluation of laryngeal ventricle anterior commissure upper; subglottic region. Used mainly with smaller TVC or FVC lesions.

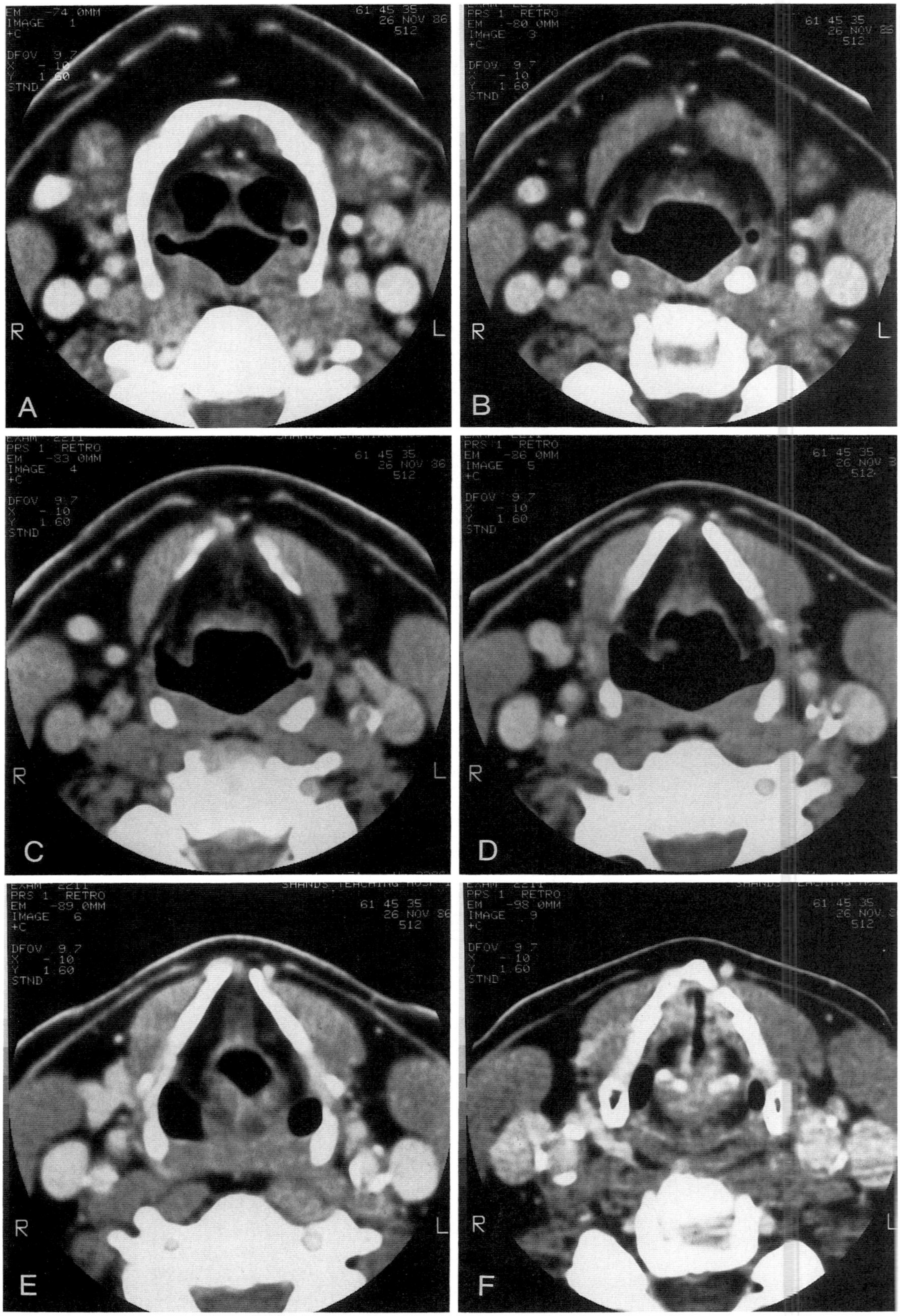

Figure 8.1*A–F*

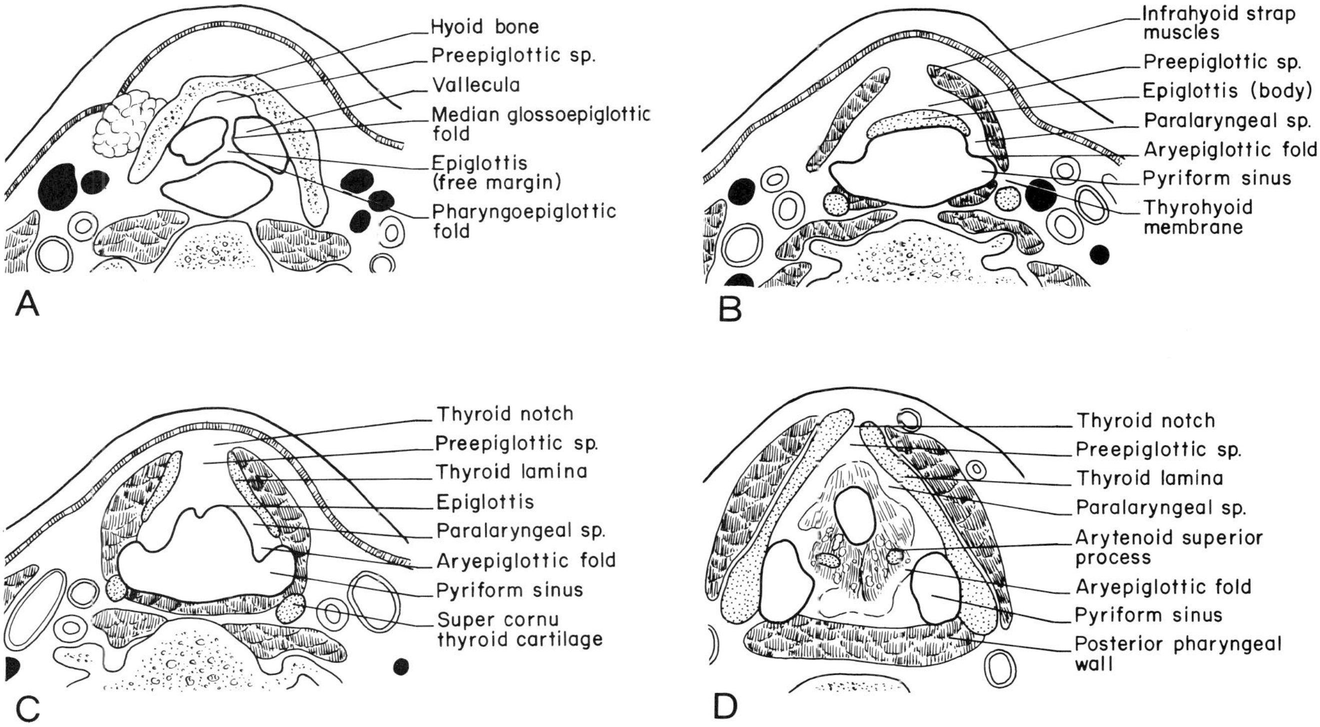
Hyoid bone
Preepiglottic sp.
Vallecula
Median glossoepiglottic fold
Epiglottis (free margin)
Pharyngoepiglottic fold
A
Infrahyoid strap muscles
Preepiglottic sp.
Epiglottis (body)
Paralaryngeal sp.
Aryepiglottic fold
Pyriform sinus
Thyrohyoid membrane
B
Thyroid notch
Preepiglottic sp.
Thyroid lamina
Epiglottis
Paralaryngeal sp.
Aryepiglottic fold
Pyriform sinus
Super cornu thyroid cartilage
C
Thyroid notch
Preepiglottic sp.
Thyroid lamina
Paralaryngeal sp.
Arytenoid superior process
Aryepiglottic fold
Pyriform sinus
Posterior pharyngeal wall
D

Figure 8.2*A–D*

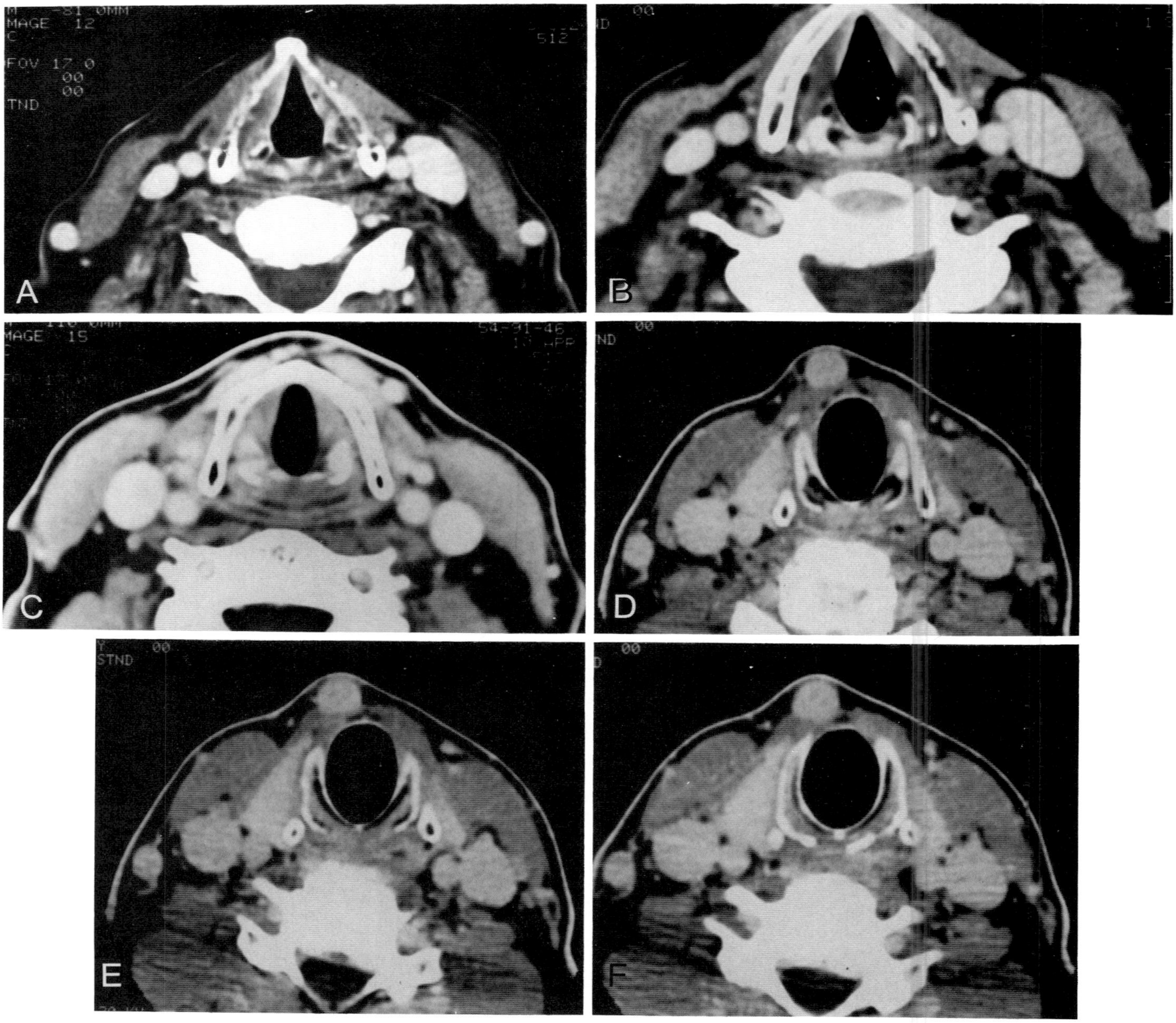

Figure 8.3*A–F*

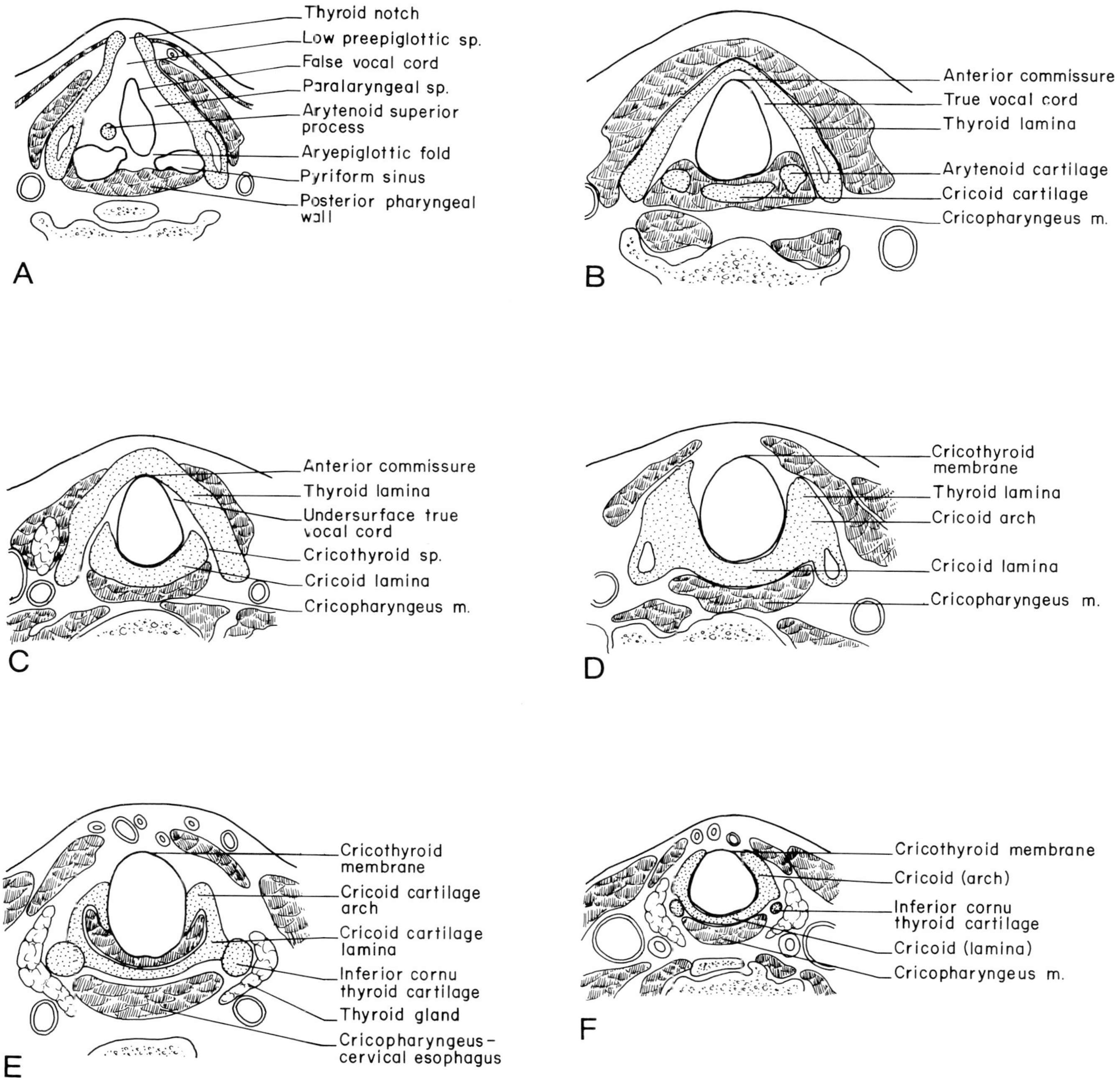

Thyroid notch
Low preepiglottic sp.
False vocal cord
Paralaryngeal sp.
Arytenoid superior process
Aryepiglottic fold
Pyriform sinus
Posterior pharyngeal wall
A
Anterior commissure
True vocal cord
Thyroid lamina
Arytenoid cartilage
Cricoid cartilage
Cricopharyngeus m.
B
Anterior commissure
Thyroid lamina
Undersurface true vocal cord
Cricothyroid sp.
Cricoid lamina
Cricopharyngeus m.
C
Cricothyroid membrane
Thyroid lamina
Cricoid arch
Cricoid lamina
Cricopharyngeus m.
D
Cricothyroid membrane
Cricoid cartilage arch
Cricoid cartilage lamina
Inferior cornu thyroid cartilage
Thyroid gland
Cricopharyngeus-cervical esophagus
E
Cricothyroid membrane
Cricoid (arch)
Inferior cornu thyroid cartilage
Cricoid (lamina)
Cricopharyngeus m.
F

Figure 8.4*A–F*

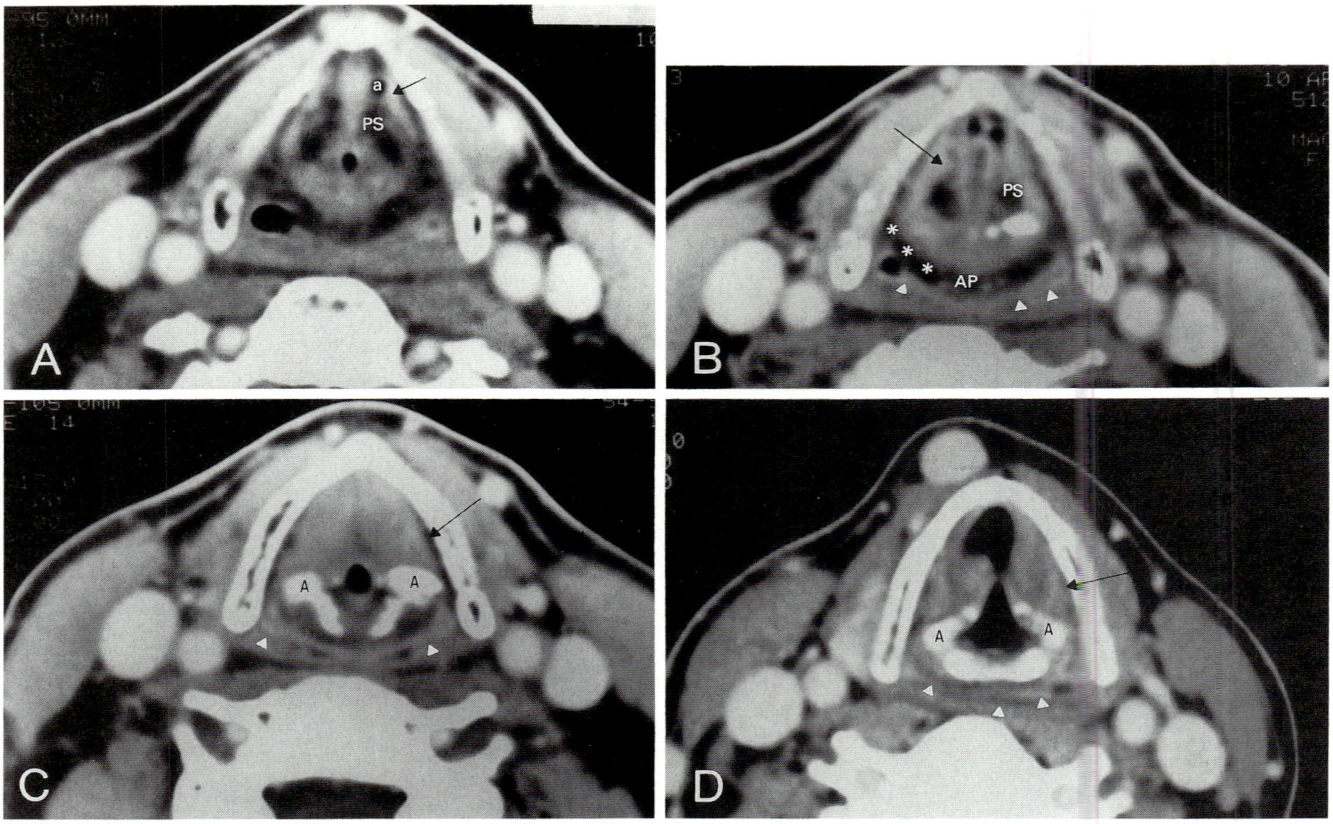

Figure 8.5*A–D*

Figure 8.5 CT of the larynx is done during breath-holding to reduce motion artifacts. Sometimes this causes the false cord, ventricular, and true cord sections to appear as seen above. One must become familiar with these appearances for reasons outlined in the text. *A*, false vocal cords are apposed in midline. Deeper structures including the appendix of the laryngeal ventricle *(a)*, fat in the paralaryngeal space *(PS)*, and intrinsic laryngeal musculature *(arrow)* are clearly visible. *B*, at the level of the ventricle-undersurface of the false vocal cord the intrinsic laryngeal musculature *(arrow)* occupies a larger proportion of the paralaryngeal space *(PS)*. Fat within the arytenoid pad *(AP)* is plainly visible; its continuity with the fat in the aryepiglottic fold and paralaryngeal space can be appreciated by following the course of this deep tissue plane on this and the section part in *A* (***). The posterior pharyngeal mucosa *(arrowheads)* can be seen as separate from the mucosa overlying the arytenoid pad here and in part *A*. The musculature of the posterior pharyngeal wall lies just posterior to this thin band of mucosal enhancement. *C* and *D*, the true cords lie apposed in the midline so that the anterior commissure cannot be evaluated. The arytenoids *(A)* are rotated medially. The paralaryngeal space *(arrow)* is now only a thin band of fat lying between the muscles of the true cord and thyroid lamina. The muscle and staining mucosa of the upper postcricoid region *(arrowheads)* are now visible.

CASES

Use checklists in Appendix A to analyze the following cases.

Problem I

(Case histories and questions on p. 182

Case 8.1 (Fig. 8.6 *A–D*)

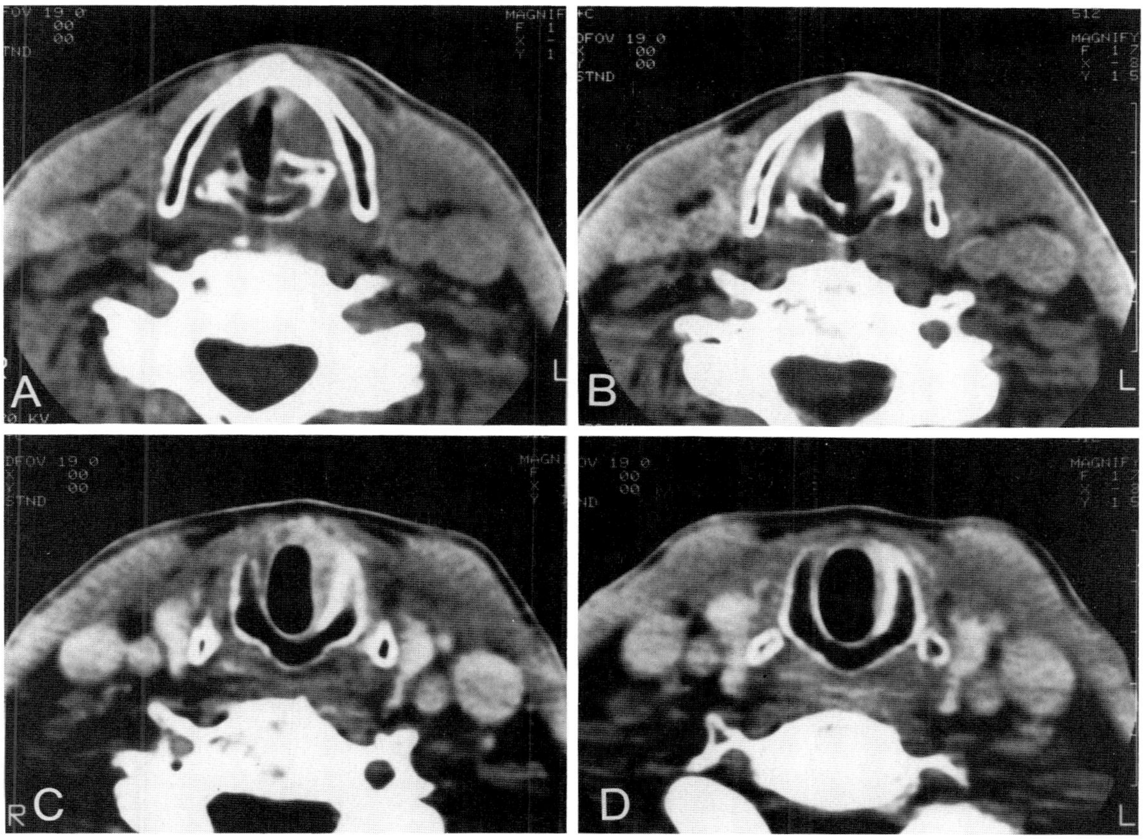

Figure 8.6*A–D*

Case 8.2 (Fig. 8.7*A–C*)

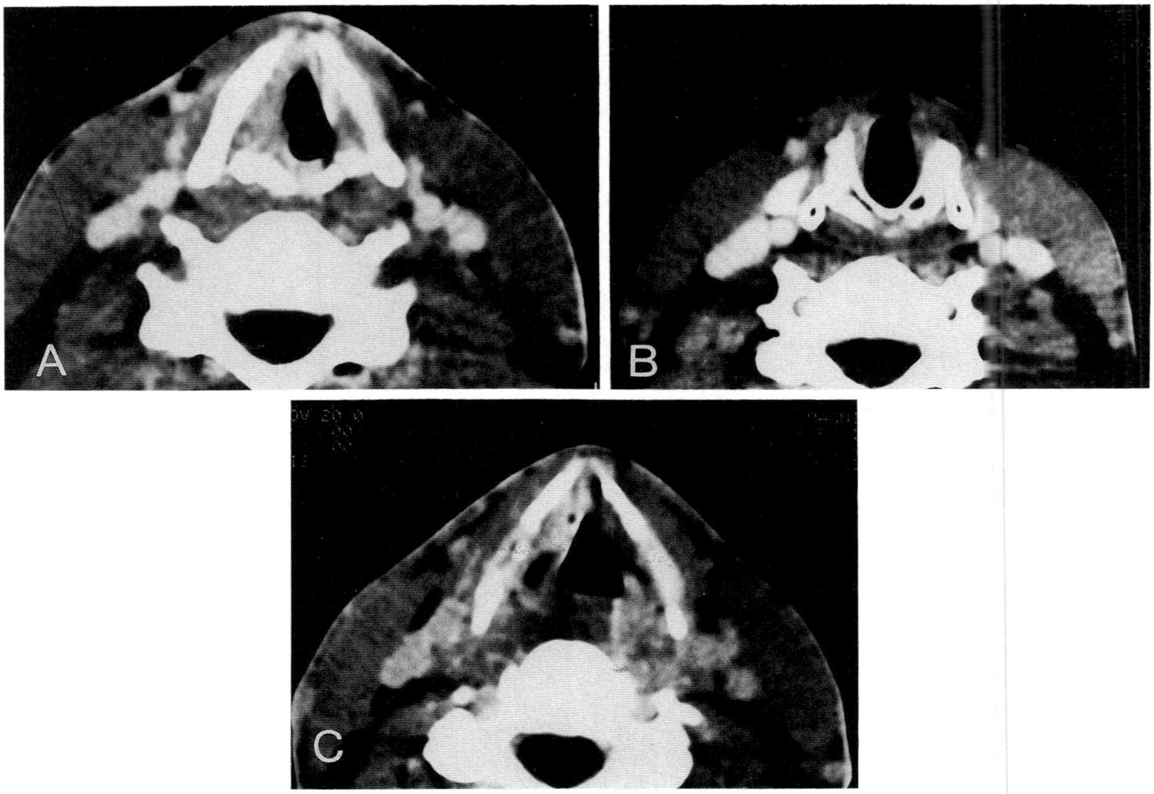

Figure 8.7*A–G*

Case Histories

Case 8.1 Patient with clinically T3 laryngeal carcinoma being considered for extended hemilaryngectomy or radiotherapy with salvage laryngectomy if radiation therapy does not control primary site. There was "minimal" subglottic spread noted at direct laryngoscopy.

Case 8.2 Patient with tumor clinically localized to the true vocal cord with diminished mobility but not fixation (T2). There was a question of spread to the laryngeal ventricle and no evidence of subglottic spread.

Questions

1. Are the treatment options in Case 8.1 viable considering the CT findings?
2. Does sclerosis of ossified cartilage mean that the cartilage is invaded? Is there another finding present that suggests cartilage invasion (i.e., other than obvious erosion or sclerosis)?
3. What is a "transglottic" cancer? Is this a good and useful term? Is a T2 lesion that involves the false cord and true cord and has 10 to 12 mm of posterolateral subglottic spread suitable for hemilaryngectomy? Radiotherapy? How does this change if the cord is fixed (T3)?
4. Anatomic issue: What must one do in order to properly evaluate the laryngeal ventricle on axial CT?

Discussion

Problem I–Locally Advanced Cancer of the True Vocal Cord Radiation therapy is certainly not a viable option for the patient in Case 8.1 since obvious cartilage invasion is present (see checklist for Case 8.1). It is quite likely that this patient would both fail locally and experience at least a localized chondronecrosis as a result of attempted radiation therapy. Vertical extended or near-total hemilaryngectomy *may* be used by experienced surgeons in selected vocal cord cancers where the true cord is fixed. In this patient the cartilage invasion and extensive (greater than 10 to 12 mm) posterolateral subglottic spread would be contraindications to extended hemilaryngectomy. Total laryngectomy perhaps followed by postoperative radiotherapy is the choice of therapy for T4 glottic cancer (Question 1).

Frank erosion of the thyroid or cricoid cartilage is the best sign of invasion, and thin section (3 to 4 mm or less), high-resolution CT is the best way to detect such invasion. Tumor adjacent to ossified cartilage may induce a sclerotic reaction without invasion; however, if sclerosis is present one can suspect but not prove that microinvasion is present. In well-ossified cartilages tumor can be seen spreading within the fatty marrow between the "cortical" surfaces; however, this is usually present in conjunction with obvious areas of erosion (Question 2).

The term "transglottic cancer" is *not* a good one mainly because its definition varies from author to author and because it takes us out of the accepted classification of laryngeal cancer into supraglottic, glottic, and subglottic categories. Definitions vary, but in general these are tumors that cross the laryngeal ventricle to involve the false cord and the true cord. Most authors agree that the subglottis must also be involved and some say that the true cord must be fixed in order to call a lesion "transglottic." The chance for ambiguity in the use of the term should be readily apparent (Question 3).

Some would argue that extended hemilaryngectomy can be done in a lesion such as that described in Question 3 and shown in Case 8.2. Others would argue that radiation therapy had a reasonable chance for primary site control. However, one must realize that both surgical and radiotherapeutic attempts to conserve the larynx in such cases have a high chance of failure. Such patients should be followed very carefully clinically and with imaging so that salvage can be instituted while recurrence is still confined to the larynx. The patient in Case 8.2 also had interarytenoid disease and subtle findings suggestive of cricoarytenoid joint involvement. Following radiation therapy he had focal cricoarytenoid necrosis and recurrent tumor on follow-up scan. He was successfully salvaged by total laryngectomy.

Anatomic Issue: Evaluation of the Laryngeal Ventricle The laryngeal ventricle lies between the true and false cords. Sections *must* be made parallel to the ventricle or vocal cords. These should be no more than 3 or 4 mm thick. Assuming good technique one can then routinely identify the level of the ventricle on axial sections. Coronal sections are *not* necessary to evaluate the ventricle or subglottic spread if axial scans are done with proper technique and one learns the anatomic landmarks of the region.

CHECKLIST—LARYNX AND HYPOPHARYNX (CASE 8.1)

	Seen	Nl	Abnl	Remarks
SUBGLOTTIS Soft tissues adjacent to cricoid			√	5 mm left lateral subglottic spread
Cricothyroid membrane			√	Thickened left and midline
Cricoid—anterior ring	No			
Cricoid—lamina		√		
Cricoid—arches			√	Left sclerotic margin marrow space dense
Thyroid cartilages—inferior cornua		√		
Cricothyroid joint		√		
Cricopharyngeus/esophageal verge		√		
Course of recurrent laryngeal nerves		√		
Thyroid gland		√		
GLOTTIS Undersurface of True Cords Infrahyoid strap muscles		√		
Thyroid cartilage			√	Left eroded posterolaterally
Right cord (position/thickness)		√		
Left cord (position/thickness)			√	Entire cord thickened
Anterior commissure			?	Probably involved
Right arytenoid (body/vocal process)		√		
Left arytenoid (body/vocal process)			√	Medially displaced
Cricoid lamina		√		
Posterior commissure			√	Thickening
Cricothyroid space			√	Widened
Paralaryngeal space			√	Left probably infiltrated
Postcricoid soft tissues		√		
Apex of pyriform sinus		√		
Soft tissues of neck		√		
Midplane of True Cords Infrahyoid strap muscles		√		
Thyroid cartilage		√		See above
Right cord (position/thickness)		√		
Left cord (position/thickness)			√	Entire cord thickened
Anterior commissure			?	Probably involved
Right arytenoid (body/vocal process)		√		
Left arytenoid (body/vocal process)			√	Medially displaced
Cricoid lamina		√		
Posterior commissure			√	Thickened
Cricothyroid space			√	Widened
Paralaryngeal space			√	Probably infiltrated
Postcricoid soft tissues		√		
Apex of pyriform sinus		√		
Soft tissues of neck		√		

Case 8.3 (Fig. 8.8)

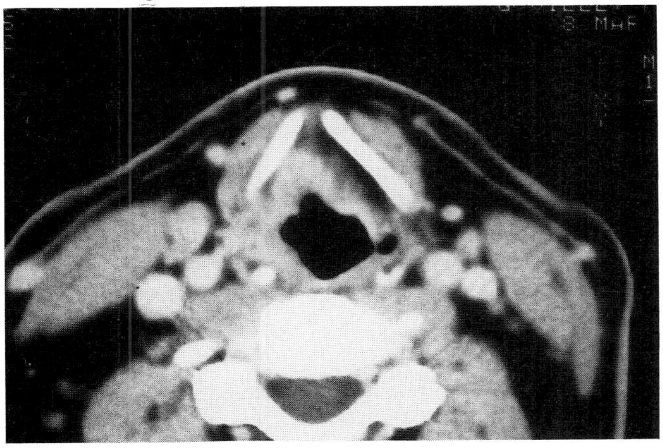

Figure 8.8

Case 8.4 (Fig. 8.9)

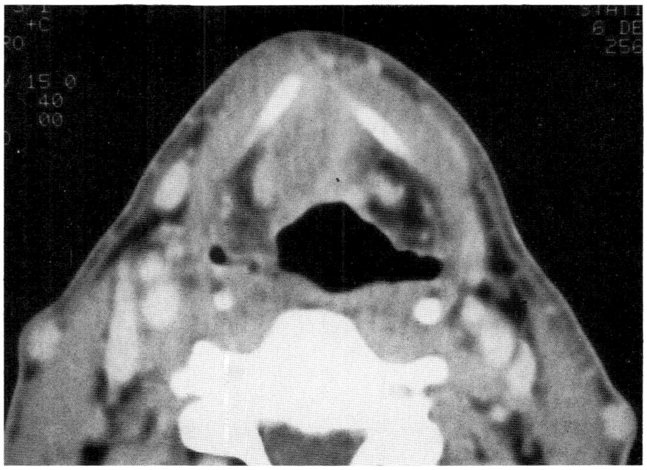

Figure 8.9

Case Histories

Case 8.3 Patient with exophytic and ulcerative-appearing squamous cell carcinoma of the epiglottis. No palpable mass or tenderness over the thyroid cartilage.

Case 8.4 Patient with bulky, exophytic squamous cell carcinoma of the epiglottis who does not want surgery. No palpable mass or tenderness over the thyroid cartilage.

Questions

1. Do the patients in Cases 8.3 and 8.4 have a reasonable chance for primary site control with radiation therapy alone?
2. Does the observed mucosal growth pattern in laryngeal cancer predict the likelihood of deep invasion? Does minimal or even moderate (up to 75%) invasion of the preepiglottic space seen on CT justify classifying a lesion as T3 rather than T2 by current AJC criteria?
3. Anatomic issue: What is the relationship of the paralaryngeal and preepiglottic spaces?

Discussion

Problem II—Supraglottic Cancer and the Preepiglottic Space Both patients (Cases 8.3 and 8.4) have extensive preepiglottic space (PES) involvement on the section shown and at every other level in the supraglottic sections (see checklists for Cases 8.3 and 8.4). In Case 8.3 the tumor was mainly one of the infrahyoid epiglottis with some spill onto the aryepiglottic fold, and the tumor was controlled with radiation therapy despite virtually complete involvement of the PES. The patient in Case 8.4, however, has cartilage invasion and spread into the anterior soft tissues of the neck (infrahyoid strap muscles). This is a T4 lesion and must *not* be irradiated (Question 1).

In general, ulcerative mucosal spread suggests a lesion that may also be deeply infiltrating; however, a bulky, nonulcerative lesion may also show extensive submucosal and other deep spread. Computed tomography and MRI are much better than any clinical parameter for demonstrating deep disease, and these mucosal growth patterns can be misleading (Question 2). It has been our experience that PES spread is present in the vast majority of infrahyoid epiglottic and marginal supraglottic cancers. At the University of Florida this alone does not seem to reduce the chances for local control by radiation therapy alone. Therefore it is our impression that CT evidence of moderate PES invasion may not carry with it the prognostic implications of upgrading the lesion from T2 to T3 as suggested in AJC guidelines. Recall that these guidelines were established in an era during which palpation of the neck and plain lateral radiographs were the main means of establishing relatively gross PES involvement (Question 2).

Anatomic Issue: Relationship of the Paralaryngeal and Preepiglottic Spaces The paralaryngeal space is in direct continuity with the PES. In fact the paired, lateral paralaryngeal spaces may be thought of as appendages of the PES. There are no serious boundaries restricting spread of tumor between these spaces. A fairly high volume of tumor can lie submucosally within these spaces and not be appreciated on indirect or direct laryngoscopy.

CHECKLIST—LARYNX AND HYPOPHARYNX (CASE 8.3)

	Seen	Nl	Abnl	Remarks
SUPRAGLOTTIS AND HYPOPHARYNX Mid Infrahyoid strap muscles		√		
Thyroid laminae		√		
Thyrohyoid membrane		√		
Paralaryngeal space: Right			√	Infiltrated
Left		√		
Pyriform sinus: Right		√		
Left		√		
Body of epiglottis			√	Thickened, infiltrated
Preepiglottic space			√	50% infiltrated, mainly on right
Posterior pharyngeal wall		√		
Soft tissues of neck		√		

CHECKLIST—LARYNX AND HYPOPHARYNX (CASE 8.4)

	Seen	Nl	Abnl	Remarks
SUPRAGLOTTIS AND HYPOPHARYNX Mid Infrahyoid strap muscles			√	Thickened, probably invaded on right
Thyroid laminae		√		
Thyrohyoid membrane			?	Probably invaded anteriorly
Paralaryngeal space: Right			√	Infiltrated
Left		√		
Pyriform sinus: Right		√		
Left		√		
Body of epiglottis			√	Completely infiltrated
Preepiglottic space			√	100% infiltrated
Posterior pharyngeal wall		√		
Soft tissues of neck			√	Possibly infiltrated in midline and on the right

Case 8.5 (Fig. 8.10)

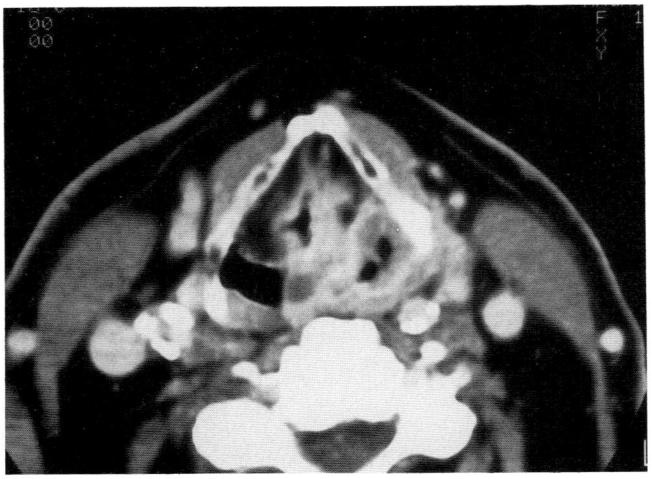

Figure 8.10

Case 8.6 (Fig. 8.11*A–D*)

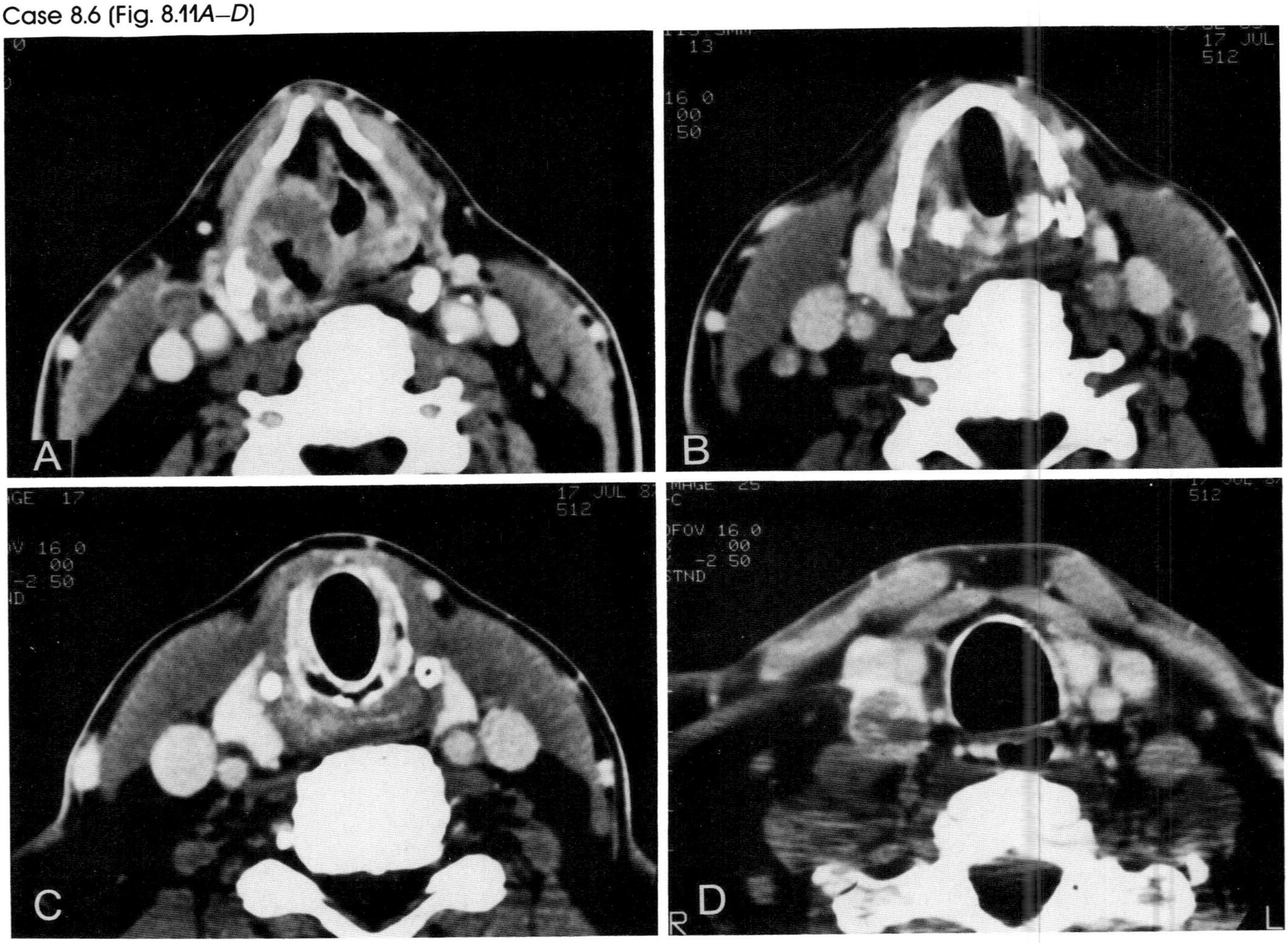

Figure 8.11*A–D*

Case Histories

Case 8.5 Patient with clinical T2 squamous cell carcinoma of the pyriform sinus.

Case 8.6 Patient with squamous cell carcinoma of the pyriform sinus; the apex and postcricoid region were thought to be involved. Clinical stage is T3N0 before CT exam.

Questions

1. Is the patient in Case 8.5 suitable for radiation therapy?
2. How would you stage the patient in Case 8.6 based on CT findings? What is the lower limit of the tumor and extent of postcricoid disease?
3. Anatomic issue: What are the three parts of the hypopharynx? Define the postcricoid portion of the hypopharynx and its relationship to the esophageal verge. How might tumor spread to this region affect therapy?

Discussion

Problem III—Spread Patterns of Hypopharyngeal Cancer The patient in Case 8.5 has gross cartilage invasion and is not suitable for radiation therapy; the patient would be at very high risk for a gross thyroid cartilage necrosis as well as failure of local control (Question 1).

The patient in Case 8.6 should be staged T3N2c, not T3N0 (see checklist for Case 8.6). There are bilateral abnormal nodes present making the neck overall N2e. There are at least two positive nodes on the right making it N2b; the left neck is N1. Both mid and low neck nodes are involved, with a positive scalene node on the right with evidence of capsular involvement but no definite capsular penetration. Low neck adenopathy significantly worsens prognosis and suggests increased risk for distant metastases. The primary site was staged T3 clinically because of cord fixation. The CT confirmed involvement of the postcricoid region extending to the midline. Moreover, spread to the esophageal verge was noted, allowing for preoperative anticipation of a gastric pull up to reconstruct the pharynx (Question 2). All findings were confirmed at surgery and pathologically.

Anatomic Issue: Parts of the Hypopharynx and Tumor Spread to Postcricoid Portion The hypopharynx is made up of the pyriform sinuses, posterior pharyngeal wall, and postcricoid region. The postcricoid region is defined by the lamina of the cricoid cartilage anteriorly and the cricopharyngeus muscle posteriorly and laterally. This part of the hypopharynx is a relatively flat ellipsoid as seen on cross-section. The esophageal verge is the junction of the postcricoid portion of the hypopharynx and the esophagus seen on endoscopy. The corresponding level on cross-sectional imaging is at the bottom of the cricoid cartilage. Here the flat ellipsoid of the postcricoid region assumes a more rounded shape. The esophagus lies posterior to the trachea and often slight to the left.

CHECKLIST—LARYNX AND HYPOPHARYNX (CASE 8.6)

	Seen	Nl	Abnl	Remarks
SUBGLOTTIS				
Soft tissues adjacent to cricoid		√		
Cricothyroid membrane		√		
Cricoid—anterior ring		√		
Cricoid—lamina		√		
Cricoid—arches		√		
Thyroid cartilages—inferior cornuc		√		
Cricothyroid joint		√		
Cricopharyngeus/esophageal verge			√	Tumor at postcricoid esoph. verge junction
Course of recurrent laryngeal nerves		√		
Thyroid gland		√		
GLOTTIS				
Undersurface of True Cords				
Infrahyoid strap muscles		√		
Thyroid cartilage		√		
Right cord (position/thickness)			√	Thickened
Left cord (position/thickness)		√		
Anterior commissure		√		
Right arytenoid (body/vocal process)	No			
Left arytenoid (body/vocal process)	No			
Cricoid lamina		√		
Posterior commissure			?	Thickened
Cricothyroid space			√	Widened
Paralaryngeal space			√	Infiltrated
Postcricoid soft tissues			√	Involved to just right of midline
Apex of pyriform sinus			√	Involved with tumor
Soft tissues of neck			√	Note positive nodes
SUPRAGLOTTIS AND HYPOPHARYNX				
Low				
Infrahyoid strap muscles		√		
Thyroid notch		√		
Arytenoids (superior process)	No			
False cords (position/thickness): Right			√	Posterior deep infiltration
Left		√		
Paralaryngeal space: Right			√	Infiltrated
Left		√		
Appendix/ventricle: Right	No			
Left	No			
Inferior epiglottis		√		
Preepiglottic space		√		
Aryepiglottic fold: Right			√	Thickened, infiltrated
Left		√		

CHECKLIST—LARYNX AND HYPOPHARYNX (CASE 8.6) *(continued)*

	Seen	Nl	Abnl	Remarks
Pyriform sinus: Right			√	Circumferential infiltration
Left		√		
Posterior pharyngeal wall		√		
Soft tissues of neck			√	Note positive nodes

Problem 4

Case 8.7 (Fig. 8.12 *A* and *B*)

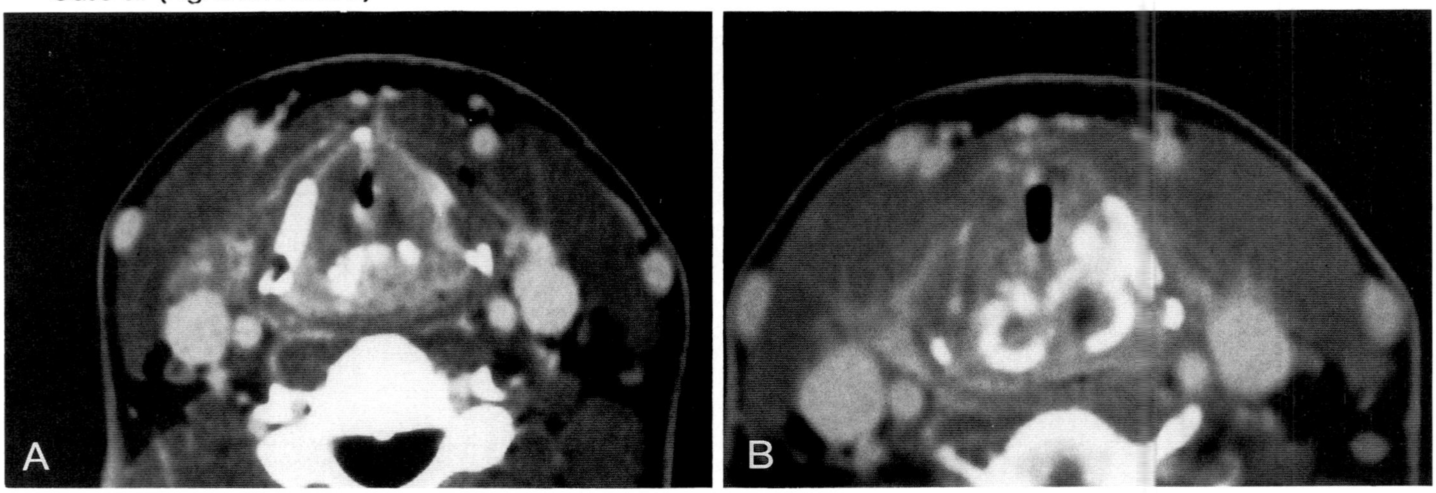

Figure 8.12*A* and *B*

Case History

Case 8.7 Patient found to be hoarse and stridorous 3 weeks after treatment at another institution for life-threatening head and chest injuries sustained in a motor vehicle accident.

Questions

1. What are the most important things to determine in imaging an injured larynx?
2. What is the most important prognostic factor in injury to the laryngeal skeleton?
3. Anatomic issue: Name three common normal variants in the contours of the cricoid cartilage.

Discussion

Problem IV—Laryngeal Trauma The main aim of imaging the acutely injured larynx is to show displaced fractures of the thyroid or cricoid cartilages (Question 1). Occasionally one can demonstrate evidence of a false passage. One can also show arytenoid dislocation, avulsion of the epiglottis, and the status of the airway. The key to prognosis and repair of laryngeal fractures is the status of the cricoid cartilage (Question 2). The patient in Case 8.7 had unrecognized, displaced fractures of the cricoid and thyroid cartilages, fracture dislocation of the cricothyroid joint, and dislocation of the arytenoid (see checklist for Case 8.7). Even with prompt repair restoration of entirely normal glottic function would be difficult. With the delay in diagnosis it becomes even less likely. Unfortunately such patients often have other life-threatening injuries that impede early detection and/or treatment.

Anatomic Issue: Cricoid Cartilage Contours The cricoid cartilage always has a slight "dip" in the midline along its superior margin. The lamina usually protrudes slightly in the midline. Sometimes a gap can be seen in the lamina in the midline or paramedian along its posterior surface. It is important to become familiar with these variations of normal so as not to interpret them as abnormalities in some clinical situations.

CHECKLIST—LARYNX AND HYPOPHARYNX (CASE 8.7)

	Seen	Nl	Abnl	Remarks
SUBGLOTTIS Soft tissues adjacent to cricoid			√	Marked subglottic edema
Cricothyroid membrane			?	Probably disrupted
Cricoid—anterior ring	No			
Cricoid—lamina			√	Comminuted displaced fracture
Cricoid—arches	No			
Thyroid cartilages—inferior cornua			√	Relationship to cricoid abnormal
Cricothyroid joint			?	Probably dislocated
Cricopharyngeus/esophageal verge	No			
Course of recurrent laryngeal nerves	No			
Thyroid gland	No			
GLOTTIS Midplane of True Cords Infrahyoid strap muscles			√	Thickened, edematous
Thyroid cartilage			√	Intact but displaced
Right cord (position/thickness)			√	Swollen, paramedian
Left cord (position/thickness)			√	Swollen paramedian
Anterior commissure			√	Grossly thickened
Right arytenoid (body/vocal process)			√	Probably posteriorly dislocated
Left arytenoid (body/vocal process)		?		Probably normal
Cricoid lamina			√	See subglottis
Posterior commissure			√	Grossly thickened
Cricothyroid space			√	Widened bilaterally
Paralaryngeal space			√	Edematous
Postcricoid soft tissues			?	Excessive enhancement ? inflammation
Apex of pyriform sinus			?	See above
Soft tissues of neck			√	Diffuse swelling

SUGGESTED READINGS

Books, Chapters, Reviews

Mancuso AA, Hanafee WN: Larynx and hypopharynx. In: *Computed Tomography and Magnetic Resonance Imaging of the Head and Neck*. Baltimore, Williams & Wilkins, 1985, pp 241–357.

Articles

On laryngeal and hypopharyngeal cancer:

Biller HF, Lawson W: Partial laryngectomy for transglottic cancers. *Laryngoscope* 93:297–300, 1984.

Biller HF, Lawson W: Partial laryngectomy for vocal cord cancer with marked limitation or fixation of the vocal cord. *Laryngoscope* 96:61–64, 1986.

Kirchner JA: Pathways and pitfalls in partial laryngectomy. *Ann Otol Rhinol Laryngol* 93:301–305, 1984.

Kirchner JA: Two hundred laryngeal cancers: patterns of growth and spread as seen in serial sections. *Laryngoscope* 87:474–482, 1977.

Oloffsson J, van Nostrand AWP: Growth and spread of laryngeal and hypopharyngeal carcinoma with reflections on the effect of preoperative irradiation. 139 cases studies by whole organ serial sectioning. *Acta Otolaryngol Suppl* 308:1–84, 1973.

Silverman PM: Medullary space involvement in laryngeal carcinoma. *Arch Otolaryngol* 111:541–542, 1985.

Tucker GF: The anatomy of laryngeal cancer. *Can J Otolaryngol* 3:417–427, 1974.

On MRI:

Castellijns JA, Gerritsen GJ, Kaiser MC, et al: MRI of normal or cancerous laryngeal cartilages: histopathologic correlation. *Laryngoscope* 97:1085–1093, 1987.

Lufkin RB, Hanafee WN, Wortham D, et al: Larynx and hypopharynx: MR imaging with surface coils. *Radiology* 158:747–754, 1986.

McArdle CB, Bailey BJ, Amparo EG: Surface coil magnetic resonance imaging of the normal larynx. *Arch Otolaryngol Head Neck Surg* 112:616–622, 1986.

On laryngotracheal trauma:

Gussack GS, Jurkovich GJ, Luterman A: Laryngotracheal trauma: a protocol approach to a rare injury. *Laryngoscope* 96:660–665, 1986.

Mancuso AA, Hanafee WN: Computed tomography of the injured larynx. *Radiology* 133:139–144, 1979.

9

Neck, Including Thyroid and Parathyroid Glands and Thoracic Inlet

INDICATIONS

The mainstay of physical diagnosis in the neck is palpation. In nonpulsatile masses fine-needle aspiration biopsy has assumed an important role in directing further clinical and imaging evaluation where a highly experienced cytopathologist is available. Computed tomography, MRI, and ultrasound are complimentary to these clinical and laboratory methods of evaluation, and their relative value varies greatly from patient to patient. Clinical triage of patients with a neck mass of uncertain etiology to specific imaging algorithms will improve the efficiency and economy of the diagnostic evaluation. Careful imaging and sophisticated interpretation of those findings can often redirect the management of these patients and sometimes avoid needless morbidity or diagnostic uncertainty. General indications for imaging the neck are presented in Table 9.1. Suggestions for triage and conduct of the imaging evaluation for neck masses as well as differential diagnosis are outlined in Tables 9.2 through 9.4. Tables 9.5 through 9.7 deal with the same issues in the thyroid and parathyroid region.

Table 9.1
Indications for Neck Imaging (Excluding Cervical Spine, Spinal Cord, Thyroid, Parathyroid)

- By disease category
  - Congenital—diagnosis and extent of branchial anomalies, lymphangioma/cystic hygroma, thyroglossal duct cyst (CT or MRI)
  - Inflammatory—cellulitis abscess, extent of abscess, adenopathy-reactive vs. suppurative (CT)
  - Benign tumor—? site of origin, etiology, extent, differential diagnosis (CT); possible brachial plexus, epidural, other neural involvement (MRI)
  - Malignant tumor
    - Sarcoma—? site of origin, extent, differential diagnosis (CT); possible brachial plexus, epidural, other neural involvement (MRI)
    - Carcinoma—direct extension (CT/MRI)
    - Nodes—? etiology (CT); lymphoma—? extent (CT); carcinoma (usually squamous cell carcinoma)—staging extranodal extent (CT)
  - Trauma—mainly for cervical spine, laryngeal injury, post-traumatic aneurysm (CT)
  - Vascular—jugular thrombosis, thrombophlebitis; aneurysm—mycotic, post-traumatic (CT/MRI)
- By presenting problem
  - Neck mass—uncertain etiology (CT)
  - Vocal cord paresis (MRI)
  - Horner's syndrome (MRI)
  - Brachial plexopathy (MRI)

In general CT is the primary tool for evaluating the neck, but MRI will be used initially in some situations. Ultrasound may be done first in thyroid or parathyroid region masses. Computed tomography is preferred in many cases because of its superiority to MRI in evaluating cervical metastatic disease (see Chapter 1). It also suffers less from motion degradation than does MRI, resulting in a consistently better rendering of the larynx and hypopharynx (see Chapter 8). Contrast-enhanced CT also provides a clearer depiction of the nature of inflammatory masses than does MRI and at times a better feeling for the extent of early extranodal spread of cervical metastases. The vascular nature of a mass can be suggested by CT; however, very enhancing lesions may be inflammatory (e.g., metastatic node with secondary infection) or just concentrating iodine (e.g., thyroid related), and supplemental dynamic CT with semiquantitative analysis or angiography may be necessary for complete evaluation (see Chapter 1). Qualitative, flow-related MRI data, especially with gradient echo techniques, can be used to judge vascularity of a lesion (e.g., aneurysm or paraganglioma), thrombosis (e.g., jugular thrombophlebitis), or intraluminal extension of tumor (e.g., paraganglioma). Magnetic resonance imaging is particularly useful if a lesion likely originates from or involves the brachial plexus, epidural space, or cervical cord; however, the need for bone detail may require adjunctive CT. Magnetic resonance imaging is particularly useful at the thoracic inlet because coronal sections are done with great ease. Lesions here also have a high rate of involvement of the brachial plexus and neural axis, and MRI can help establish the relationship of lesions to these structures as well as to the upper mediastinum and brachiocephalic vessels.

Table 9.6
Basic Imaging for Thyroid-Related Masses

Clinical triage[a] leading to a well-formulated issue in which imaging may alter clinical disposition				
1) Screen for nodule 2) ? palpable nodule, solitary or multiple 3) Low neck mass, ? thyroid origin 4) Cystic vs. solid	Solitary nodule, probably benign, ? hypofunctioning	Solitary nodule, probably malignant, ? extent	Diffuse enlargement, probably benign?, ? extent prior to surgery	Diffuse enlargement, probably malignant, ? extent prior to surgery
Ultrasound	Radionuclide imaging	CT (MRI supplemental in selected cases)	MRI	CT (MRI supplemental in selected cases)

[a]See Table 9.5. Imaging use varies greatly with needs and practices of referring clinicians.

Table 9.7
Imaging Options in Patients with Suspected Parathyroid Adenoma

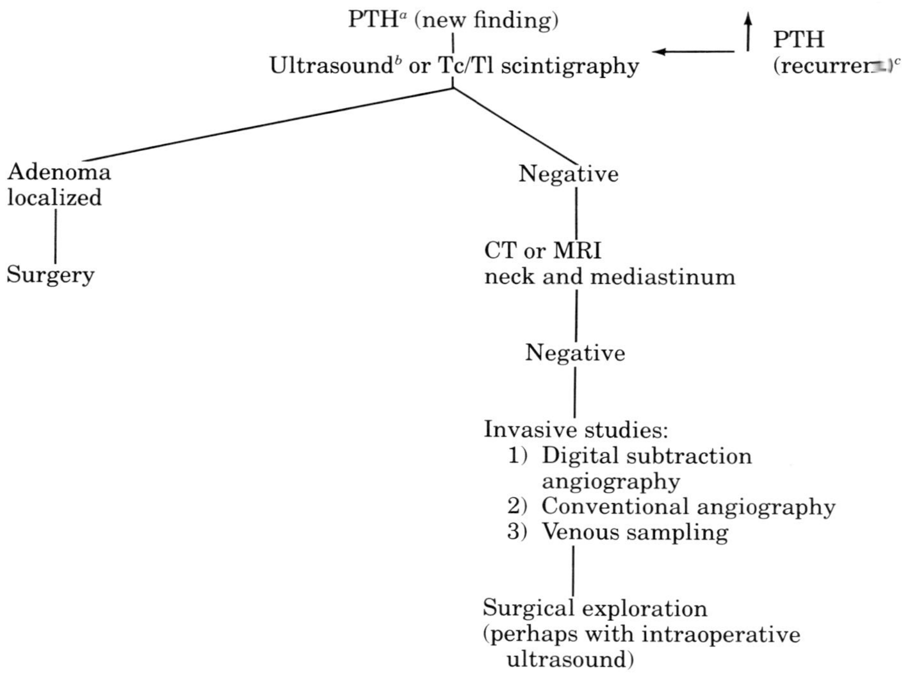

[a]Parathyroid hormone.
[b]Ultrasound preferred for cost and convenience.
[c]Move down algorithm until two exams are positive *and* correlate anatomically.

in Chapter 1. Precontrast scans are almost never done. Reformations are rarely more informative than axial sections. If coronals through the thoracic inlet are necessary MRI is used adjunctively or primarily.

Magnetic resonance study of the neck is best accomplished with a localized receiver coil. A volume-type coil is preferred but the changing contours of the head-neck and neck-shoulder junctions make it difficult to design an optimal geometry for all cases. Flat receiver coils can be useful in selected cases if they can be easily suspended over the area of interest, otherwise they may prove difficult to use. The problems with receiver coil design also may complicate studies needing to survey the neck. For instance, an optimal study of the upper neck and related aerodigestive tract usually requires a volume head coil, and the designs of most volume head coils do not adapt well to examining the mid to lower neck and thoracic inlet. This means that a neck survey might require a coil change. At present such changes slow throughput significantly. Coils designed for spine studies usually do not adapt well to studies of the rest of the neck. Improvements in receiver design are to be expected, and this problem should diminish somewhat over the next several years.

Patients are studied with 2DFT, Rf-refocused spin echo pulse sequences as a general rule. Gradient echo techniques will undoubtedly assume an increasingly important role in this region because of their capacity to reduce motion artifacts (fast scanning). The flow sensitivity of gradient echo techniques may also prove useful in the neck because of this need to specifically identify the normal neck vasculature relative to pathology. These pulse sequences, whatever their potential, remain adjunctive at present. Gadolinium-DTPA may prove useful for selected indications and make MRI even more competitive with CT for neck studies; its potential is currently under study.

Axial views are used most frequently. Coronals are particularly helpful for evaluating the thoracic inlet, supraclavicular region, and brachial plexus, and showing the relationship of laterally situated masses to the neural axis. Sagittals are occasionally helpful for masses that are near the midline and/or affect the spine or spinal cord.

A general approach to imaging neck problems would be as follows:

FOV: 18 to 24 cm
SLT: 5 mm (3 mm in selected region of interest)
Acquisition matrix: 160 to 192 × 256 or 256 × 256

Upper and mid neck—neural axis involvement unlikely
- Acquisition 1: Axial, single echo 500 to 700/20 to 30 or 600 to 700/45-msec pulse (repeat if necessary to cover entire region of interest)
- Acquisition 2: Axial, dual echo 2000/30 to 100*
- Acquisition 3: Axial single echo with pulse sequence optimized for desired contrast through pathology of interest
- Acquisition 4: Another plane, gradient echo, etc., as needed.

Low neck, thoracic inlet, brachial plexus
- Acquisition 1: Axial, single echo 500 to 700/20 to 30 or 600 to 700/45
- Acquisition 2: Coronal, single echo 500 to 700/20 to 30 or 600 to 700/45
- Acquisition 3: Axial or coronal single or dual echo 2000/30 to 100* if single echo TE $\geq$ 60
- Acquisition 4: Optional gradient echo, sagittal, etc.

Neck—neural axis likely involved
- Acquisition 1: Axial, single echo 500 to 700/20 to 30
- Acquisition 2: Depends on position of mass on #1—if midline sagittal 500 to 700/20 to 30; if paramedian coronal 500 to 700/20 to 30
- Acquisition 3: Repeat most informative plane with single or dual echo 2000/30 to 100* if single echo TE $\geq$ 60
- Acquisition 4: Optional plane, pulse sequence, gradient echo.

*TE range allows for selection of spin density–T_2-weighted pair or "mixed" and T_2-weighted pair as desired.

Table 9.8
CT Protocols—Neck

Area under Study	Extent of Study	Gantry Angle	Slice Thickness	FOV (cm)	Coronals	Algorithm	Contrast/Comment
a) Staging cervical metastases	a) Tip of clivus, C_{1-2} level to sternal notch in general. More limited exams possible with some primary sites	a) Variably parallel to IOML, mandibular body, true vocal cord (TVC) depending on primary site (see site-specific protocols)	a) 3 or 5 mm, depending on primary and relative node location (see site-specific protocols). 3 mm thick by 5-mm increments usual.	a) 14–18	a) Never	a) Soft tissue (ST); bone occasionally for skull base, subtle vertebral spread	a) I.V. contrast must be used; if not possible, MRI may be better choice; N.B.—exact approach depends on primary site; in recurrent disease always cover retropharyngeal nodes (C_1–C_2)
b) Upper-mid neck mass—unknown etiology (fine-needle biopsy can often help direct study)	b) Highly dependent on clinical situation; "safe" study is from skull base (foramen ovale level) to sternal notch. If likely squamous cell carcinoma node, must search for primary (see next column, comments and cancer protocols)	b) Nasopharynx–skull base parallel to IOML; oropharynx parallel to mandibular body; may continue through neck or angle parallel to TVC beginning at hyoid	b) 3 mm skull base to hard palate to hyoid. 3 mm by 5-mm increments from hyoid to thoracic inlet	b) 14–18	b) Rarely, if mass actually turns out to be arising in parapharyngeal space	b) ST; bone only retrospectively if involved or bony origin is noted	b) I.V. contrast essential. May begin by studying mass and then extending or limiting exam based on location, morphology of mass, and associated findings. Do MRI if relationship of mass to neural axis is uncertain on CT
c) Low neck mass—unknown etiology; consider ultrasound, fine-needle biopsy first	c) C_2 to sternal notch usually suffices, but mediastinum and upper neck even to skull base may be necessary	c) Parallel to TVC (or C_{4-5} or C_{5-6} disk space alternatively)	c) 3 mm through mass, thyroid region and low neck—3 mm by 5-mm increments above and below	c) 14–18	c) Rarely—use MRI if truly necessary	c) As in (a) and (b)	c) I.V. contrast essential; if thyroid etiology likely always consider MRI for coronals, also for neural axis relationship as needed. Search for primary other than thyroid above clavicles usually not fruitful. *Hyperextend neck, get shoulders relaxed and down*

Table 9.9
CT Protocols—Thyroid and Parathyroid

Area under Study	Extent of Study	Gantry Angle	Slice Thickness	FOV	Coronals	Algorithim	Contrast/ Comment
THYROID							
a) Probable benign mass—? extent. Consider MRI instead	a) Top to bottom of mass; usually midneck to upper mediastinum	a) Parallel to true vocal cord; C_{4-5} or C_{5-6} disk space alternatively	a) 3 or 5 mm depending on questions asked	a) 14–18 cm, perhaps wider at thoracic inlet	a) Do MRI if necessary	a) Soft tissue (ST)	a) I.V. contrast essential; get shoulders down and extend neck. Consider MRI as replacement or for supplemental coronal
b) Cancer	b) C_{1-2} to carina	b) As in (a)	b) 3 mm through thyroid region, 3 mm by 5-mm increments above and below	b) 14–18 cm in neck; may be slightly larger at thoracic inlet and below	b) Do MRI as needed	b) ST	b) See (a); neck and mediastinal survey for nodes almost always included
PARATHYROID							
a) Adenoma—nonoperated	a) Thyroid region, low neck; mediastinum as needed	a) as above	a) 3 mm thyroid and low neck; 5 mm mediastinum	a) 14–18 cm	a) No	a) ST	a) See above; consider ultrasound as initial screen; do mediastinum only if thyroid region and low neck are negative
b) Adenoma—recurrent; will usually be one of 2 or 3 studies for confirmation	b) Carotid bifurcation to subcarinal region	b) As above	b) 3 mm thyroid region and low neck; 5 mm above and below	b) 14–18 cm	b) No	b) ST	b) See thyroid for technical points; mediastinum high yield in this setting, parathyroid adenoma at carotid bifurcation *rare* but possible

Normal Anatomy
(use checklists in Appendix A as a study aid)

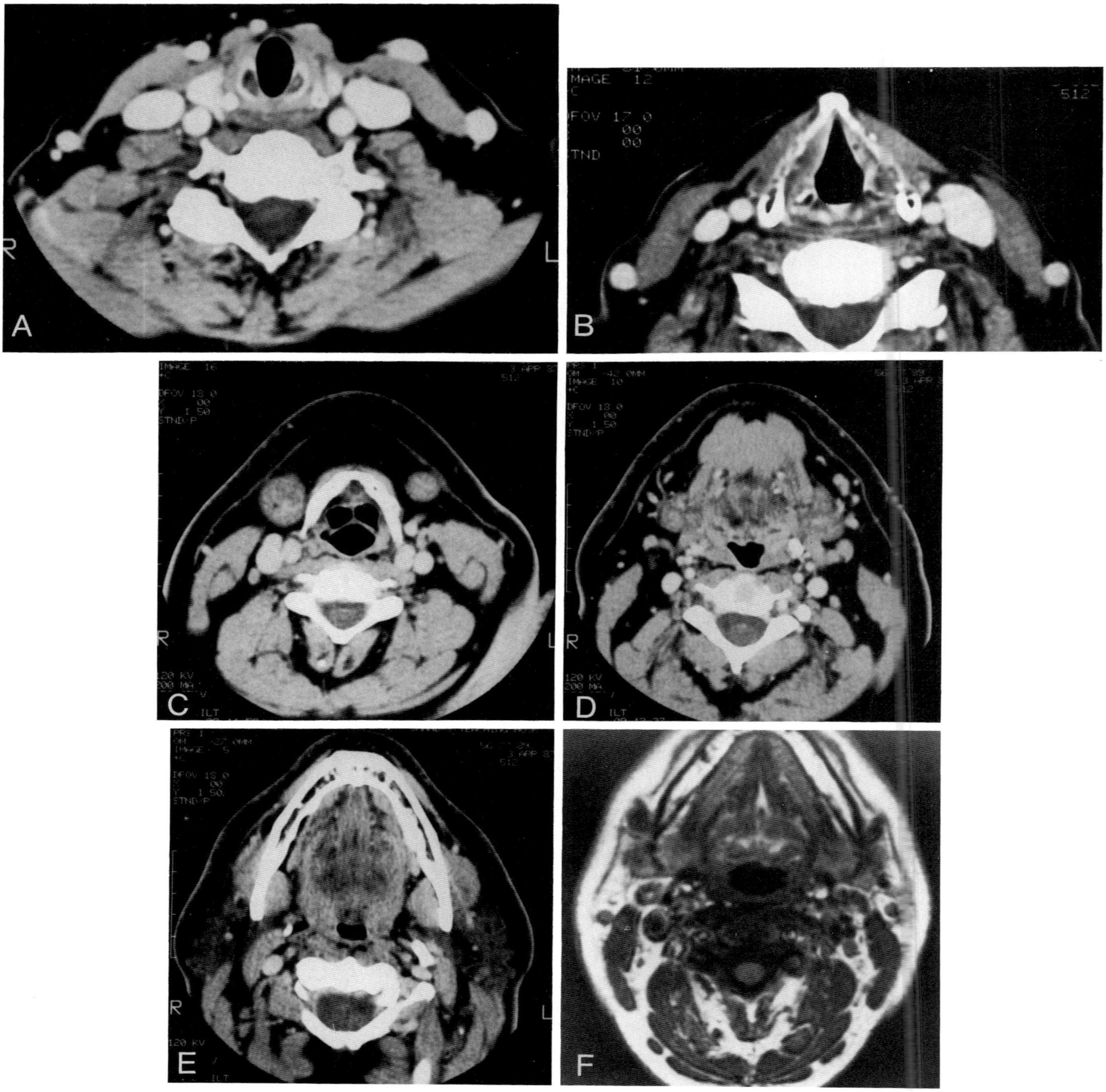

Figure 9.1*A–F*

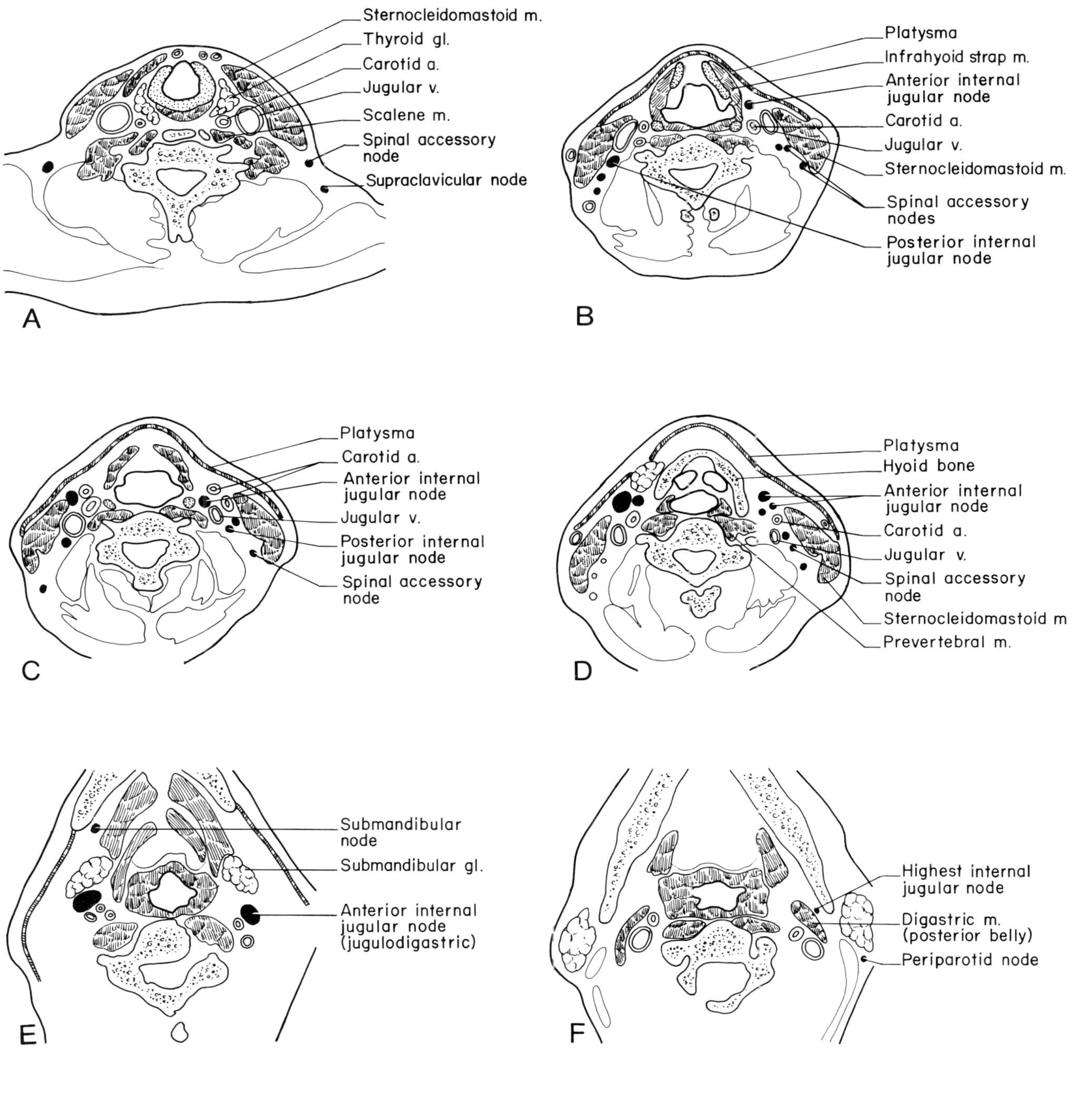
Sternocleidomastoid m.
Thyroid gl.
Carotid a.
Jugular v.
Scalene m.
Spinal accessory node
Supraclavicular node
A
Platysma
Infrahyoid strap m.
Anterior internal jugular node
Carotid a.
Jugular v.
Sternocleidomastoid m.
Spinal accessory nodes
Posterior internal jugular node
B
Platysma
Carotid a.
Anterior internal jugular node
Jugular v.
Posterior internal jugular node
Spinal accessory node
C
Platysma
Hyoid bone
Anterior internal jugular node
Carotid a.
Jugular v.
Spinal accessory node
Sternocleidomastoid m.
Prevertebral m.
D
Submandibular node
Submandibular gl.
Anterior internal jugular node (jugulodigastric)
E
Highest internal jugular node
Digastric m. (posterior belly)
Periparotid node
F

gologist? Why are these tumors sometimes hidden from view?

4. Anatomic issue: How do you decide if variation of the superficial contours of the tonsillar tissues in the upper aerodigestive tract is significant?

Discussion

Problem I—Neck Masses of Uncertain Etiology The mass in Case 9.1 cannot be a lymph node because it lies within the musculature of the deep neck well away from the lymph node–bearing area surrounding the jugular vein. Small nodes can be found between the more posterior neck muscles (e.g., suboccipital nodes) but not within the scalene-levator scapulae group where this mass is located (Question 1). Judging from its position this should be a mass of neural origin or a sarcoma of some other origin (e.g., rhabdomyosarcoma, malignant fibrous histiocytoma, liposarcoma). Given this set of circumstances, the diagnostic imager must suggest that the gross morphology and position of the lesion does not fit with the pathologic diagnosis and that the tissue should be restudied and if necessary rebiopsied (Question 1). Reevaluation of the original histology and repeat biopsy in this patient revealed sarcoma.

At the University of Florida we prefer, in general, CT for the initial evaluation of neck masses of uncertain etiology in an adult. This is because in our hands it is much more definitive for staging cervical adenopathy secondary to squamous cell carcinoma and it remains a more efficient means for "surveying" the head and neck region. Also, the presence of calcification and gross morphologic features such as cystic change, wall morphology, and enhancement can aid in differential diagnosis. We also believe strongly that the imaging workup should be integrated with needle biopsy. If needle biopsy suggests an etiology other than metastatic squamous cell carcinoma, MRI certainly may be used as a first choice, perhaps even more effectively than CT if the mass is likely to involve or arise from neural elements on structures at the thoracic inlet. Also, MRI may certainly be used in noninflammatory pediatric neck masses.

In Case 9.2 there is a subtle but definite infiltrating mass penetrating the right glossotonsillar sulcus–tongue base region (Fig. 9.5*B*). This was not visible endoscopically, but speculative biopsies at this site, directed by the CT finding, revealed squamous cell carcinoma. The hypertrophic tonsillar tissue seen in both Figure 9.5*A* and *B* is a normal variant; the tumor is indicated only by the more subtle mass penetrating the intrinsic muscles on the right.

In patients in whom a needle biopsy of a neck mass reveals squamous cell carcinoma and there is no apparent primary following careful head and neck exam by an experienced otolaryngologist, CT or MRI will demonstrate a "submucosal" primary about 20 to 25% of the time. This is very important to the patient since it will focus the therapy of the primary tumor, with both an improved chance for local control and reduction in morbidity of therapy.

Anatomic Issue: Significance of Superficial Contour Variation of Tonsillar Tissues The lymphoid tissue of the nasopharynx, faucial tonsils, tongue base, and posterior pharyngeal wall creates a great deal of *superficial* asymmetry in the upper airway. These contours vary greatly among individuals and this tissue may be present throughout life. One must look to the *deep* tissue planes as evidence of significant pathology to avoid overcalling mass lesions. A mass penetrating the intrinsic muscles of the tongue base (as in Case 9.2) is highly significant, whereas the remainder of the lymphoid tissue in this particular patient has no significance in predicting the primary site. Learn to look at the parapharyngeal space, intrinsic muscles of the tongue base, carotid sheath, and, on MRI, superior constrictor muscle for evidence of deep infiltration (see Case 7.1, Chapter 7). Use the superficial asymmetry only to identify areas where you will check for deep spread. Do *not* use *superficial* asymmetry alone as an indication of significant mass lesions. Such overinterpretation will cause clinicians to get the mistaken impression that CT and MRI lack value in clinical situations in which they can be of tremendous clinical benefit when done and interpreted correctly.

Problem II

Case 9.3 (Fig. 9.6*A–C*)

(Case histories and questions on p. 210)

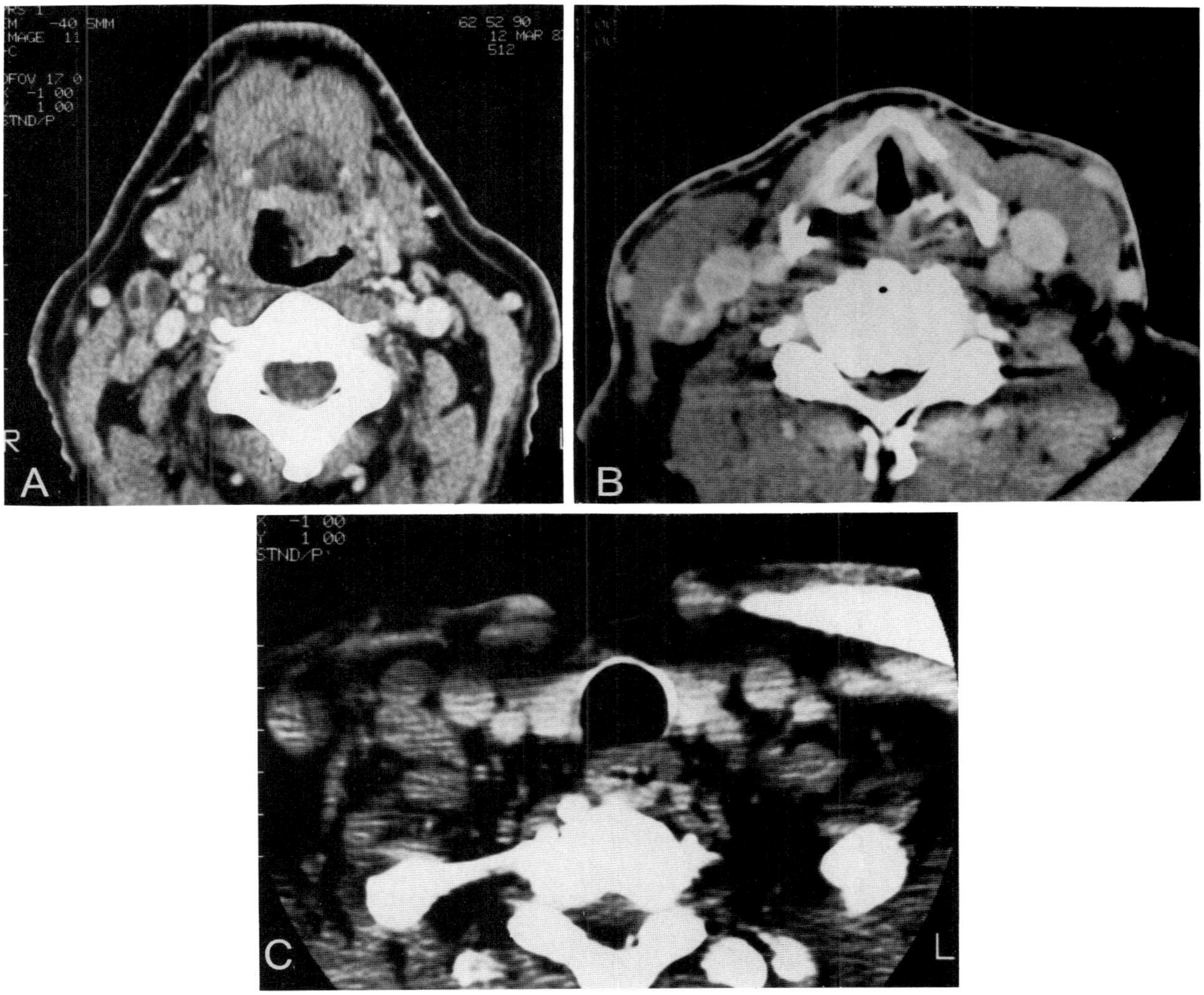

Figure 9.6*A–C*

Case 9.4 (Fig. 9.7*A* and *B*)

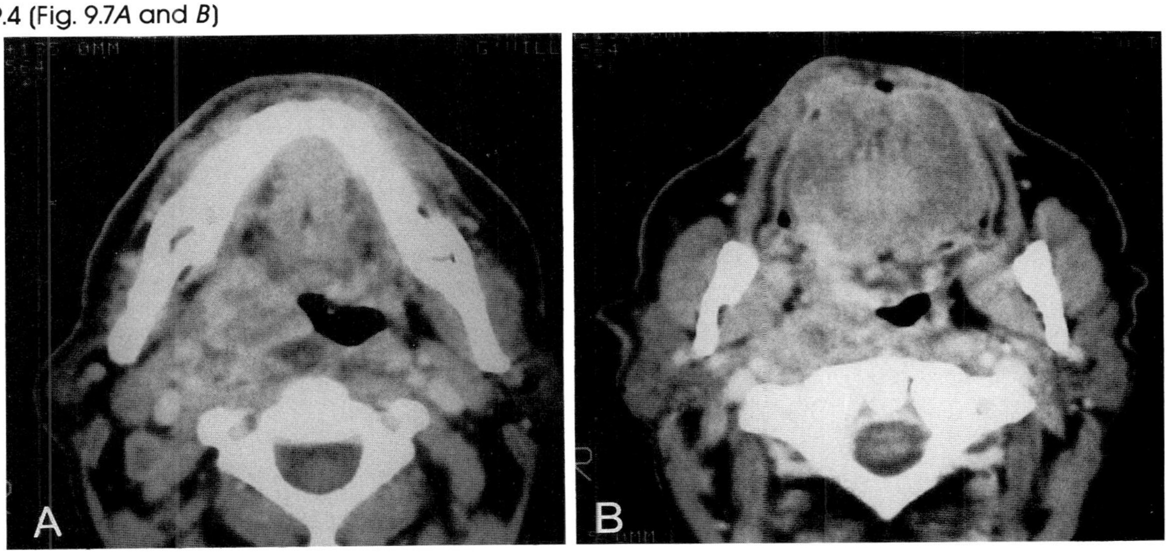

Figure 9.7*A* and *B*

Case 9.5 (Fig. 9.8*A* and *B*)

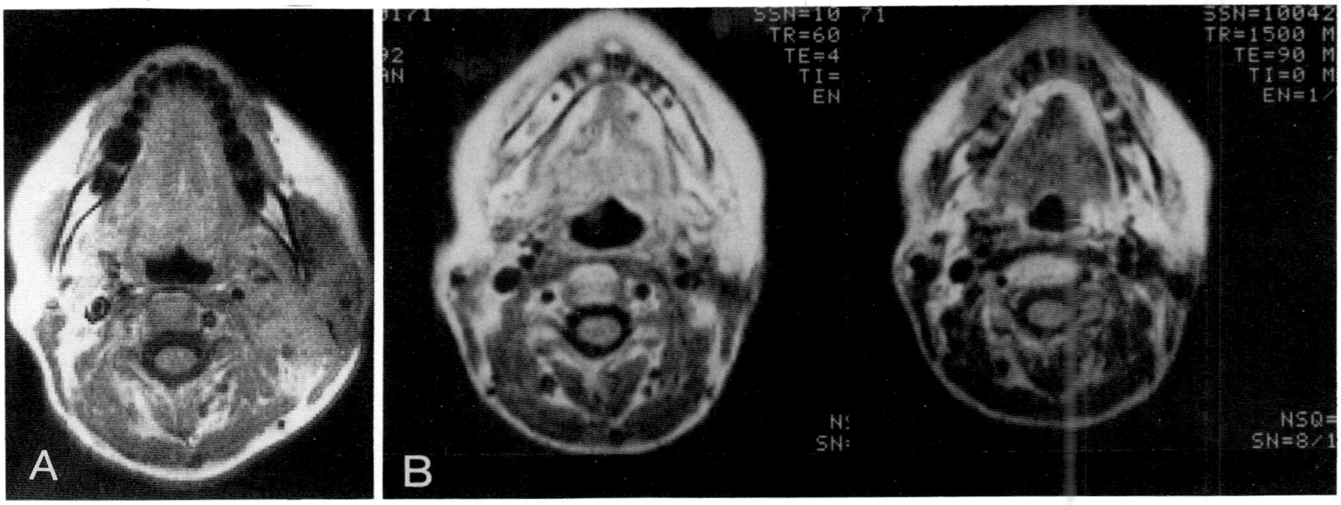

Figure 9.8*A* and *B*

Case Histories

Case 9.3 This patient with squamous cell carcinoma of the tongue base was staged T2N1.

Case 9.4 A patient with tonsillar carcinoma is being considered for primary surgical management and postoperative radiation therapy. Lesion was staged T2N2b clinically.

Case 9.5 A 35-year-old female with N3a neck secondary to T1 carcinoma of the tongue base. One scan (Fig. 9.8*A*) is done before and the other (Fig. 9.8*B*) after high-dose radiation therapy to the primary and neck.

Questions

1. What is the correct nodal staging in Case 9.3 based on CT findings. Is there evidence of capsular penetration of the nodal metastases?
2. Name three normal variations or technical factors that can produce a real or apparent focal lucency in a node that could be erroneously interpreted as a metastasis.
3. Is the course of action chosen in Case 9.4 reasonable based on the CT findings?
4. What are the chances of gross total resection of the nodal mass in Case 9.5 without preoperative radiation therapy?
5. Anatomic issue: Describe the position, number, and degree of normal variation of the retropharyngeal nodes in adults and children.

Discussion

Problem II—Staging Cervical Metastatic Disease The correct nodal staging in Case 9.3 would be N2c rather than the N1 stage given following palpation. This patient has unequivocally positive nodes bilaterally. Note that the clinically positive upper internal jugular node on the right contains two metastatic deposits. This patient was difficult to scan because of his short, thick neck but there are midjugular nodes on each side (Figure 9.6*B*) and a positive right "scalene" node at the thoracic inlet (Figure 9.6*C*). The neck is overall staged N2c; the right is N2b and the left N1 by CT (Question 1). With all three levels involved on the right this patient is at relatively high risk for distant metastases, and a complete metastatic workup (chest, bone, liver) would seem to be in order. There is no extranodal spread (Question 1). With these data a precise highly informed management plan for the neck disease can be developed. This patient had bilateral neck dissections following radiation therapy. Spinal accessory nerve was saved on both sides. Sternocleidomastoid muscle and jugular vein were preserved on the left.

The finding of a focal lucency in a node is highly specific in the proper clinical setting. Recognizing these as metastatic deposits can markedly improve on palpation alone for staging of cervical lymph node metastases in patients with squamous cell carcinoma of the upper aerodigestive tract. In fact, such findings are much more useful than size criteria. Lucent foci may, however, be produced by volume averaging with adjacent fat, normal fatty accumulations in the hilus of a node, or folding of a node. The latter finding is especially common in the upper internal jugular group when the nodes fold over the posterior belly of the digastric muscle (Question 2).

In Case 9.4 the patient not only has an advanced primary tumor and neck disease but also has grossly positive retropharyngeal nodes. There is both extranodal spread of tumor and gross disease above the posterior belly of the digastric muscle. Surgery done before radiation would likely leave the patient with less than a gross total resection above the posterior belly of the digastric as well as the gross disease in the retropharyngeal group. Frankly, radiation therapy alone also has little chance of controlling retropharyngeal adenopathy beyond 1.5 cm in size with evidence of capsular penetration when the primary is outside of the nasopharynx. The combination of CT findings in this patient indicates an extraordinarily poor prognosis. If treatment for cure is contemplated it would seem to be ill-advised to begin with surgery since chances for radiation therapy control of a grossly positive surgical bed are near nil in this setting (Question 3).

Case 9.5 is a case of massive adenopathy with a small primary. The neck disease wraps around the posterior belly of the digastric and is likely fixed to the carotid (Fig. 9.8*A*); there would be little chance of complete gross total resection without sacrifice of the carotid artery (Question 4). Post–radiation therapy MRI (Fig. 9.8*B*) shows that the tumor has "backed off" the carotid and formed a dense fibrous "pseudocapsule" that served as a plane of surgical resection. Patient is disease free 3 years following therapy. Pathologic review of neck specimen showed no residual tumor and dense fibrous pseudocapsule. Considerable experience and judgment must be used in determining the extent of extranodal spread of tumor. If done correctly this can help greatly in directing the treatment of neck disease.

Anatomic Issue: The Retropharyngeal Nodes The lateral retropharyngeal nodes lie *medial* to the carotid artery from the C_1 to the C_3 level. There are normally one to three nodes on each side. These tend to be largest near the skull base, frequently measuring 10 to 15 mm in children. In young adults (up to 30 to 35 years old) these nodes normally measure 5 to 8 mm in diameter; they measure 3 to 5 mm in older individuals. The median (medial) retropharyngeal nodes are in fact intercalated lymph nodules along the posterior wall of the nasopharynx. The medial retropharyngeal nodes appear to be anterior to the prevertebral strap muscles, and the lateral retropharyngeal nodes are located in the groove between these muscles and the internal carotid artery.

CHECKLIST—STAGING CERVICAL AND RETROPHARYNGEAL NODES (CASE 9.3)

	Number of Discreet Nodes over 1.5 cm or Any Size If They Have Focal Defects[a]	Largest Dimensions of Conglomerate Nodal Mass and Approximate Number of Nodes in Mass	? Capsular Penetration ("Yes" or "No")	Tumor Likely Fixed to: Carotid, Scalene, Sternocleidomastoid, Other	Comments
Retropharyngeal C_1–C_3 levels	Not seen				
Highest internal jugular (at and just above posterior belly of digastric)	Not seen				
Periparotid	Not seen				
Submandibular and submental	—				
Upper internal jugular (posterior belly of digastric to hyoid)	15-mm node with two focal defects	—	No	No	
Middle internal jugular (hyoid to midcricoid)	Right—15-mm internal jugular node two focal defects Left—15-mm internal jugular node—necrotic	—	No	No	
Lower internal jugular	2.6-cm node anterior to anterior scalene on right	—	No	No	2nd 1-cm node also
Spinal accessory (also state level in column 1)	—				
Other (tracheo-esophageal groove, supraclavicular, occipital)	Low internal jugular node(s) could be considered supraclavicular				

[a]Indicate side of neck for any abnormally noted. Also, be sure that focal defect is *not* due to volume averaging of adjacent fat, folding of a normal node, or fat in the hilus of the node.

CHECKLIST—STAGING CERVICAL AND RETROPHARYNGEAL NODES (CASE 9.4)

	Number of Discreet Nodes over 1.5 cm or Any Size If They Have Focal Defects[a]	Largest Dimensions of Conglomerate Nodal Mass and Approximate Number of Nodes in Mass	? Capsular Penetration ("Yes" or "No")	Tumor Likely Fixed to: Carotid, Scalene, Sternocleidomastoid, Other	Comments
Retropharyngeal C_1–C_3 levels	2 or 3	2.5 × 2 cm	Highly likely	Carotid not encased focal/ adherence possible	
Highest internal jugular (at and just above posterior belly of digastric)	Posterior belly thickened but no nodes above muscle except those noted above				
Periparotid	—				
Submandibular and submental	—				
Upper internal jugular (posterior belly of digastric to hyoid)	Not seen				
Middle internal jugular (hyoid to midcricoid)	Not seen				
Lower internal jugular	Not seen				
Spinal accessory (also state level in column 1)	1 cm with focal defect adjacent to nerve at posterior belly of digastric				
Other (tracheo-esophageal groove, supraclavicular, occipital)					

[a]Indicate side of neck for any abnormally noted. Also, be sure that focal defect is *not* due to volume averaging of adjacent fat, folding of a normal node, or fat in the hilus of the node.

CHECKLIST—NECK: MISCELLANEOUS USES (CASE 9.6)

	Seen	Nl	Abnl	Remarks
UPPER (C_1 TO HYOID)				
Subcutaneous fat and platysma		√		
Sternocleidomastoid muscle			√	Displaced posteriorly
Parotid tail		√		
Submandibular gland			√	Edematous
Mandible		√		
Mylohyoid muscle		√		
Posterior belly digastric	No			
Carotid sheath			√	Entire region edematous; left greater than right
Internal jugular nodes			√	Enlarged, reactive
Spinal accessory nodes			√	Enlarged, reactive
Submandibular nodes			√	Enlarged, reactive
Retropharyngeal nodes			√	2.5–3-cm necrotic, suppurative on right
Visceral compartment			√	Retrovisceral space edema vs. fluid
Prevertebral muscles			√	Edematous
Paraspinous muscles			?	Edematous on right
Spine		√		
Spinal canal and contents		√		

Case 9.7 (Fig. 9.10*A* and *B*)

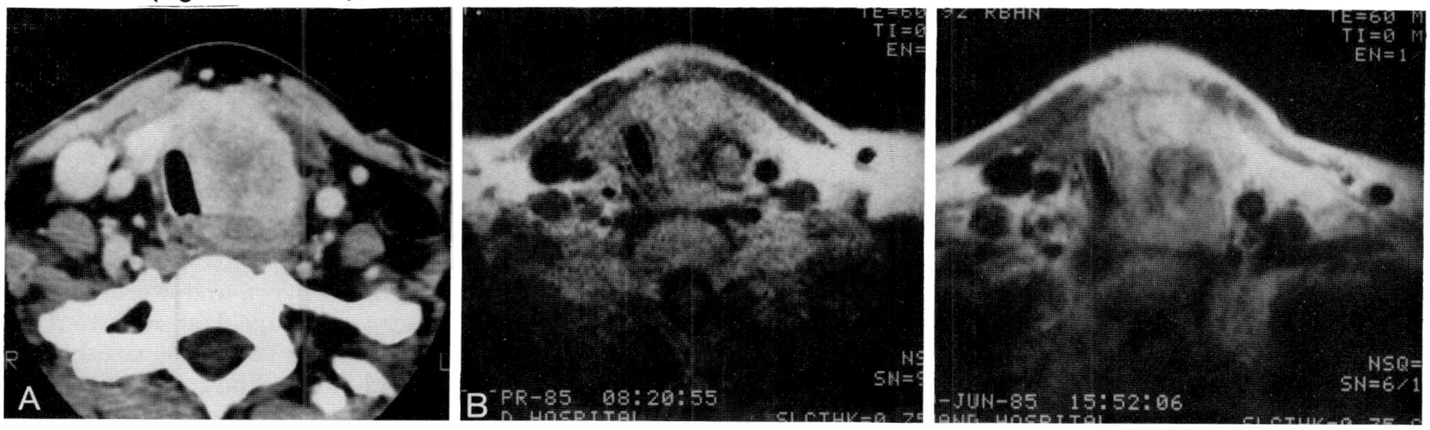

Figure 9.10*A* and *B*

Case 9.8 (Fig. 9.11*A* and *B*)

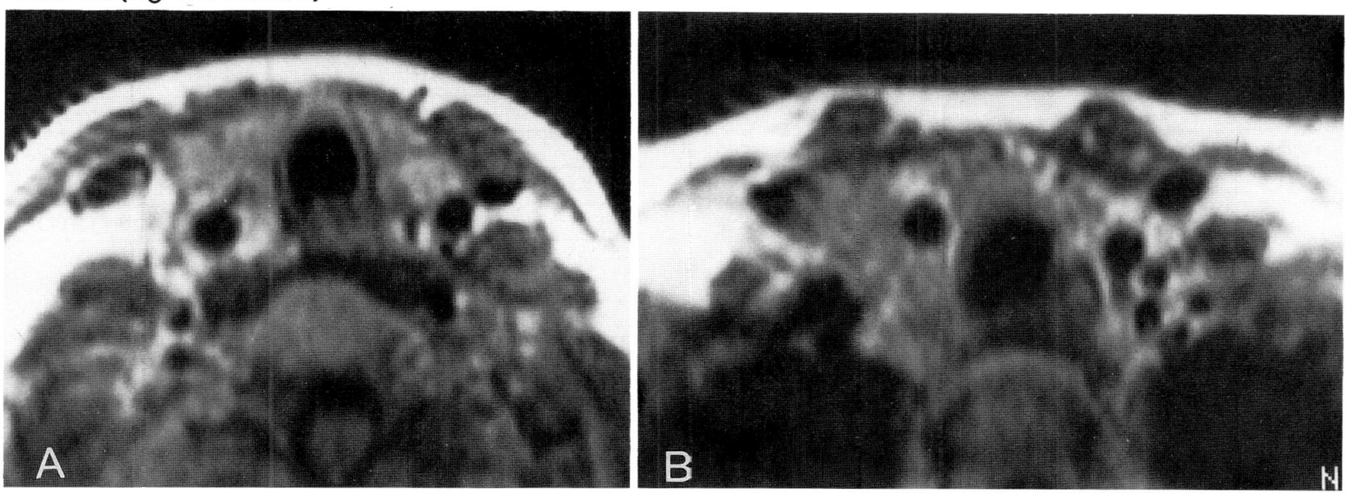

Figure 9.11*A* and *B*

Case Histories

Case 9.7 A 40-year-old male with medullary carcinoma of the thyroid gland has been told that surgery would require resection of trachea and esophagus.

Case 9.8 A 25-year-old female with needle biopsy of neck mass showing papillary-follicular carcinoma of the thyroid gland. The study was done to determine local extent of tumor prior to surgery.

Questions

1. Do the MRI findings support the surgical plans in Case 9.7?
2. Is tumor invading the trachea in Case 9.8? Is the tumor a locally aggressive or relatively nonaggressive in its morphology? Why?
3. Anatomic issue: What clinically important structures lie in the region of the tracheoesophageal groove?

Discussion

Problem IV—Imaging the Local and Regional Extent of Extraglandular Thyroid Carcinoma Magnetic resonance imaging and CT have important, complimentary roles to play in patients with thyroid cancer that has spread beyond the capsule of the gland. In Case 9.7 the CT shows tracheal compression and suggests esophageal involvement, but it required MRI to confirm invasion of the muscular wall of the esophagus as well as the tracheal ring of that level. These findings would support the surgical plan if ... resection is desired (Question 1) ... invasion indicates a very aggressive tumor (Question 2). All findings were confirmed at surgery. In addition, two positive 10-mm mediastinal nodes were resected in a combined cervicothoracic operation. This operative approach was undertaken because of the CT and MRI findings at the jugulosubclavian junction.

Anatomic Issue: Structures in the Tracheoesophageal Groove The tracheoesophageal groove is bordered by the carotid artery, thyroid gland, and prevertebral muscle, as well as the trachea and esophagus. The recurrent laryngeal nerve and a group of

SUGGESTED READINGS

Books, Chapters, Reviews

Mancuso AA, Hanafee WN: The neck. In: *Computed Tomography and Magnetic Resonance Imaging of the Head and Neck.* Baltimore, Williams & Wilkins, 1985, pp 169–240.

Reede DL, Bergeron RT, Osborn AG: CT of the soft tissues of the neck. In Bergeron RT, Osborn AG, Som PM (eds): *Head and Neck Imaging—Excluding the Brain.* St. Louis, CV Mosby, 1984, pp 491–530.

Rouviere H: *Anatomy of the Human Lymphatic System* (ed 1). Ann Arbor, MI, Edwards Brothers, 1938, pp 1–82.

Articles

On cervical and retropharyngeal nodal metastases:

Ballantyne AJ: Significance of retropharyngeal nodes in cancer of the head and neck. *Am J Surg* 108:500, 1964.

Cachin Y, Sancho-Garnier H, Micheau C, Marandas P: Nodal metastasis from carcinomas of the oropharynx. *Otolaryngol Clin North Am* 12:145–154, 1979.

Friedman M, Shelton VK, Mafee M, et al: Metastatic neck disease. Evaluation of computed tomography. *Arch Otolaryngol* 110:443–447, 1984.

Mancuso AA, Harnsberger HR, Muraki AS, Stevens MH: Computed tomography of cervical and retropharyngeal lymph nodes: normal anatomy, variants of normal and applications in staging head and neck cancer. Part II: pathology. *Radiology* 148:715–723, 1983.

Mancuso AA, Maceri D, Rice D, Hanafee WN: CT of cervical lymph node cancer. *AJR* 136:391–395, 1981.

McGavran MH, Bauer WC, Ogura JH: The incidence of cervical lymph node metastases from epidermoid carcinoma of the marynx and the relationship to certain characteristics of the primary tumor. *Cancer* 14:55–66, 1961.

Richard JM, Sancho-Garnier H, Micheau C: Prognostic factors in cervical lymph node metastasis in upper respiratory and digestive tract carcinomas: study of 1,712 cases during a 15-year period. *Laryngoscope* 97:97–101, 1987.

On neck masses of uncertain etiology:

Feldman PS, Kaplan MJ, Johns ME, et al: Fine-needle aspiration in squamous cell carcinoma of the head and neck. *Arch Otolaryngol* 109:735–642, 1983.

Mancuso AA, Hanfee WN: Elusive head and neck carcinomas beneath intact mocusa. *Laryngoscope* 93:133–139, 1983.

Martin H, Morfit HM: Cervical node metastasis as the first symptom of cancer. *Surg Gynecol Obstet* 76:133–159, 1944.

Miller D, Ervin T, Weichselbaum R, Fabian RL: The differential diagnosis of the mass in the neck. A fresh look. *Laryngoscope* 91:140–145, 1981.

Muraki AS, Mancuso AA, Harnsberger HR Metastatic cervical adenopathy from tumors of unknown origin: the role of CT. *Radiology* 152:749–754, 1984.

On MRI of the neck:

Glazer HS, Niemeyer JH, Balfe DM, et al: Neck neoplasms: MR imaging. Part I. Initial evaluation. *Radiology* 160:343–348, 1986.

Glazer HS, Niemeyer JH, Balfe DM, et al: Neck neoplasms: MR imaging. Part II. Posttreatment evaluation. *Radiology* 160:349–354, 1986.

Stark DD, Moss AA, Gamsu G, et al: Magnetic resonance imaging of the neck. I. Normal anatomy. *Radiology* 150:447–454, 1984.

Stark DD, Moss AA, Gamsu G, et al: Magnetic resonance imaging of the neck. II. Pathologic findings. *Radiology* 150:445–461, 1984.

On MRI in thyroid masses and thyroid cancer:

Gefter WB, Spritzer CE, Eisenberg B, LiVolsi VA, et al: Thyroid imaging with high-field strength surface-coil MR. *Radiology* 164:483–490, 1987.

Lawson VG: The management of airway involvement in thyroid tumors. *Arch Otoarlyngol* 109:86–90, 1983.

McShane DP, Freeman JL, Noyek AM, et al: A review of conventional and CT imaging in the evaluation of thyroid malignancies. *Otolaryngol* 16:4–9, 1987.

Noma S, Nishimura K, Togashi K, et al: Thyroid gland: MR imaging. *Radiology* 164:495–499, 1987.

Tytor M, Olofsson J: Thyroid tumors invading the larynx and trachea. *Otolaryngol* 15:7–79, 1986.

On imaging of the parathyroid glands:

Gooding GAW, Okerlund MD, Stark DD: Parathyroid imaging: Comparison of double-tracer (T1-201, Tc-99m) scintigraphy and high resolution use. *Radiology* 161:57–64, 1986.

Miller DL, Doppman JL, Shwaker TH, et al: Localization of parathyroid adenomas in patients who have undergone surgery. Parts I and II. *Radiology* 162:137–141, 1987.

Peck WW, Higgins CB, Fisher MR, et al: Hyperparathyroidism: comparison of MR imaging with radionuclide scanning. *Radiology* 162:143–146, 1987.

Stark DD, Gooding GAW, Moss AA: Parathyroid imaging: comparison of high-resolution CT and high-resolution sonography. *AJR* 141:633–638, 1983.

Appendix A

Checklists

CHECKLIST—ORBIT

	Seen	Nl	Abnl	Remarks
UPPER				
Preseptal soft tissues				
Globe				
Intra/extraconal fat				
Optic nerve and sheath				
Ophthalmic artery				
Optic canal				
Anterior clinoid process				
Levator palpebrae and superior rectus muscles				
Superior ophthalmic vein				
Lacrimal fossa and gland				
Orbital process frontal bone				
Trochlea/superior oblique muscle/tendon				
Crista galli				
Cribriform plate				
Planum sphenoidale				
Tuberculum sellae				
Suprasellar cistern and contents				
MID				
Orbital septum				
Preseptal soft tissues				
Globe				
Lens/anterior chamber				
Posterior chamber				
Intraconal fat				
Optic nerve and sheath				
Superior orbital fissure/orbital apex				
Cavernous sinus				
Sella and contents				
Medial rectus muscle				
Lateral rectus muscle				
Extraconal orbital fat				
Medial wall orbit/ethmoids				
Greater wing sphenoid				

continued

CHECKLIST—ORBIT *(continued)*

	Seen	Nl	Abnl	Remarks
LOWER Preseptal soft tissues				
Globe				
Intraconal fat				
Inferior rectus muscle				
Inferior orbital fissure				
Foramen rotundum				
Floor orbit				
Infraorbital canal/groove				
Cavernous sinus				
Sphenoid sinus				
Extraconal orbital fat				
Medial wall orbit/ethmoids				
Lacrimal bone/nasolacrimal fossa				
Maxillary sinus				
Greater wing of sphenoid				

CHECKLIST—VISUAL PATHWAYS BEYOND ORBITS

	Seen	Nl	Abnl	Remarks
Optic nerve to optic canal				
Optic nerve in optic canal				
Optic chiasm				
Optic tract				
Lateral geniculate body				
Optic radiations				
Visual cortex				
Cavernous sinus nerves (III, IV, VI)				
Quadrigeminal plate–tectum and pretectal regions				
Midbrain ventral to acqueduct				
Nucleus III				
Nucleus IV				
Median longitudinal fasiculus (MLF)				
Pontomedullary junction, floor of 4th ventricle nucleus VI, lower MLF				

CHECKLIST—PARANASAL SINUSES, NASAL CAVITY, FACIAL BONES
(also see orbits if applicable)

	Seen	Nl	Abnl	Remarks
UPPER				
Soft tissues of scalp				
Frontal sinus—outer table				
Frontal sinus—inner table				
Frontal sinus—contents				
Intracranial structures, spaces				
Nasofrontal duct (frontal recess)				
Cribriform plate				
Ethmoids (contents, walls)				
Perpendicular plate (ethmoid)				
Frontal bone—general				
Frontal bone—orbital process				
Orbital roof				
Optic canals				
Planum sphenoidale and clinoids				
Greater wing sphenoid				
Superior orbital fissure				
Orbital contents (orbital checklist as needed)				
MID				
Preseptal and other soft tissues				
Nasal bone				
Frontal process maxilla				
Lacrimal bone and fossa/sac				
Lower ethmoids (contents, walls)				
Perpendicular plate (of ethmoids)				
Vomer				
Nasal cavity				
Middle meatus				
Middle conchae/turbinate				
Ethmoidal bullae				
Uncinate process (of ethmoid)				
Maxillary sinus (ostia, contents, bony walls)				
Sphenoethmoidal recess				
Sphenoid sinus (ostia, contents, bony walls)				
Greater wing sphenoid				
Inferior orbital fissure				
Cavernous sinus				
Zygoma				

continued

CHECKLIST—PARANASAL SINUSES, NASAL CAVITY, FACIAL BONES
(continued)

	Seen	Nl	Abnl	Remarks
LOWER Soft tissue of face (fat, muscles)				
Nasal bones				
Nasolacrimal canal				
Nasal septum				
Middle meatus (lower)				
Inferior meatus				
Inferior concha/turbinate				
Maxillary sinus (contents, walls)				
Groove for posterior superior alveolar nerve				
Posterior choanae				
Nasopharynx (nasopharynx checklist as needed)				
Clivus				
Sphenopalatine foramen				
Pterygopalatine fossa				
Pterygoid plates				
Infratemporal fossa (retroantral fat)				
Distal maxillary neurovascular bundle				
Hard palate (greater and lesser palatine foramina)				
Maxillary alveolar ridge				
Maxillary (anterior nasal) spine				
Maxillary tuberosity				
Buccinator muscle				
Buccinator space				
Zygomatic arch				
Mandible				

CHECKLIST—PAROTID REGION

	Seen	Nl	Abnl	Remarks
UPPER Pinna				
Pretragal soft tissues and nodes				
Zygomatic arch				
Masseter muscle				
Mandible—head				
Mandible—condyle				
Condylar fossa–temporomandibular joint				
External auditory canal—cartilaginous portion				
External auditory canal—bony portion				
Mastoid portion of temporal bone				
Facial canal—descending portion				
Stylomastoid foramen				
Styloid process				
Fat pad below stylomastoid foramen				
Digastric groove				
Insertion of posterior belly of digastric muscle				
Tragal pointer				
Prestyloid parapharyngeal space				
Carotid artery				
Jugular vein				
MID Subcutaneous fat				
Masseter muscle				
Mandible—ramus				
Buccinator space				
Parotid duct				
Parotid tissue—accessory lobe				
Parotid gland—superficial portion				
Parotid gland—deep portion				
Retromandibular vein				
External carotid artery				
Expected course of facial nerve				
Intraparotid nodes				
Mastoid tip				
Styloid process				
Posterior belly of digastric muscle				
Prestyloid parapharyngeal space				
Carotid artery				
Jugular vein				
Medial pterygoid muscle				
Course of mandibular nerve				

continued

CHECKLIST—PAROTID REGION *(continued)*

	Seen	Nl	Abnl	Remarks
LOWER Subcutaneous fat				
Masseter muscle				
Mandible—body/angle				
Parotid—tail (*below* plane of main trunk of facial nerve)				
Retromandibular vein				
External carotid artery				
Sternocleidomastoid muscle				
Posterior belly of digastric muscle				
Intraparotid nodes				
Prestyloid parapharyngeal space				
Carotid artery				
Jugular vein				
Medial pterygoid muscle				
Upper internal jugular nodes				
Submandibular gland				

CHECKLIST—SUBMANDIBULAR REGION

	Seen	Nl	Abnl	Remarks
UPPER Subcutaneous fat				
Platysma				
Mandible—angle/body				
Parotid tail				
Mylohyoid muscle				
Submandibular space				
Submandibular gland—deep process				
Medial pterygoid muscle				
Sublingual space				
Posterior belly of digastric muscle				
Tongue base				
MID Subcutaneous fat				
Platysma				
Mandible body				
Anterior belly of digastric muscle				
Submental space				
Mylohyoid muscle				
Submandibular space				
Submandibular gland				
Submandibular nodes				
Facial artery and vein				
Geniohyoid muscle				
Tongue base				
Internal jugular nodes				
LOWER Subcutaneous fat				
Platysma				
Anterior belly of digastric muscle				
Geniohyoid muscle				
Hyoid bone				
Submental space				
Submandibular space				
Submandibular gland				
Internal jugular nodes				

CHECKLIST—TEMPORAL BONE

	Seen	Nl	Abnl	Remarks
UPPER Mastoid—periantral air cells				
Epitympanic recess—upper antrum				
Koerner's septum				
Otic capsule bone (arcuate eminence)				
Arcuate tunnel				
Superior semicircular canal				
Inferior semicircular canal (superior limb)				
Common crus				
Lateral semicircular canal				
Vestibular aqueduct				
Internal auditory canal				
Facial canal—labyrinthine segment				
Bill's bar				
Facial canal—anterior genu				
Petrous apex				
UPPER-MID Mastoid—periantral air cells				
Sigmoid plate				
Epitympanic recess				
Lateral wall epitympanic recess (scutum)				
Aditus ad antrum				
Mastoid antrum				
Koerner's septum				
Malleus—head				
Incus—body and short process				
Facial canal—tympanic (horizontal) segment				
Facial canal—posterior genu				
Pyramidal eminence				
Tensor tympani semicanal				
Otic capsule bone				
Vestibule				
Oval window niche				
Posterior semicircular canal				
Vestibular aqueduct				
Cochlea including modiolus				
Internal auditory canal				
Petrous apex				

continued

CHECKLIST—TEMPORAL BONE *(continued)*

	Seen	Nl	Abnl	Remarks
MID-LOWER Mastoid air cells				
Sigmoid plate				
External auditory canal—bony portion				
External auditory canal—cartilaginous portion				
Tympanic membrane				
Mesotympanum				
Malleus—long process				
Incus—long process				
Stapes—crura				
Tensor tympani semicanal				
Tensor tympani muscle and tendon				
Facial canal—descending portion				
Sinus tympani				
Otic capsule bone				
Vestibule				
Posterior semicircular canal				
Cochlea				
Petrous apex				
Cochlear aqueduct				
LOWER Mastoid air cells				
Sigmoid plate				
External auditory canal—bony portion				
External auditory canal—cartilaginous portion				
Tympanic membrane				
Hypotympanum				
Malleus—long process				
Incus—long process				
Eustachian tube—bony portion				
Facial canal—descending portion				
Stylomastoid foramen				
Fat pad below stylomastoid foramen				
Sinus tympani				
Otic capsule bone				
Cochlea				
Round window				
Cochlear aqueduct				
Petrous apex				
Carotid canal				
Jugular fossa (pars nervosa, venosum, spur)				
Jugular tubercle				

Pterygoid plates				
Pterygopalatine fossa				

continued

CHECKLIST—TOPOGRAPHIC ANATOMY OF POSTERIOR FOSSA RELATED TO TEMPORAL BONE VII AND VIIIth NERVE

	Seen	Nl	Abnl	Remarks
Prepontine cistern				
Basilar artery				
Pons				
Cerebellum				
Pontomedullary junction				
Flocculus				
Cerebellopontine angle cistern				
Trigeminal nerve				

CHECKLIST—NASOPHARYNX *(continued)*

	Seen	Nl	Abnl	Remarks
Other Nasal cavity				
Maxillary sinuses				
Mandible				
Deep portion of parotid				
Clivus				
Stylomastoid foramen				
Mastoid tip				
Foramen magnum				
LOWER Superficial Soft Tissues Soft palate				
Adenoidal tissue				
Deep Structures and Spaces Levator veli palatini and pharyngeal wall musculature				
Parapharyngeal space				
Infratemporal fossa and masticator space (medial pterygoid muscle)				
Pterygoid plates				
Buccinator space				
Carotid sheath				
Prevertebral muscles				
Retropharyngeal nodes				
Other Parotid (deep and superficial portions)				
Maxillary sinuses				
C_1 and spinal canal				
Mandible				

CHECKLIST—LOWER CRANIAL NERVES (IX–XII) AND UPPER SYMPATHETIC TRUNK[a]

	Seen	Nl	Abnl	Remarks
Pontomecullary junction and upper medulla (IX, X, XII)				
Upper cervical cord (XI)				
Medullary cisterns				
Jugular fossa (IX, X, XI)				
Hypoglossal canal (XII)				
Lower clivus				
Inferior petrous portion of temporal bone				
Carotid sheath region to posterior belly of digastric muscle (all)				
Carotid sheath region to bifurcation (all but XI)				
Carotid sheath region to thorax (X, sympathetics)				

[a]Associated symptoms are important determinants of how cranial nerve imaging workup should proceed. Consult diagnostic algorithms for guidance.

CHECKLIST—Vth CRANIAL NERVE[a]

	Seen	Nl	Abnl	Remarks
Pontomesencephalic junction to medulla (sensory and motor nuclei)				
Midpons—ventrolateral (origin of nerve)				
Upper cerebellopontine angle				
Petrous apex				
Meckel's cave and cistern of trigeminal ganglion				
Cavernous sinus				
Sphenoid bone—all parts				
Paranasal sinuses				
Nasopharynx				
Superior orbital fissure (V_1)				
Supraorbital soft tissues				
Foramen rotundum (V_2)				
Pterygopalatine fossa (V_2)				
Infraorbital groove and canal (V_2)				
Inferior orbit (V_2)				
Skin of cheek (V_2)				
Foramen ovale (V_3)				
Upper infratemporal fossa masticator space (pterygoid muscle) (V_3)				
Between mandible and pterygoid insertions (V_3)				
Mandibular formen (V_3)				
Mandibular alveolar canal and marrow space (V_3)				
Mental foramen (V_3)				

[a]Associated symptoms and presentations vary. See imaging algorithms for details of how workup should proceed.

CHECKLIST—ORAL CAVITY, OROPHARYNX, FLOOR OF MOUTH, TONGUE BASE, MANDIBLE
(if lesion extends cephalad use nasopharynx checklist as well)

	Seen	Nl	Abnl	Remarks
UPPER Superficial Soft Tissues Uvula				
Soft palate				
Tonsillar fossa (faucial tonsils)				
Upper gingivobuccal sulcus				
Deep Soft Tissues Parapharyngeal space				
Infratemporal fossa/masticator space				
Oral tongue				
Buccinator muscle				
Buccinator space				
Carotid sheath				
Prevertebral muscles				
Retropharyngeal nodes				
Bones Hard palate				
Palatine foramina				
Pterygoid processes				
Maxillary alveolar ridge				
Maxillary tuberosity				
Mandible (condyle, ramus, coronoid)				
Upper cervical spine				
Other Parotid gland				
MID Superficial Soft Tissues Uvula (tip)				
Level of circumvallate papillae				
Anterior ⅔ (oral) tongue				
Mid-lower tonsillar fossa				
Upper glossotonsillar sulcus				
Lower gingivobuccal sulcus				
Deep Soft Tissues Parapharyngeal space				
Pterygomandibular space (lingual nerve)				
Infratemporal fossa/masticator space				
Carotid sheath				
Prevertebral muscles				
Retropharyngeal nodes				
Bones Mandibular alveolar ridge				
Mandibular ramus, body, foramen				
Upper cervical spine				
Other Parotid (superficial and deep)				

continued

CHECKLIST—ORAL CAVITY, OROPHARYNX, FLOOR OF MOUTH, TONGUE BASE, MANDIBLE *(continued)*

	Seen	Nl	Abnl	Remarks
LOWER Superficial Soft Tissues				
Lower glossotonsillar sulcus				
Lingual tonsils				
Valleculae				
Pharyngoepiglottic folds				
Deep Soft Tissues Mylohyoid muscle				
Genioglossus-geniohyoid muscles				
Lingual septum				
Sublingual space (lingual vessels)				
Hyoglossus-styloglossus muscles				
Intrinsic tongue muscles (base)				
Anterior belly digastric				
Posterior belly digastric				
Carotid sheath (nodes)				
Prevertebral muscles				
Preepiglottic space				
Bones Mandible (body/angle)				
Mental foramen				
Hyoid				
Other Submandibular gland and space				
Submandibular-submental nodes				
Parotid—tail				

CHECKLIST—LARYNX AND HYPOPHARYNX

	Seen	Nl	Abnl	Remarks
SUPRAGLOTTIS AND HYPOPHARYNX Mid Infrahyoid strap muscles				
Thyroid laminae				
Thyrohyoid membrane				
Paralaryngeal space: Right				
Left				
Pyriform sinus: Right				
Left				
Body of epiglottis				
Preepiglottic space				
Postpharyngeal wall				
Soft tissues of neck				
High Infrahyoid strap muscles				
Thyrohyoid membrane				
Hyoid bone				
Superior cornua thyroid cartilages				
Paralaryngeal space: Right				
Left				
Aryepiglottic folds: Right				
Left				
Pyriform sinus: Right				
Left				
Free margin of epiglottis				
Preepiglottic space				
Pharyngoepiglottic folds				
Valleculae				
Tongue base				
Posterior pharyngeal wall				
Soft tissues of neck				
Low Infrahyoid strap muscles				
Thyroid notch				
Arytenoids (superior process)				
False cords (position/thickness): Right				
Left				
Paralaryngeal space:				
Right				
Left				

continued

CHECKLIST—LARYNX AND HYPOPHARYNX *(continued)*

	Seen	Nl	Abnl	Remarks
Appendix/ventricle: Right				
Left				
Inferior epiglottis				
Preepiglottic space				
Aryepiglottic fold:				
Right				
Left				
Pyriform sinus: Right				
Left				
Posterior pharyngeal wall				
Soft tissues of neck				
GLOTTIS Undersurface of True Cords				
Infrahyoid strap muscles				
Thyroid cartilage				
Right cord (position/thickness)				
Left cord (position/thickness)				
Anterior commissure				
Right arytenoid (body/vocal process)				
Left arytenoid (body/vocal process)				
Cricoid lamina				
Posterior commissure				
Cricothyroid space				
Paralaryngeal space				
Postcricoid soft tissues				
Apex of pyriform sinus				
Soft tissues of neck				
Midplane of True Cords Infrahyoid strap muscles				
Thyroid cartilage				
Right cord (position/thickness)				
Left cord (position/thickness)				
Anterior commissure				
Right arytenoid (body/vocal process)				
Left arytenoid (body/vocal process)				
Cricoid lamina				
Posterior commissure				
Cricothyroid space				
Paralaryngeal space				
Postcricoid soft tissues				
Apex of pyriform sinus				
Soft tissues of neck				

continued

CHECKLIST—LARYNX AND HYPOPHARYNX *(continued)*

	Seen	Nl	Abnl	Remarks
SUBGLOTTIS Soft tissues adjacent to cricoid				
Cricothyroid membrane				
Cricoid—anterior ring				
Cricoid—lamina				
Cricoid—arches				
Thyroid cartilages—inferior cornua				
Cricothyroid joint				
Cricopharyngeus/esophageal verge				
Course of recurrent laryngeal nerves				
Thyroid gland				

CHECKLIST—STAGING CERVICAL AND RETROPHARYNGEAL NODES

	Number of Discreet Nodes over 1.5 cm or Any Size If They Have Focal Defects[a]	Largest Dimensions of Conglomerate Nodal Mass and Approximate Number of Nodes in Mass	? Capsular Penetration ("Yes" or "No")	Tumor Likely Fixed to: Carotid, Scalene, Sternocleidomastoid, Other	Comments
Retropharyngeal C_1–C_3 levels					
Highest internal jugular (at and just above posterior belly of digastric)					
Periparotid					
Submandibular and submental					
Upper internal jugular (posterior belly of digastric to hyoid)					
Middle internal jugular (hyoid to midcricoid)					
Lower internal jugular					
Spinal accessory (also state level in column 1)					
Other (tracheoesophageal groove, supraclavicular, occipital)					

[a]Indicate side of neck for any abnormally noted.

CHECKLIST—NECK: MISCELLANEOUS USES

	Seen	Nl	Abnl	Remarks
UPPER (C_1 TO HYOID) Subcutaneous fat and platysma				
Sternocleidomastoid muscle				
Parotid tail				
Submandibular gland				
Mandible				
Mylohyoid muscle				
Posterior belly of digastric				
Carotid sheath				
Internal jugular nodes				
Spinal accessory nodes				
Submandibular nodes				
Retropharyngeal nodes				
Visceral compartment				
Prevertebral muscles				
Paraspinous muscles				
Spine				
Spinal canal and contents				
MID (HYOID TO CRICOID) Subcutaneous fat and platysma				
Sternocleidomastoid muscle				
Carotid sheath				
Internal jugular nodes				
Spinal accessory nodes				
Visceral compartment				
Prevertebral muscles				
Paraspinous muscles				
Spine				
Spinal canal and contents				
LOWER (CRICOID TO THORACIC INLET) Subcutaneous fat and platysma				
Sternocleidomastoid muscle				
Carotid sheath				
Internal jugular nodes				
Spinal accessory nodes				
Other nodes				
Thyroid				
Esophagus				
Tracheoesophageal groove/trachea				
Prevertebral muscles				
Scalene muscles				
Roots of brachial plexus				
Paraspinous muscles				
Spine				
Spinal canal and contents				

continued

CHECKLIST—NECK: MISCELLANEOUS USES *(continued)*

	Seen	Nl	Abn	Remarks
Supraclavicular fossa				
Clavicle				
Sternum				
Jugulosubclavian junction				
Left brachiocephalic vein				
First and second ribs				
Lung apicies				

Appendix B

TNM Classifications and Definitions

TNM Classification	Definitions[a]
Primary Tumor (T)	
TX	Tumor that cannot be assessed by rules
T0	No evidence of primary tumor
Nasopharynx	
TIS	Carcinoma in situ
T1	Tumor confined to one site of nasopharynx or no tumor visible (positive biopsy only)
T2	Tumor involving two sites (both posterosuperior and lateral walls)
T3	Extension of tumor into nasal cavity or oropharynx
T4	Tumor invasion of skull or cranial nerve involvement, or both
Oropharynx	
TIS	Carcinoma in situ
T1	Tumor 2 cm or less in greatest diameter
T2	Tumor more than 2 cm but not more than 4 cm in greatest diameter
T3	Tumor more than 4 cm in greatest diameter
T4	Massive tumor more than 4 cm in diameter with invasion of bone, soft tissues of neck, or root (deep musculature) of tongue
Supraglottis	
TIS	Carcinoma in situ
T1	Tumor confined to site of origin with normal mobility
T2	Tumor involving adjacent supraglottic site(s) or glottis without fixation
T3	Tumor limited to larynx with fixation and/or extension to involve postcricoid area, medial wall of pyriform sinus, or preepiglottic space
T4	Massive tumor extending beyond the larynx to involve oropharynx, soft tissues of neck, or destruction of thyroid cartilage
Glottis	
TIS	Carcinoma in situ
T1	Tumor confined to vocal cord(s) with normal mobility (including involvement of anterior or posterior commissures)
T2	Supraglottic and/or subglottic extension of tumor with normal or impaired cord mobility
T3	Tumor confined to the larynx with cord fixation
T4	Massive tumor with thyroid cartilage destruction and/or extension beyond the confines of the larynx
Subglottis	
TIS	Carcinoma in situ
T1	Tumor confined to the subglottic region
T2	Tumor extension to vocal cords with normal or impaired cord mobility
T3	Tumor confined to larynx with cord fixation
T4	Massive tumor with cartilage destruction or extension beyond the confines of the larynx, or both
Nodal Involvement (N)	
NX	Nodes cannot be assessed
N0	No clinically positive node
N1	Single clinically positive ipsilateral node 3 cm or less in diameter
N2	Metastasis in single ipsilateral lymph node, more than 3 cm but not more than 6 cm in greatest dimension, or in multiple ipsilateral nodes, none more than 6 cm in greatest dimension, or in bilateral or contralateral lymph nodes, none more than 6 cm
N2a	Metastasis in a single ipsilateral lymph node more than 3 cm but not more than 6 cm in greatest dimension
N2b	Metastasis in multiple ipsilateral lymph nodes, none more than 6 cm in greatest dimension
N2c	Metastasis in bilateral or contralateral lymph nodes, none more than 6 cm in greatest dimension
N3	Metastasis in lymph node more than 6 cm in greatest dimension

[a]From Manual for Staging of Cancer ed 3. American Joint Committee on Cancer.

APPENDIX C

Spread Patterns of Head and Neck Malignancies

Primary Site and Critical Anatomy	Suggested Imaging Plane(s)	Spread Pattern: Deep Spaces	Spread Pattern: Muscle Bundles	Spread Pattern: Bone	Spread Pattern: Neurovascular Bundles	Nodes
ETHMOID						
Cribriform plate Fovea ethmoidalis Olfactory tracts, frontal lobes Vertical plate ethmoid-midline Medial wall orbit Periorbital fat Muscle cone Orbital apex Pterygopalatine fossa (IOF)	C C C A,C A,C A,C A,C A A			All sites direct and via natural ostia	Olfactory neuroepithelium	Rare; retropharyngeal at risk if nasal cavity is involved
Cavernous sinus	A,C				Via orbital apex or infraorbital nerve (f. rotundum)	
Antroethmoidal septum Sphenoid Floor of orbit Maxillary antrum Nasal cavity Septum-midline	C A,C C A,C A,C A,C					
MAXILLARY ANTRUM						
Floor of orbit Infraorbital nerve Periorbital fat Muscle cone Orbital apex	C C C C A			All sites by direct spread and natural ostia		Unusual except in advanced lesions or those through anterior wall to skin
Pterygopalatine fossa (IOF) Cavernous sinus	A A,C	Via orbital apex or infraorbital nerve (f. rotundum) or via distal internal maxillary vessels				Retropharyngeal at risk if nasal cavity, nasopharynx, or infratemporal fossa involved
Antroethmoidal septum Ethmoids Medial wall septum	C	See ethmoid spread pattern if involved				
Nasal cavity Hard palate Nasopharynx	A,C C A,C					
Posterior wall Retroantral fat Infratemporal fossa	A A A			At groove for posterior superior alveolar nerves, arteries, veins	Via posterior-superior alveolar nerves, arteries, veins can go to pterygomaxillary fossa	
Anterior wall—skin, subcutaneous fat Nasolacrimal canal	A A,C					
NASOPHARYNX						
Roof Sphenoid sinus	C,S A,C			Direct		Retropharyngeal; always positive
Cavernous sinus	A,C	Via parapharyngeal space; pterygopalatine fossa		Direct along f. rotundum, ovale	Via V_2 or V_3	
Clivus	A,S			Direct		
Inferior petrous apex Floor middle cranial fossa Brain	C,A C,A C,A	Via parapharyngeal space	Via tensor, levator palatini	Via tensor, levator, pharyngeal space, fossa of Rosenmuller	Via carotid Via V_3	Usually bilateral; internal jugular and spinal accessory nodes very frequently involved

continued

Spread Patterns of Head and Neck Malignancies *(Continued)*

Primary Site and Critical Anatomy	Suggested Imaging Plane(s)	Spread Pattern: Deep Spaces	Muscle Bundles	Bone	Neurovascular Bundles	Nodes
Lateral wall Pterygoid plates	A,C A		Via tensor palatini m. Via pterygoid m.	Direct		
Infratemporal fossa (masticator space)		Via parapharyngeal space	Via pterygoid m.			
Pterygopalatine fossa	A	Via infratemporal fossa		Via pterygoid processes	Via V_2	Nodal staging less critical in management decisions than in lower aerodigestive tract lesions (e.g., orophyarynx, larynx)
Inferior orbital fissure Superior orbital fissure	A A	Via pterygopalatine fossa From infratemporal fossa		Via base pterygoid process	Via V_2	
Orbital apex	A	From pterygopalatine fossa via IOF and SOF		Via pterygoid plates and basisphenoid	Via V_1, V_2	
Nasal cavity	A,S					
Oropharynx Parapharyngeal space Posterior pharyngeal wall Soft palate	A A A C,S	Via parapharyngeal space	Via tensor, levator palatini to soft palate then via palatopharyngeus			
Ethmoid sinuses	A,C			From sphenoid sinus nasal cavity (vomer) direct		
Maxillary sinus	A,C	From pterygopalatine fossa, orbital apex–IOF		Pterygoid plates	Via V_2; posterosuperior alveolar neurovascular bundle	
SOFT PALATE						
Palatoglossus Palatopharyngeus Tensor/levator palatini Parapharyngeal space	All are suboptimal alone, axial best overall	To NP via parapharyngeal space	Palatoglossus to tongue Palatopharyngeus to PPW tensor/levator to NP	Hard palate, pterygoid plates (direct)		Internal jugular Spinal accessory Retropharyngeal
TONSILLAR FOSSA[b]						
Palatoglossus muscle Superior constrictor muscle Palatopharyngeus muscle Parapharyngeal space Styloglossus, stylohyoid, stylopharyngeus Supratonsillar recess Soft palate Soft tissues—neck	A A A A A A A A	Via parapharyngeal space to soft tissues of neck, muscles attaching to styloid, carotid sheath, and nasopharynx Via supratonsillar recess to soft palate and NP	Via palatoglossus to soft palate; via styloid group of muscles to soft tissues of neck, carotid sheath, upper cranial nerves, and other cephalocaudal spread deep to pharyngeal walls	In very advanced lesions direct spread to mandible, skull base (via styloid) and pterygoid plates possible	Direct spread to carotid sheath possible, also to cranial nerves IX–XII and sympathetics	Internal jugular Spinal accessory Retropharyngeal
BASE OF TONGUE AND GLOSSOTONSILLAR SULCUS						
Intrinsic tongue muscles Geniohyoid, genioglossus mm Mylohyoid muscle Sublingual space Submandibular space Parapharyngeal space Preepiglottic space Soft tissues—neck	A,S A,C A,C A,C A,C A A,S A	Anterior spread FOM via sublingual (may be clinically occult) Via submandibular and parapharyngeal space to soft tissue of neck To preepiglottic space via intrinsic tongue muscle	Via intrinsic tongue mm to sublingual space, mylohyoid m, genioglossus, geniohyoid; this spread in FOM may not be palpable	Hyoid via myohyoid muscle and mandible is possible in very advanced lesions	Rarely direct spread to carotid sheath, cranial nerves IX–XII when extensive spread into soft tissue of neck is present; this occurs more in GTS lesions than tonsillar fossa	Internal jugular submandibular, submental, spinal accessory, retropharyngeal
UPPER GINGIVOBUCCAL SINUS						
Infratemporal fossa Buccinator muscle Maxillary tubercle Maxillary alveolar ridge	A A A A(?C)	Low infratemporal fossa	Via buccinator insertion on maxilla	Maxillary alveolar ridge, inferior maxilla, maxillary tubercle, low pterygoid plates by direct extension	Via posterior-superior alveolar nn; retroantral potentially to pterygopalatine fossa	Buccinator (deep facial) rarely; submandibular; internal jugular

continued

Primary Site and Critical Anatomy	Suggested Imaging Plane(s)	Spread Pattern: Deep Spaces	Muscle Bundles	Bone	Neurovascular Bundles	Nodes
RETROMOLAR TRIGONE AND LOWER GBS						
Infratemporal fossa Maxillary tubercle	A A	Low infratemporal fossa (retroantral)	Via buccinator + superior constrictor attachment to pterygomandibular raphe	Maxillary tubercle; pterygoid plates via attachment of pterygomandibular raphe	Via posterior-superior alveolar nn to retroantral region and potential pterygopalatine fossa	Buccinator (rarely); submandibular; internal jugular
Pterygoid plates Pterygomandibular raphe Buccinator muscle	A A A	Pterygomandibular space	Medial pterygoid	RMT, mandibular alveolar ridge via tooth sockets		
Pterygomandibular space Parapharyngeal space Medial pterygoid muscle Mylohyoid muscle Mandible	A A A A A	Parapharyngeal space from pterygomandibular space; medial to pterygomandibular raphe	Mylohyoid muscle via pterygomandibular raphe then potentially along FOM (see below)	Lingual surface mandible	Lingual nerve via pterygomandibular space; inferior alveolar nerve in or along mandible	
HARD PALATE	C,A			Direct invasion potentially to nasal cavity, maxilla, pterygoid plates	Potentially along incisive and palatine foramina (greater and lesser)	Retropharyngeal if soft palate or posterior nasal cavity involved; internal jugular
FLOOR OF MOUTH	A	Sublingual—deep FOM; neck via submandibular space; deep oral tongue	Mylohyoid—anteriorly and over posterior edge to neck via submandibular space; in very advanced lesions to hyoid bone and suprahyoid neck	Mandible—lingual surface via mylohyoid m	Lingual aa, nn; hypoglossal nn	Submental, submandibular internal jugular
Mylohoid muscle Genioglossus-geniohyoid muscle Sublingual space Submandibular space Suprahyoid neck Mandible	C sometimes A(?C) A,C A A A	To submandibular space and neck via mylohyoid muscle and sublingual space	Via genioglossus-geniohyoid to deep anterior FOM, tongue base, oral tongue	Hyoid—in advanced lesions via mylohyoid m	Submandibular duct	
ORAL TONGUE[c]						
Intrinsic muscles Palatoglossus muscle (ATP) Lingual septum	A A A	See FOM	Free spread with intrinsic muscles, can go from posterior oral tongue to BOT	See FOM	See FOM	Submandibular internal jugular; bilateral possible
ANTERIOR TONSILLAR PILLAR (ATP)[d]						
Palatoglossus–superior construction m. Pterygomandibular raphe Pterygomandibular space Soft palate	A A A A,C	From pterygomandibular and parapharyngeal space can begin to mimic RMT but spread will be mainly medial to pterygomandibular raphe and more anterior than tonsillar fossa lesion; via supratonsillar recess to NP possible	Via palatoglossus and superior constrictor to tongue and soft palate From soft palate to NP possible along tensor/levator palati	See FOM	Possible lingual nn via pterygomandibular space	Internal jugular mainly

continued

Primary Site	Plane of Section	Deep Spread[a]: Spaces: Preepiglottic Paralaryngeal	Cartilage Invasion	Subglottic	Exolaryngeal	Other	Nodes
SUPRAGLOTTIC							
Suprahyoid epiglottis (SHE)	A,S	PES via vallecula or through epiglottic cartilage if upper infrahyoid epiglottis involved	Epiglottis—always		Tongue base via vallecula or PES		Bilateral internal jugular; spinal accessory
Infrahyoid epiglottis (IHE)	A,S	PES through epiglottic cartilage common PS submucosal via PES or direct if AEF involved	Epiglottis—always Thyroid—rarely, usually via thyroepiglottic ligament, point of attack just above anterior commissure	Only in lesions that have spread to anterior commissure and continue inferiorly along cricothyroid membrane	Lesions showing thyroid cartilage destruction can continue into anterior infrahyoid strap muscles		Bilateral internal jugular; spinal accessory occasionally
Aryepiglottic fold (AEF)	A	PS from posteriorly via AEF; this may go submucosal to FVC from here; PES from PS or directly through IHE	Thyroid cartilage via PS (unusual) Cricoarytenoid joint via base of AEF	When they become transglottic—usually posterolateral via cricoarytenoid joint		Spill into pyriform sinus common	Usually ipsilateral; internal jugular Occasionally spinal accessory
False vocal cord and ventricle (FVC)	A,C	PS main deep mode of spread; often become transglottic from here; often have large submucosal component	Thyroid via PS Cricoid via cricoarytenoid joint	Via PS deep to conus frequently occurs—these are transglottic lesions; TVC usually fixed but may not be	May occur via thyroid cartilage or cricothyroid space in advanced lesions		Internal jugular; spinal accessory midneck common
HYPOPHARYNX							
Pyriform sinus (PYS)	A	PS via anterior wall PYS; PES via PS	Thyroid—inferior portion or lamina, inferior cornu, superior cornu all commonly invaded cricoid via lateral surface of cricoarytenoid joint	Deep to conus not infrequently and may not be visible clinically	Via thyrothyoid membrane, via foci of cartilage destruction frequently present; via cricothyroid space	Postcricoid spread is important and imaging may be best way to see this area in bulky lesions Postcricoid Esophageal verge to esophagus	Internal jugular and spinal accessory mid to low neck nodes commonly involved; tracheoesophageal nodes at risk when postcricoid region or esophageal verge involved
TRUE VOCAL CORD (TVC)	A,C	PS to ventricle, FVC as well as subglottic space deep to conus elasticus	Thyroid—at anterior commissure; at lamina (unusual); cricoarytenoid joint	Often circumferential; laterally may be deep and/or superficial to conus elasticus	Anteriorly through the cricothyroid membrane or through the thyroid cartilage at the anterior commissure to prelaryngeal soft tissues	If extensive subglottic spread tracheal involvement possible	Internal jugular nodes; spinal accessory occasional
SUBGLOTTIC	A	Lower paralaryngeal to TVC, may be curcumferential, quite extensive and not clinically obvious	Cricoid—unusual, probably via cricoary-tenoid joint or direct	By definition	Anteriorly through the cricothyroid membrane to prelaryngeal soft tissues	Tracheal spread possible	Internal jugular; spinal accessory; tracheoesophageal groove; mid, low neck at high risk

[a]PES, preepiglottic space; PS, paralaryngeal space.

[a]Abbreviations: *A*, axial; *C*, coronal; *IOF*, inferior orbital fissure; *SOF*, superior orbital fissure; *s*, sagittal; *NP*, nasopharynx; *m(m)*, muscle(s); *a(a)*, artery(ies); *v(v)*, vein(s); *n(n)*, nerve(s); *PES*, preepiglottic space; *PS*, paralaryngeal space; *PYS*, pyriform sinus; *PPW*, posterior pharyngeal wall; *TVC*, true vocal cord; *FVC*, false vocal cord; *FOM*, floor of mouth; *BOT*, base of tongue; *GTS*, glossotonsillar sulcus; *GBS*, gingivobuccal sulcus; *RMT*, retromolar trigone; V_1,V_2,V_3, supraorbital, maxillary, and mandibular divisions of trigeminal nerve.

[b]See also soft palate, nasopharynx, and glossotonsillar sulcus.

[c]See also floor of mouth and base of tongue.

[d]See also floor of mouth, retromolar trigone, oral tongue, tonsillar fossa, and soft palate.